Methods and Concepts in Hand Surgery

Butterworths International Medical Reviews

Orthopaedics

Methods and Concepts in Hand Surgery

Edited by

Neil Watson, MA, FRCS
Consultant Hand and Orthopaedic Surgeon, Milton Keynes District General Hospital,
Buckinghamshire, UK

and

Richard J. Smith, MD
Clinical Professor Orthopaedic Surgery, Harvard Medical School, Chief of Hand Surgery,
Department of Orthopaedics, Massachusetts General Hospital, Boston, Massachusetts,
USA

Butterworths
London Boston Durban Singapore Sydney Toronto Wellington

First published 1986

© Butterworth & Co. (Publishers) Ltd. 1986

British Library Cataloguing in Publication Data

Methods and concepts in hand surgery.
   1. Hand—Surgery
   I. Watson, Neil   II. Smith, Richard J.
   617'.575059   RD559

   ISBN 0-407-00428-9

Photoset by Butterworths Litho Preparation Department
Printed and bound in England by Robert Hartnoll Ltd, Bodmin, Cornwall

Preface

Hand surgery as a sub-specialty is still in the maturation phase. Such is the demand for experienced hand surgeons that the future of the specialty is assured. At present the number of surgeons whose practice is entirely devoted to hand surgery remains relatively small but is growing all the time. We have planned this volume with this in mind. We appreciate that, for the majority of surgeons, be they orthopaedic, plastic or general, hand surgery is an area of special interest and represents only a part of their work.

This volume in the Butterworths International Medical Review Series sets out to cover some important aspects of hand surgery which remain controversial.

We have gathered together contributors who we consider to be experienced practitioners in their own specific areas of interest, within the specialty.

They have been asked to give their views on the 'state of the art' in their subject. Necessarily, these views are those of the respective contributors and may not be those of the editors. Readers may find some of the ideas and concepts to be either at variance with their own views, or even a little dogmatic.

However, this book does not set out to be a standard textbook of hand surgery; several good examples of these already exist. Rather, it seeks to complement them, perhaps to question some 'standard' practices, and to provoke comment and discussion. If it succeeds by doing so, then the editors and their contributors will have achieved their aim.

It is not an easy task to coordinate a multi-author book, particularly when the authors are widely scattered. We have been greatly helped by Charles Fry and his colleagues at Butterworths and for this we are extremely grateful.

Neil Watson
Richard J. Smith

Contributors

James B. Bennett, MD
Chief, Hand Surgery Section, Division of Orthopaedic Surgery, Baylor College of
Medicine and the Methodist Hospital; Hand Surgery Consultant, Shriner's
Hospital for Crippled Children; Consultant, the Institute for Rehabilitation (Hand
Surgery) and Research, Houston, Texas, USA

Danny L. Bennett, MD
Former Christine Kleinert Fellow in Hand Surgery, University of Louisville School
of Medicine; Assistant Professor of Plastic Surgery, University of Missouri, Kansas
City, Missouri, USA

David M. Evans, FRCS
Consultant Plastic Surgeon, Wexham Park Hospital, Slough, Buckinghamshire,
UK

Jesse B. Jupiter, MD
Assistant Orthopaedic Surgeon, Massachusetts General Hospital; Assistant
Professor of Orthopaedic Surgery, Harvard Medical School, Boston,
Massachusetts, USA

Joseph E. Kutz, MD
From the Louisville Institute for Hand and Microsurgery;
Associate Clinical Professor of Surgery, University of Louisville School of
Medicine, Louisville, Kentucky, USA

D. Angus McGrouther, MSc, FRCS
Consultant Plastic Surgeon, Canniesburn Hospital, Glasgow, Scotland

Clayton A. Peimer, MD
Associate Professor, Department of Orhopaedic Surgery, School of Medicine,
State University of New York at Buffalo; Chief, Division of Hand Surgery,
Department of Orthopaedics, Millard Fillmore Hospitals and the Erie County
Medical Center, Buffalo, New York, USA

Robert H. C. Robins, FRCS
Consultant Orthopaedic Surgeon, Royal Cornwall Hospital, Truro, Cornwall, UK

Richard J. Smith, MD
Clinical Professor Orthopaedic Surgery, Harvard Medical School, Chief of Hand Surgery, Department of Orthopaedics, Massachusetts General Hospital, Boston, Massachusetts, USA

John K. Stanley, MCh.Orth, FRCS(Ed)
Consultant Hand Surgeon, Wrightington Hospital, Wigan, Lancashire, UK

Thomas E. Trumble, MD
Hand Surgery Service, Department of Orthopaedic Surgery, Massachusetts General Hospital, Harvard Medical School, Boston, Massachusetts, USA

Neil Watson, MA, FRCS
Consultant Hand and Orthopaedic Surgeon, Milton Keynes District General Hospital, Milton Keynes, Buckinghamshire, UK

Paul M. Weeks, MD
Professor and Chairman, Plastic Surgery, Washington University School of Medicine, St Louis, Missouri, USA

Kit Wynn Parry, MBE, DM, FRCP, FRCS
Director of Rehabilitation, Royal National Orthopaedic Hospital, Stanmore, Middlesex, UK

Contents

1
Treatment of the hand in cerebral palsy

Richard J. Smith and Thomas E. Trumble

INTRODUCTION

Cerebral palsy is a permanent, non-progressive abnormality of muscle function caused by injury to the immature brain. This injury occurs during the perinatal period or early in infancy. In addition to the abnormal muscle function, there are often associated abnormalities of sensibility and of subcortical or cerebellar function. The severity and nature of these abnormalities is determined by the cause of the brain injury.

CAUSES OF CEREBRAL PALSY

Cerebral palsy may be due to anoxia, cerebral bleeding, hydrocephalus or viral infection. With these patients large areas of the brain will be affected. There will be diffuse spastic and flaccid muscle involvement and abnormalities of both sensibility and intellectual ability.

If cerebral injury is caused by pressure of forceps during a difficult labor, the deficit is more likely to be well localized, resulting in hemiplegia and asymmetrical muscle involvement.

Prematurity is often associated with cerebral palsy. With premature infants the walls of the vessels deep to the anterior fontanelle are particularly fragile, and are therefore highly susceptible to rupture from sudden increase of intracranial pressure during delivery. These vessels are located in the central area of the brain, the area that controls the motor efferents to both lower limbs. Thus, cerebral palsy following premature birth is often associated with spasticity of the lower limbs and little involvement of the upper limbs. Intelligence is usually not affected.

Erythroblastosis is often the cause of damage to the internal capsule of the brain. Cerebral palsy patients with erythroblastosis are therefore more likely to have athetosis and oculomotor abnormalities with relatively little spasticity, flaccidity or defect in intelligence.

EARLY DIAGNOSIS OF CEREBRAL PALSY

Diagnosing cerebral palsy in the newborn may be difficult. Abnormal muscle function is most likely to become apparent first in the upper limb. The diagnosis should be suspected if there is paucity of spontaneous movement during the first few months of life, or if motion of both upper limbs is not symmetrical. Although some athetoid motion of the fingers and arms is seen in normal infants at birth, such motion should subside as the central nervous system matures and should disappear by 1 month of age. Persistence of athetosis past one or two months suggests subcortical cerebral injury. The normal newborn often has tremor of the upper limbs during the first few days of life; however, if tremor is seen after one month one should suspect cerebral damage.

By six months of age various immature reflexes such as the Moro reflex, the grasp reflex and tonic neck reflexes should have disappeared. In patients with cerebral palsy these reflexes persist.

Still later, the diagnosis of cerebral palsy may be diagnosed by delay of maturation and abnormal posture and muscle tone. By one year the normal infant should have developed fairly sophisticated motor control of upper and lower limbs with increased voluntary activity. However, with cerebral palsy, tonic neck reflexes and hypertonicity of the flexors and/or the extensors may remain. Abnormal motor reflex activity is prolonged throughout childhood and may never become completely inhibited because of incomplete maturation of the cerebral cortex.

CLASSIFICATION

There are many methods by which cerebral palsy has been classified. Some have categorized cerebral palsy into cases that are 'spastic' and those that are 'extrapyramidal'. Other classifications are based on the principal areas affected by motor abnormality. With this method patients are described as having hemiplegia, or paraplegia. Probably the most useful classification is that of Phelps (1957), who classified cerebral palsy according to the predominant type of motor abnormality:

(1) tremor,
(2) athetosis,
(3) ataxia,
(4) flaccid paralysis,
(5) spastic paralysis,
(6) rigidity.

Tremor, athetosis and ataxia

Tremor, athetosis and ataxia result from lesions in the extrapyramidal subcortical cerebral centers. Athetosis and tremor usually involve the internal capsule. Ataxia principally involves the cerebellum. Patients with these extrapyramidal types of cerebral palsy usually have neither sensory abnormalities nor defects of intellect. With athetosis, adjacent muscle groups contact sequentially so that the limb will writhe with any voluntary activity. Athetoid motion may even occur at rest. Patients with athetosis may be improved by operations that stabilize the joints.

Tendon transfers are usually unsuccessful. Patients with tremor or ataxia cannot be helped by upper extremity surgery.

Flaccid paralysis

Flaccid paralysis may be due to loss of voluntary muscle control because of a defect in the alpha efferent system. Cerebral palsy patients with extensive flaccid paralysis usually have severe brain involvement and quadriplegia. Although flaccid muscles may be replaced by tendon transfers these patients are usually not candidates for reconstructive surgery. However, if some muscle groups have become flaccid because of continued stretching by their spastic antagonists, their tone may improve and they may regain excellent voluntary control once they are allowed to regain the normal resting length. Splinting the affected joints or releasing the spasticity may restore function to these muscles.

Spastic paralysis

Spastic paralysis is characterized by maximal resistance to passive lengthening shortly after motion has begun. Resistance diminishes rapidly with continued lengthening. Patients with spasticity have hyperactive deep tendon stretch reflexes and clonus. The neuromuscular abnormality of spasticity is partly affected by the abnormality of the gamma neurone system which supplies the intrafusal fibers of the muscle spindles. Normally, the gamma neurones alter the length of the muscle spindles in response to change in the efferent discharge of the spindles. They thereby permit opposing muscle groups to achieve smoothly integrated muscle contraction. The gamma neurone system thus sets the level at which the stretch reflex is hyperactive. Without a gamma system muscles become hypotonic. Patients with spasticity have a cerebral lesion that renders the gamma system uninhibited and causes muscle hypertonia. The tone of spastic muscles is influenced by many factors including excitement, nervousness, fatigue and sensory stimulation. Thus the extent of muscle spasticity is variable from both hour to hour and day to day.

Rigidity

A rigid muscle is one that exerts constant resistance to stretch throughout its entire range of passive motion. Regardless of the speed at which the muscle is stretched, resistance will remain approximately the same. Unlike the springy tone of a limb with spasticity, passively flexing a limb with rigidity feels more like attempting to bend a lead pipe.

EVALUATION OF THE PATIENT WITH SPASTIC CEREBRAL PALSY

Muscle examination

Muscle examination of the upper limbs must specifically test the ability of the patient to contract and relax each muscle group with the intercalary joints placed in varying positions. Usually with spastic cerebral palsy the deformity of the upper extremity includes internal rotation of the shoulder, flexion of the elbow, pronation of the forearm, flexion and ulnar deviation of the wrist, finger flexion and thumb-in-palm deformity. Occasionally there may be swan-neck deformities of the fingers. In order to determine whether the muscles of the upper limb are under voluntary control the examiner must relax the spasticity of one group of muscles in order to test their antagonists. The influence of intercalary joint position on muscle function should be noted. For example, in testing finger extensors, the examiner may note that there is full active finger extension 'with 20° wrist flexion' or 'with 40° wrist flexion' or 'with 70° wrist flexion'. In each case, finger extensors may contract fully. However, the position in which the intercalary joints must be placed to achieve extension may well determine the type of operative procedure to be performed.

Although electromyography has been used to evaluate muscle function in the cerebral palsy patient, valid quantitative data cannot be obtained by this means. For example, one cannot accurately judge the force of muscle contraction by electromyographic readings of a cerebral palsy patient. However, according to Hoffer, Perry and Melkonian (1979) the involved muscles of cerebral palsy usually do not change phase after they are transferred; it often is helpful to demonstrate the phases during which a muscle contracts before selecting a plan of tendon transfer. The best results of tendon transfer for the cerebral palsy patient probably occur when the muscles that are transferred are active prior to surgery in the same phase as their recipients.

Sensory evaluation

Tachdijian and Minear (1958) have shown that the sensory abnormalities associated with spastic cerebral palsy are usually those of higher cortical discriminatory functions such as stereognosis, position sense and two-point discrimination. The more primitive types of sensibility such as pain, light touch, and temperature depend principally on thalamic function and usually remain intact since they are mostly unaffected by insult to the cerebral cortex.

Sensory evaluation must be totally atraumatic. The child is never asked to turn her head away, nor are the mother's hands placed over the eyes. To test stereognosis a key, pencil, coin, bottle cap and paper clip are shown. The child is asked to identify each by feeling it with the normal hand. The objects are then covered and the patient is allowed to manipulate them in the affected hand, and asked to identify each one. The child will be much more cooperative if she thinks a game is being played rather than being forced to sit blindfolded in what may well be perceived as a potentially hostile environment.

Proprioception is tested by holding each finger at its sides so that the child is not cued by increased pressure on the volar or dorsal skin. 'Up' and 'down' is first identified and then the child is asked to guess the position of the finger each time it is moved. Again, the other hand is used to obstruct the child's vision. Two-point discrimination is tested using a caliper or paper clip (but be sure these instruments are not sharp). The child must 'guess' each time she is touched.

Another useful test is the 'nickel–quarter' test. The milled edge of a quarter is run downward or the smooth edge of a nickel longitudinally along the side of the finger and the patient is asked to 'guess' which it is. This is a game easily played by most children and indentifies their ability to synthesize and interpret spatial and temporal sensibility. The nickel–quarter test may be considered a type of moving two-point discrimination test. The cost of the testing materials is always 30 cents.

Evaluation of intelligence

To some extent, what is called intelligence is dependent upon the integration of sensory input to form appropriate responses. Sensory deprivation can adversely affect the ability of children to arrive at these responses if they have been placed in an environment where their lifetime experience is limited. They will appear 'unintelligent'. To a large extent, this may be due to lack of sensory input rather than inability to synthesize the input into appropriate responses. Children who have been sheltered or institutionalized because of the muscular abnormalities of spastic cerebral palsy may score poorly on standard 'intelligence tests'. These scores may not reflect whether or not the patients can be educated, but rather the background to which the child has been exposed.

In addition, most standard intelligence tests are partly based on motor responses that may prove difficult to perform by a child with motor abnormalities. A patient with oculomotor defects may be unable to read instructions and questions and to visualize the pictures shown to him. Poor eye/hand coordination may be responsible for slow and incorrect response on an examination paper. Emotional problems may alter ability to score well in the highly stressful environment of an examination. All these factors must be considered when interpreting the relevance of an 'intelligence test' in judging the suitability of the cerebral palsy patient for surgery.

Functional evaluation

Before deciding on a treatment plan, the patient with cerebral palsy should be seen on several occasions and under different circumstances. He should be observed at play, when relaxing and when eating, dressing and attending to other activities of daily living. Both the child's teachers and family should watch carefully and report on what is done well, or poorly, and with which activity use of the hand is avoided completely.

A most important part is to study video-tapes of the patient as part of the motor evaluation. The taping is done in the Department of Rehabilitation and not in the doctor's office. The patient is there with his mother and siblings in a room filled with other people doing other things. The television camera is run by a therapist without the use of any floodlights and the tape remains on throughout the entire session. There are no doctors around. There are no needles or syringes. Nothing is in view to threaten the child during the taping session, as it is well understood that surgeons, residents and medical students who crowd the clinics, conferences and the doctors' offices are people that children usually like to avoid. They mean trouble and no child can be at ease when they are around.

The video-tape is reviewed at another time by the surgeon and therapist, and later by the family and patient. Then is determined what functions are most in need of improvement, and the activities for which the affected limb is used are evaluated. How can it be used better? For what activities is the limb totally ignored?

NON-OPERATIVE TREATMENT FOR SPASTIC CEREBRAL PALSY

Orthotics

Orthotics has a place in the management of the patient with cerebral palsy. Static braces and splints may prevent contractures. For example, wrist splints in younger children may stretch wrist flexors and the volar wrist capsule for several hours each day, keeping the joints supple. Usually these splints are best worn during sleep when there is less spasticity.

Splints may also be used to prejudge planned surgical procedures. For example, if an operation is being planned to dorsiflex the wrist, the use of a wrist cock-up splint while the child performs activities of daily living may help determine whether the new position would improve hand function. It is possible that bringing the wrist into a more normal position may make it more difficult to release an object that is grasped and may render the hand more awkward. The wrist splint helps identify these problems prior to surgery.

On occasion, a wrist splint may assist hand function. It has been found, however, that most patients find the splint awkward and few patients will use it for long. In patients with spasticity, persistence of immature reflexes such as the grasp reflex may result in a palmar splint merely increasing digital flexion tone.

Hand therapy

Other than splints, non-operative treatment of the cerebral palsy patient may include attempts to establish patterns of normal muscle use. With spasticity, the stretch reflex may be released by encouraging slow reciprocal motions of the opposing muscle groups. Stretching exercises, however, are of little value if muscle contractures are usually not a significant feature of spastic hemiplegia. When there is rigidity, the speed of reciprocal motion between antagonists is increased. Relaxation training has successfully diminished the unwanted motion of athetosis or tremor in many patients with cerebral palsy.

Medications and injections

Various drugs have been used in the treatment of cerebral palsy with generally indifferent success. Among the medications that have proved successful are prostigmine, reserpine, dramamine and various sedatives. Valium may be effective in decreasing postoperative muscle spasm and pain.

The use of anesthetics, alcohol, or phenol nerve blocks are of limited value. However, anesthetic blocks may be of use in testing limb function prior to proposed neurectomy or tenotomy, or in order to evaluate muscles whose function is masked by overactive antagonists.

SURGICAL TREATMENT OF THE UPPER LIMB IN PATIENTS WITH SPASTIC CEREBRAL PALSY

Surgical treatment of the patient with cerebral palsy may have as its goals improvement of function or appearance.

In order to improve function limited goals must be set. The surgeon should attempt to improve the hand so that it can act better as an assistive hand. No attempt should be made (except in the most mildly affected limbs) to restore fine prehension or versatile, independent motion of the fingers and thumb. If the hand functions effectively with 'spring grip' it may be a disservice to balance the hand for improved release. For example, some patients are able to place an object into a tightly clenched fist so that the affected limb holds the object firmly. The less affected limb, as the dominant limb, is then free to perform more difficult motor tasks. The spastic limb holds the wood while the dominant limb hammers the nail; the spastic limb holds the jar while the dominant limb unscrews the jar cap; the spastic limb holds the trumpet while the less affected limb depresses the stops. When the activity is completed, the object must be retrieved from the clenched hand by the less affected limb.

For these patients the eager surgeon may be tempted to rebalance the hand so that flexion is weaker and release is more easily achieved. However, this 'balanced hand' may be less functional than the 'spring grip' hand as grip is weaker. Thus, assistive function is not as effective. The awkward release of an object from the spring grip hand may be less of a penalty in the patient with cerebral palsy than is the weakened grip of the balanced and more aesthetic hand.

Yet another patient with an identical deformity of his right hand may wish the hand to be better positioned so that it looks more normal, and so that he can shake hands in greeting customers and friends. He may not use the hand for prehension. If his goals are clearly defined, reconstructive efforts to permit better finger release and wrist dorsiflexion and improved appearance probably are justified.

Rarely will the authors operate on a patient when he is less than five years of age. The patterns of deformity may change during the early years of childhood. In addition, functional evaluation is difficult as manual habit patterns are just beginning to form. Some surgeons set limits as to the minimal intelligence necessary to achieve a good result from surgery. However, because of the difficulties of interpreting the validity of the intelligence test of a cerebral palsy patient, no IQ level is set as a prerequisite for surgery. Indeed, the authors have operated on many patients with Stanford Binet IQ scores below 50 who have gained improved function following a smooth postoperative course. Sensibility has also been used as a criterion for surgery. If a limb with poor sensation is ignored by the patient it is unlikely to be used regardless of the muscle balance obtained by surgery. However, Zancolli and Zancolli (1981) have noted that, regardless of its critical sensibility, a hand used for assistive purposes will continue to be used after successful reconstructive surgery regardless of its sensibility.

Surgical techniques in the treatment of spastic cerebral palsy

In planning the surgical reconstruction in the hand with spastic cerebral palsy, there are many alternative procedures that may be considered. These include tendon transfer, tenotomy, tendon lengthening, muscle slide, neurotomy and neurectomy, bone shortening, tenodesis, capsulodesis and arthodesis. The choice of which procedure to use depends upon the deformity, the functional disability and the goals of surgery. Most frequently, more than one procedure is performed simultaneously.

Tendon transfers

When performing a tendon transfer for cerebral palsy, success is most frequently achieved if *augmentation* and *release* are performed simultaneously (*Figure 1.1 (a)*, (*b*) *and* (*c*); *Figure 1.2 (a) and (b)*). For example, the excellent success usually achieved by transferring flexor carpi ulnaris (FCU) to extensor carpi radialis longus (ECRL) or brevis (ECRB) to correct wrist palmar flexion/ulnar deviation

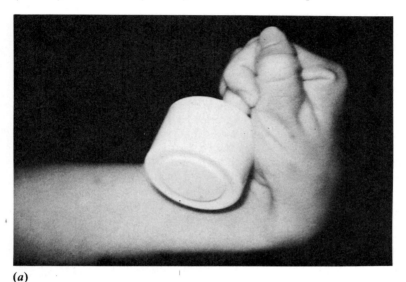

(*a*)

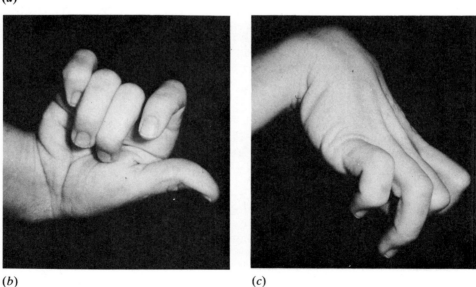

(*b*)   (*c*)

Figure 1.1 (a), (b) and (c) This patient with cerebral palsy has spasticity of the flexors of the wrist, fingers and thumb. The varying patterns of deformity are seen in these photographs taken within a few minutes of each other

deformity described by Green (1942) is due to the simultaneous *release* of the deforming force (of the flexor carpi ulnaris) and *augmentation* of the weakened side of the joint (ECRL and ECRB). If the first metacarpal is acutely fixed with swan-neck deformity of the thumb, transfer of brachioradialis (BR) into abductor pollicis longus (APL) has a better chance of correcting the deformity if the tight metacarpal flexors are released simultaneously. Therefore, with brachioradialis transfer to *augment* metacarpal extension, the adductor pollicis is simultaneously *released* from its origin. If thumb-in-palm deformity is caused by tight flexor pollicis longus, the flexor pollicis longus is released and transferred to the radial side of the thumb in order to *augment* abduction while *releasing* flexion.

As noted above, electromyographic studies have shown that frequently tendons transferred to correct deformities in patients with spastic cerebral palsy do not change phase. Thus, one would expect that flexor carpi ulnaris transferred to the extensor side of the wrist may not contract spontaneously when the patient wants to bring the wrist into dorsiflexion. Yet the transfer usually succeeds in rebalancing the wrist. No doubt this is due in large measure to *release* of the deforming force of the flexor carpi ulnaris and the *augmented* extensor tone at the dorsum of the wrist.

When performing tendon transfers for peripheral nerve palsy it is often best to transect the recipient tendon proximal to the site of tendon transfer. However, when transferring a tendon in a patient with cerebral palsy, the recipient

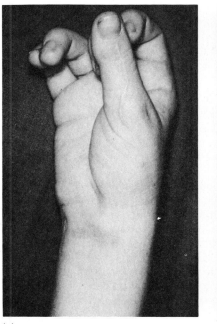
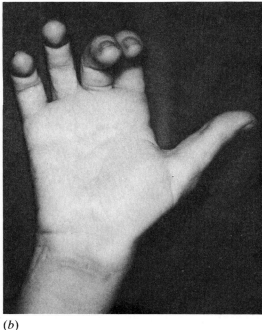

(*a*)   (*b*)

Figure 1.2 (a) and 1.2 (b) Three operations were performed. They included flexor–pronator release, flexor carpi ulnaris transfer to extensor carpi radialis longus and transfer of flexor pollicis longus to abductor pollicis brevis with interphalangeal arthrodesis of the thumb. The patient has achieved good grip, pinch and release, and was able to use the hand for assistive functions

muscle/tendon unit is allowed to remain intact, so that we may detach, loosen or tighten the transfer in the future if this proves necessary.

Multiple tendon transfers may be performed simultaneously for patients with cerebral palsy. However, the authors will not simultaneously perform a muscle slide and tendon transfer. The difficulties in selecting the appropriate length of tendon transfers are sufficiently troublesome under any circumstances. Selecting the proper length and tension is even more difficult in patients with cerebral palsy. These difficulties are further compounded if the proximal end of the muscle is detached. Under these circumstances it is impossible to judge the appropriate length and tension at which the transfer should be sutured.

When choosing tendons for a transfer one should always be aware of the effect of the tendon transfer on joints more distally. If the wrist is brought into dorsiflexion, the finger flexors will become tighter. The surgeon, the patient and the patient's family should anticipate a change in the balance of the hand that may require surgery. Thus, it is best not to do too much at once. Wait at least six months after the operative procedure before proceeding with further surgery, as it usually requires at least six months for the hand to assume its new posture.

Among the tendon transfers found useful in the treatment of cerebral palsy are the following.

TRANSFERS TO AUGMENT SUPINATION
(1) Pronator teres to radial tuberosity: this operation described by Colton, Ransford and Lloyd-Roberts (1976) releases active pronation contraction while augmenting supination. Pronator quadratus continues to function for forearm pronation.
(2) Flexor carpi ulnaris to extensor carpi radialis longus: although this transfer is done principally to correct wrist flexion/ulnar deviation, the direction in which the transfer travels will augment supination.

TRANSFERS TO AUGMENT WRIST DORSIFLEXION
(1) Flexor carpi ulnaris to extensor carpi radialis brevis: this transfer releases the deforming force while augmenting the weaker force. However, if flexor carpi radialis is weak and overcorrection occurs, extension of the fingers and thumb may be compromised. Clenched fist or thumb-in-palm deformity may become more severe.
(2) Flexor carpi ulnaris to extensor carpi radialis longus: this transfer is similar to flexor carpi ulnaris to extensor carpi radialis brevis, but achieves more radial deviation postoperatively. Also, there is more supination component to the transfer than (1) above.
(3) Brachioradialis to extensor carpi radialis brevis: this is a strong transfer as the brachioradialis is the strongest muscle of the forearm. However, no antagonist is released by this transfer. This transfer is most useful if flexor carpi radialis does not appear to be functioning or has been used for another transfer. According to McCue, Honner and Chapman (1970) it is important to release the brachioradialis up to its origin at the elbow in order to maximize its excursion.
(4) Flexor carpi ulnaris to extensor digitorum communis: Keats (1965) and Hoffer (1982) have shown that this transfer extends the wrist through its attachment to the finger extensors. If flexor carpi ulnaris is transferred to extensor digitorum communis, the risk of achieving wrist dorsiflexion at the expense of finger extension is lessened. However, there is a risk that the fingers may assume a clawed position before wrist dorsiflexion is achieved.

TRANSFERS TO AUGMENT METACARPOPHALANGEAL EXTENSION OF THE FINGERS

(1) Recession of central slip to base of the proximal phalanx: as described by Smith (1977), if the sagittal bands have migrated distally, contraction of the extensor muscle belly will have little effect on the metacarpophalangeal joint and will exert full effect on the proximal interphalangeal joint. This may gradually cause a decreased mobility of the fingers. By this transfer, the central slip is detached. Proximal interphalangeal and distal interphalangeal extension are achieved through the intrinsic muscles. The extrinsic extensor is placed at the base of the proximal phalanx to assist in metacarpophalangeal extension (*Figures 1.3, 1.4, 1.5, 1.6a and b, 1.7, 1.8a and b*).

(2) Flexor carpi ulnaris to extensor digitorum communis: as noted above, the transfer improves finger extension and may also improve wrist extension.

TRANSFERS TO AUGMENT THUMB EXTENSION

(1) Brachioradialis to abductor pollicis longus: this transfer is often performed along with either a slide or tenotomy of the adductor pollicis or ulnar neurectomy. The brachioradialis is the strongest muscle of the forearm and exerts an excellent force upon the first metacarpal when transferred into abductor pollicis longus. The transfer should be considered in 'swan-neck' deformities of the thumb. The use of the brachioradialis to augment thumb extension in cerebral palsy was first mentioned by Samilson and Morris (1964). They transferred the brachioradialis to the abductor pollicis longus and extensor pollicis longus to correct the thumb adduction deformity when a flexion contracture of the interphalangeal joint of the thumb was present as well. Inglis, Cooper and Burton (1970) also have described transferring the flexor carpi radialis to the thumb extensors. After this transfer changes in wrist position (such as recurrence of a wrist palmar-flexion deformity) will affect thumb function.

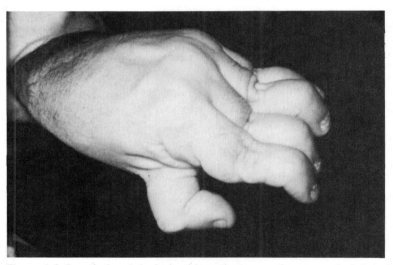

Figure 1.3 Spastic hemiplegia in this patient caused swan-neck deformities of all fingers. There was incomplete metacarpophalangeal extension because the sagittal bands had displaced distally. Excessive force of EDC was exerted on the middle phalanges causing proximal interphalangeal hyperextension

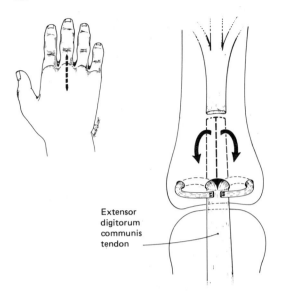

Extensor
digitorum
communis
tendon

Figure 1.4 At operation, the central slip of the EDC was transected at the dorsum of the proximal phalanx, split and passed through a drill hole at the base of the proximal phalanx. (From Smith, 1977, by courtesy of the publisher)

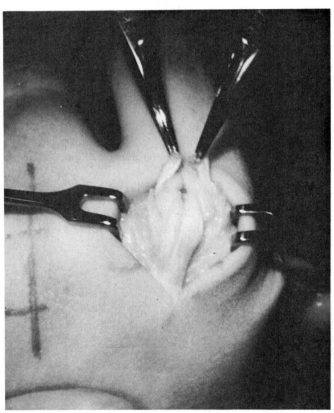

Figure 1.5 Shows recession of central slip of EDC in index finger

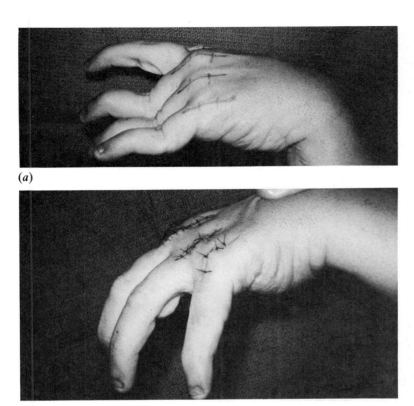

(a)

(b)

Figure 1.6 (a) Immediately after recession of the central slip of the index finger, its position is improved. Compare the index with the adjacent fingers not operated at this time. (*b*) Now all fingers have been operated. The metacarpophalangeal joints are now better extended and the proximal interphalangeal joints fall into mild flexion when the wrist is palmar-flexed

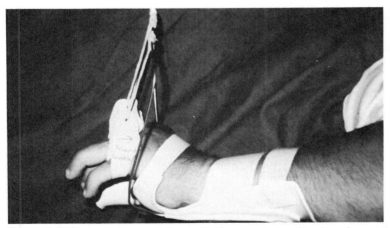

Figure 1.7 Active postoperative splinting protects the transfer and allows proximal interphalangeal joint motion

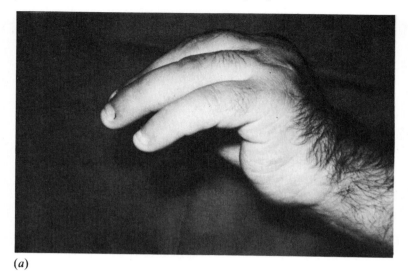

(a)

(b)

Figure 1.8 (a) *and* (b) The recession of the EDC has restored better function and appearance to the hand

(2) Flexor pollicis longus to abductor pollicis brevis: this transfer has been shown by Smith (1982) to be indicated only for patients with a tight flexor pollicis longus and thumb-in-palm deformity involving all three joints (*Figures 1.9, 1.10, 1.11 and 1.12*). Preoperatively, the deformity will be less with the wrist in palmar flexion. A deforming force (the flexor pollicis longus) is removed and brought to the lateral side of the thumb to improve abduction. The interphalangeal joint of the thumb is fused. The extensor pollicis longus then has a longer lever arm to help extend the metacarpophalangeal joint.

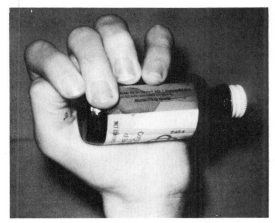

Figure 1.9 In this patient with cerebral palsy, spasticity of flexor pollicis longus has caused acute flexion of the interphalangeal joint of the thumb which interferes with grasp

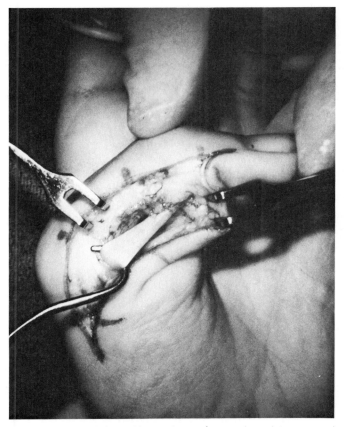

Figure 1.10 The flexor pollicis longus tendon is indentified and the interphalangeal joint of the thumb is arthrodesed

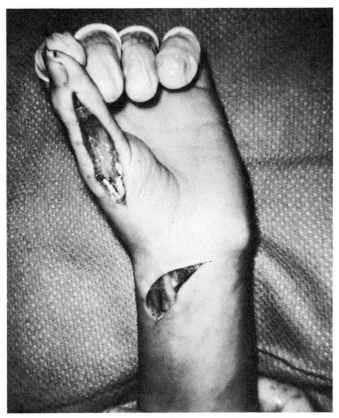

Figure 1.11 The flexor pollicis longus tendon is withdrawn at the wrist and then passed subcutaneously at the radial side of the thumb to be inserted into the tendon of abductor pollicis brevis

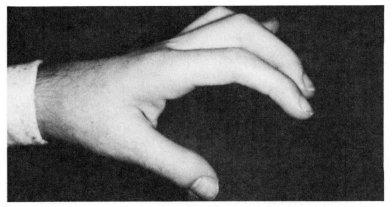

Figure 1.12 This transfer has permitted better abduction and extension of the thumb. The transfer has released the deforming force (flexion and adduction) and has augmented thumb abduction. Interphalangeal joint arthrodesis has augmented thumb extension

Tenotomy

Tenotomy is often useful as an auxiliary procedure at the same time as tendon transfer, muscle slide or capsulodesis is performed. Usually, the authors prefer to use the tenotomized muscles as a transfer or to lengthen an overactive tendon so that it may continue to function. Yet, as part of the surgical reconstructive program, tenotomies may help to restore a limb most simply and with little dissection. The following tenotomies have proven successful in appropriate cases.

TENOTOMY TO RELIEVE FOREARM PRONATION

Tenotomy of pronator teres, and/or tenotomy of pronator quadratus is used. For mild pronation deformities, a double pronator tenotomy performed at the time of flexor carpi ulnaris transfer to extensor carpi radialis brevis or longus may allow the deformity to be lessened without much risk of overcorrection. Flexor carpi radialis continues to pronate the forearm weakly.

TENOTOMY TO RELEASE WRIST FLEXION

Tenotomy of flexor carpi ulnaris or tenotomy flexor carpi radialis is used here. If there is severe wrist flexion contracture with good finger extension, better wrist dorsiflexion can be achieved by tenotomy of flexor carpi ulnaris (in patients with ulnar deviation) or flexor carpi radialis (if there is radial deviation) without transferring them dorsally. The risk of overcorrection is lessened if the tenotomized motor is not transferred to its own antagonist.

TENOTOMY TO RELEASE FINGER FLEXION

(1) Tenotomy of flexor digitorum superficialis: this release is often helpful for patients with proximal interphalangeal flexion contractures.
(2) Tenotomy of interosseous muscles: in essence this is a proximal intrinsic release and is advised for patients with swan-neck deformity and tight metacarpophalangeal flexion contractures, particularly if they are due to intrinsic muscle scarring.

TENOTOMY TO RELEASE THUMB-IN-PALM DEFORMITY

(1) Tenotomy of adductor pollicis: this procedure is only used for patients with severe flexion contracture of the metacarpophalangeal joint. More commonly, the origin of adductor pollicis is released and the muscle allowed to slide radially (*Figure 1.13a and b*).
(2) Tenotomy of flexor pollicis brevis: for severe flexion contracture of metacarpophalangeal joint; abductor pollicis brevis should not be disturbed.

Tendon lengthening and muscle slide

If spasticity of a muscle causes a disabling deformity but that muscle must be retained for function, the deforming muscle can be released by muscle slide or tendon lengthening. Unlike tenotomy, muscle function persists but it is weaker. For example, there may be overpull of the interosseous muscles causing metacarpophalangeal flexion contracture and limited ability to flex the interphalangeal joints. Yet intrinsic muscle function may be necessary to permit active metacarpophalangeal joint flexion. Interosseous muscle contraction may be weakened but preserved by interosseous muscle slide. The origin of each of the interosseous muscles is released subperiosteally and allowed to re-attach more distally (*Figure 1.14*). Tendons of the hypothenar muscles are divided. The patient

18

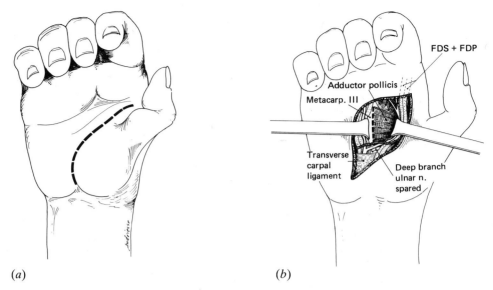

(a)   (b)

Figure 1.13 (a) and (b) Subperiosteal release of adductor pollicis from the third metacarpal and the capitate relaxes flexion/adduction contracture of the first metacarpal in patients with 'swan-neck' deformity of the thumb. (From Smith, 1977, by courtesy of the publisher)

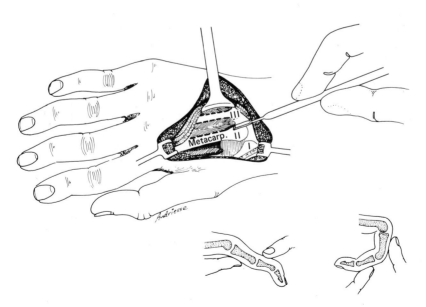

Figure 1.14 Subperiosteal release of the interosseous muscles from the metacarpals in patients with spastic intrinsic contracture preserves interosseous muscle function while it releases intrinsic muscle tightness. (From Smith, 1977, by courtesy of the publisher)

is splinted with metacarpophalangeal joints extended and interphalangeal joints flexed for several weeks. At the end of that time, the patient has increased metacarpophalangeal extension while still maintaining metacarpophalangeal flexion.

As another example, the flexor–pronator muscles may cause excessive pronation of the forearm and flexion of the wrist and fingers. Yet, for grasp and for wrist control these muscles may be necessary. Under these circumstances, tendon lengthening or muscle slide, as described by Page (1923), may relax the involved muscles sufficiently to permit better balance. With muscle slide, the origins of the spastic muscles are relaxed (*Figure 1.15a, b and c*).

As a rule, muscle slide is preferred to tendon lengthening when multiple adjacent muscles require relaxation or if the tendon of the muscle is short and would prove difficult to lengthen. For example, if all the wrist flexors and digit flexors are tight, all may be released from their origin and allowed to re-attach more distally. However, if there is significant overactivity of the flexor pollicis longus alone, lengthening of its tendon should be preferred to muscle slide. The adductor pollicis has a short tendon. If there is adduction spasticity, the adductor origin from the third metacarpal may be released and allowed to re-attach more radially.

Bone shortening and arthrodesis

Bone shortening is rarely done unless arthrodesis is performed simultaneously. For patients with a severely palmar-flexed wrist and tight flexors, radiocarpal arthrodesis in dorsiflexion or neutral position will often cause disabling tightening of all digit flexors. Excision of the proximal carpal row at the time of arthrodesis may relax the flexors sufficiently to permit improved digit extension. The surgeon must be prepared for the loss of tenodesis effect when the joint is fused. Often it is preferable to immobilize the joint by Kirschner wire fixation or with a splint as a trial prior to performing arthrodesis. For a severe pronation deformity, radio-ulnar arthrodesis may achieve the most predictable and satisfactory correction of a severe deformity that is resistant to tendon transfer or tenotomy.

Tenodesis and capsulodesis

Tenodesis or capsulodesis of the metacarpophalangeal or interphalangeal joints can stabilize the thumb or fingers, improving position and function. Rarely, however, will tenodesis or capsulodesis succeed in holding the improved position unless tendon release or tendon transfer is performed simultaneously. If a tendon imbalance persists the tenodesis or capsulodesis will gradually stretch and the deformity will recur. It is usually most effective with tenodesis or capsulodesis to suture the tendon stump or cartilaginous volar plate to the neck of the metacarpal or phalanx just proximal to the involved joint. When the distal stump of the tendon is used to stabilize a joint, the proximal tendon can be transferred to help re-balance the hand.

Neurotomy or neurectomy

Dividing a motor nerve in order to totally paralyze the muscles it supplies has been successfully used for many years to decrease deformities of the lower limbs.

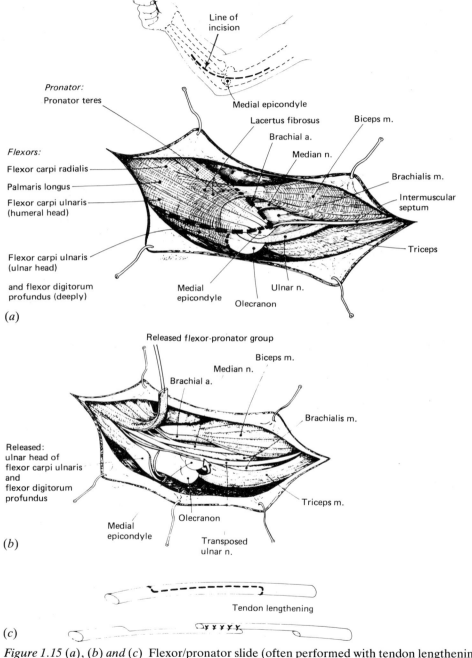

Line of incision

Pronator:
Pronator teres

Medial epicondyle

Lacertus fibrosus

Biceps m.

Brachial a.

Median n.

Flexors:

Flexor carpi radialis

Brachialis m.

Palmaris longus

Flexor carpi ulnaris
(humeral head)

Intermuscular
septum

Flexor carpi ulnaris
(ulnar head)

Triceps

and flexor digitorum
profundus (deeply)

Medial
epicondyle

Ulnar n.

Olecranon

(a)

Released flexor-pronator group

Biceps m.

Median n.

Brachial a.

Brachialis m.

Released:
ulnar head of
flexor carpi ulnaris
and
flexor digitorum
profundus

Triceps m.

Medial
epicondyle

Olecranon

Transposed
ulnar n.

(b)

Tendon lengthening

(c)

Figure 1.15 (a), (b) and (c) Flexor/pronator slide (often performed with tendon lengthening) is used to treat patients with spastic hemiplegia or quadriplegia who have tight wrist and digit flexors. Secondary supplemental augmentation of wrist or digit extension often is needed. (From Smith, 1977, by courtesy of the publisher)

Neurotomy has also proved successful in relieving spasticity of the small muscles of the hand. The short-term effects of neurotomy can be tested by injecting the appropriate nerve preoperatively. The authors prefer neurotomy to phenol or alcohol injections about the hand as the results are more long-lasting and there is less danger of injuring adjacent tissues. Thus, if excessive interosseous muscle hyperactivity which has caused swan-neck deformities is also associated with hyperactivity of the adductor pollicis, transection of the deep branch of the ulnar nerve may restore balance to the hand. Often neurotomy is performed at the same time as augmentation tendon transfer.

SELECTION OF THE APPROPRIATE PROCEDURE TO TREAT CEREBRAL PALSY OF THE UPPER LIMB

Considering the difficulty in evaluating the patient with cerebral palsy affecting the hands, the varying patterns of deformity and the limited goals that can be achieved, selection of an operative plan can be difficult. An outline of surgical reconstruction can, at best, only suggest some programs that may be considered for the treatment of any patient. A general plan for various patterns of deformities follows.

Pronation deformity

Severe pronation of the forearm

If the forearm is severely pronated and cannot be brought into neutral position passively, the distal radio-ulnar joint is arthrodesed in neutral position. Pronator teres and pronator quadratus are tenotomized at their insertions (*Figures 1.16a and b; 1.17a and b*).

Moderately severe pronation contracture permitting passive supination to the neutral position

If the passive flexion of the elbow to 90° permits increased supination (to 20–30°), the insertion of the pronator teres is released and may be transferred to the radial tuberosity. If there is no appreciable change in the rotation of the forearm with the elbow flexed, the pronator quadratus is also released.

Forearm pronation/wrist flexion/finger flexion deformity

Mild to moderate pronation of the forearm with severe flexion of the wrist and digits

For these patients, attention is directed primarily at improving the position of the digits and wrist.

(1) If the fingers remain tightly flexed while the wrist is flexed, the flexor–pronator slide is performed. If the thumb remains flexed after displacement of the

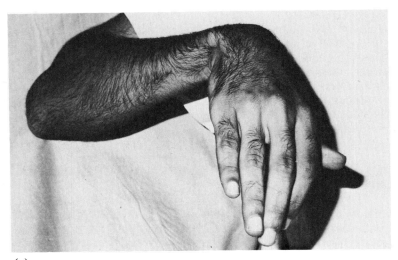

(a)

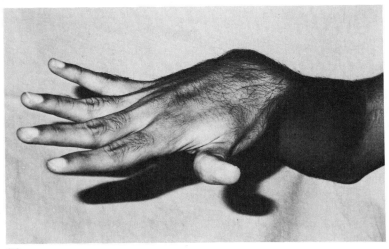

(b)

Figure 1.16 (a) and (b) This young man with spastic flexion and ulnar deviation of the wrist and pronation of the forearm was most disturbed by the appearance of his hand and his inability to shake hands at work. He was a law student

flexor–pronator origin, tendon of flexor pollicis longus is lengthened at the distal forearm. At a second operation, flexor carpi ulnaris is transferred to digit extensor if insufficient finger extension is achieved to allow satisfactory release of grasp. If grasp release is satisfactory but the wrist cannot be extended past 30° of palmar flexion, flexor carpi ulnaris is transferred to extensor carpi radialis brevis. If the patient has a pronation deformity as well as wrist flexion deformity, flexor carpi ulnaris is transferred to extensor carpi radialis rather than to extensor brevis longus in order to better improve supination.

(2) If the wrist can be actively dorsiflexed to within 30° of neutral position, and if finger extension remains adequate, flexor carpi ulnaris is transferred to extensor carpi radialis brevis. If wrist dorsiflexion to within 30° of neutral can be achieved, but finger extension is inadequate, flexor carpi ulnaris is transferred to extensor digitorum communis.

In either of these cases pronation deformity is corrected by radio-ulnar arthrodesis is severe and by pronator teres tenotomy and/or transfer if moderate.

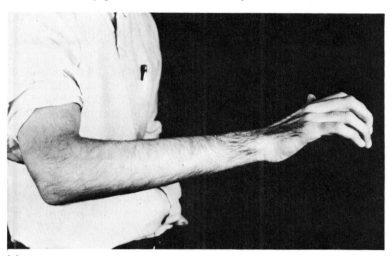

(*a*)

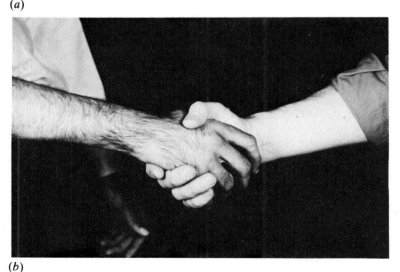

(*b*)

Figure 1.17 (a) and (b) Wrist deformity was corrected by transfer of flexor carpi ulnaris to extensor carpi radialis longus. The pronation contracture was unable to be corrected passively. It was therefore treated by distal radio-ulnar arthrodesis in neutral position. He was most pleased with the results as the limb had a better appearance and he was now able to shake hands

Mild flexion/ulnar deviation of the wrist with adequate digit extension

For these patients there is often no functional disability and nothing need be done. If there is disability because of wrist position, or if the patient wishes to improve the appearance of the hand, flexor carpi ulnaris lengthening may be considered.

Severe flexion of wrist and fingers unable to be corrected passively

Under these circumstances, the surgeon must be careful to determine whether the primary goals of surgery are to improve function, appearance or hygiene. If the patient attempts to use the hand, one might consider arthrodesis of the wrist in 30° of palmar flexion and proximal row carpectomy or even complete carpal excision as described by Hoffer (1978). Braun and Vise (1973) described relaxing the flexors by dividing flexor superficialis and profundus and suturing proximal superficialis to distal profundus ('STP' = superficialis to profundus) in the lengthened position. At the same operative procedure, flexor carpi ulnaris may be transferred to extensor carpi radialis brevis.

If surgery is to be performed for aesthetic purposes, the wrist may be arthrodesed in 30° of dorsiflexion. Flexor digitorum superficialis may be divided and flexor digitorum profundus lengthened until the fingers rest in a more natural position.

If the purpose of surgery is merely to prevent skin maceration by the tightly flexed digits, tenotomy of flexor digitorum profundus and superficialis may be all that is needed.

Thumb-in-palm deformity

Thumb-in-palm deformity is frequent with cerebral palsy and interferes with hand function in many ways. The acutely flexed thumb cannot participate in grasp. With the thumb lying clenched in the palm, it obstructs any attempt to grasp objects. In addition, the grasp reflex may be provoked by the thumb stimulating the palmar skin to increase finger flexion. Thumb-in-palm deformity may be caused by spasticity of the flexor pollicis longus, thenar muscles or the adductor. Usually there is also relative weakness of the extrinsic extensors both to the phalanges and metacarpals.

Tight flexor pollicis longus

With tight flexor pollicis longus, interphalangeal, metacarpophalangeal and trapeziometacarpal joints of the thumb are acutely flexed. This flexed position is accentuated with wrist dorsiflexion and relaxed with wrist palmar flexion. If adductor pollicis functions, the thumb may be brought out of the palm and may participate in grasp by transfer of the flexor pollicis longus subcutaneously to the abductor pollicis brevis. The interphalangeal joint of the thumb is arthrodesed or tenodesed.

Tight thenar muscles and adductor pollicis

Tight thenar muscles and adductor pollicis will flex the thumb acutely at the metacarpophalangeal joint. The interphalangeal frequently remains extended. Wrist position does not affect thumb position. Our preferred procedure is arthrodesis of the metacarpophalangeal joint of the thumb, lengthening of flexor pollicis longus and adductor pollicis muscle slide.

Acute flexion of the trapeziometacarpal joint

If adductor pollicis is the chief cause of the thumb-in-palm deformity, the first metacarpal will be acutely flexed and adducted. The preferred procedure is release of adductor pollicis from the third metacarpal and augmentation of the first metacarpal extension by transfer of brachioradialis to adductor pollicis longus.

Swan-neck deformity of the fingers

If the finger is flexed acutely at the metacarpophalangeal joint and extended at the interphalangeal joints, this may be due either to tightness of the intrinsic muscles or shift of the sagittal bands distally at the metacarpophalangeal joints. If there is spasticity of the interosseous muscles the intrinsic tightness test will be positive. When the metacarpocarpophalangeal joints are passively placed in extension, there will be increased resistance to flexion at the proximal interphalangeal joints. If the deformity is due to migration of the sagittal bands, the metacarpophalangeal joints will readily extend passively and the proximal interphalangeal joints will assume a more normal position with metacarpophalangeal extension.

(1) If there is mild intrinsic tightness interosseous muscle slide is performed. If the intrinsic tightness is severe the position is first tested by injecting the deep branch of the ulnar nerve. If this improves the position of the fingers, neurectomy is performed by complete division of the deep branch of the ulnar nerve distal to its bifurcation. Silver *et al.* (1976) described crushing a portion of the nerve rather than transecting it.
(2) If the swan-neck deformity is due to distal migration of the sagittal bands, the central slip is divided proximal to its insertion, the metacarpophalangeal joint is passively extended and the central slip sutured to the dorsal base of the proximal phalanx. The extensor tendons will then have little or no effect on the interphalangeal joints and will actively extend the metacarpophalangeal joint (*see Figures 1.3, 1.4, 1.5, 1.6, 1.7 and 1.8*).

CONCLUSIONS

Only a small percentage of all patients with cerebral palsy will require surgery. With many patients the deformities are not severe and function is satisfactory. For other patients, deformities may be too severe to allow satisfactory reconstruction. Some patients totally ignore the limb due to sensory loss, habit patterns or emotional or intellectual difficulties. For those few patients who do benefit from surgery, none can be made completely normal.

One must take care that all aspects of the problems that may affect the patient with cerebral palsy are evaluated. One must aim for limited goals and make these goals clear to the patient and to his family before surgery. If the preoperative, surgical and postoperative management are carefully planned, the rewards may be a better functioning limb and a happy patient and family.

References and further reading

BAROLAT-RAMONA, G. and DAVIS, R. (1980) Neurophysiological mechanisms in abnormal reflex activities in cerebral palsy and spinal spasticity. *Neurology, Neurosurgery and Psychiatry,* **43,** 333–342

BRAUN, R. M. and VISE, G. T. (1973) Sublimis to profundus tendon transfers in the hemiplegic upper extremity. *Journal of Bone and Joint Surgery,* **55A,** 873

CARROLL, R. E. and CRAIG, F. S. (1951) Surgical treatment of cerebral palsy — the upper extremity. *Surgical clinics of North America,* **30,** 385–396

CHAIT, L. A., KAPLAN, I., STEWART-LORD, B. and GOODMAN, M. (1980) Early surgical correction in the cerebral palsied hand. *Journal of Hand Surgery,* **5,** 122–126

COLTON, C. L., RANSFORD, A. O. and LLOYD-ROBERTS, G. C. (1976) Transposition of the tendon of pronator teres in cerebral palsy. *Journal of Bone and Joint Surgery,* **58B,** 220–223

FILLER, B. C., STARK, H. H. and BOYES, J. H. (1976) Capsulodesis of the metacarpophalangeal joint of the thumb in children with cerebral palsy. *Journal of Bone and Joint Surgery,* **58A,** 667–670

GELBERMAN, R. H. (in press). The upper extremity in cerebral palsy. In *Pediatric Upper Extremity Surgery,* edited by W. Bora. Philadelphia: W. B. Saunders Co.

GOLDNER, J. L. (1955) Reconstructive surgery of the hand in cerebral palsy and spastic paralysis resulting from injury to the spinal cord. *Journal of Bone and Joint Surgery,* **37A,** 1141–1151

GOLDNER, J. L. (1961) Upper extremity reconstructive surgery in cerebral palsy or similar conditions. *American Academy of Orthopedic Instructional Course Lectures,* **18,** 169–177

GOLDNER, J. L. (1966) Reconstructive surgery of the upper extremity affected by cerebral palsy or brain or spinal cord trauma. *Current Practice in Orthopaedic Surgery,* **3,** 125–138

GOLDNER, J. L. and FERLIC, D. C. (1966) Sensory status of the hand as related to reconstructive surgery of the upper extremity in cerebral palsy. *Clinical Orthopaedics and Related Research,* **46,** 87–92

GOLDNER, J. L. (1971) Cerebral palsy: Part I: General principles. *American Academy of Orthopaedic Surgeons Instructional Course Lectures,* **20,** 20–34

GOLDNER, J. L. (1971) Outline of operative procedures for reconstruction of the upper extremity in cerebral palsy. In *Operative Orthopaedics in Cerebral Palsy,* edited by S. Keats, pp. 50–99. Springfield, Illinois: C. C. Thomas

GOLDNER, J. L. (1974) Upper extremity tendon transfers in cerebral palsy. *Orthopaedic Clinics of North America,* **5,** 389–414

GOLDNER, J. L. (1975) The upper extremity in cerebral palsy. In *Orthopaedic Aspects of Cerebral Palsy,* edited by R. Samilson, pp. 221–257. Philadelphia: J. B. Lippincott

GOLDNER, J. L. (1979) Upper extremity surgical procedures for patients with cerebral palsy. *American Academy of Orthopaedic Surgery Instructional Course Lectures,* **28,** 37–66

GREEN, W. T. (1942) Operative treatment of cerebral palsy of spastic type. *Journal of the American Medical Association,* **118,** 434–440

GREEN, W. T. (1942) Tendon transplantation of the flexor carpi ulnaris for pronation–flexion deformity of the wrist. *Surgery, Gynecology and Obstetrics,* **75,** 337–342

GREEN, W. T. and BANKS, H. H. (1962) Flexor carpi ulnaris transplant and its use in cerebral palsy. *Journal of Bone and Joint Surgery,* **44A,** 1343–1352

HOFFER, M. M. (1978) The upper extremity in cerebral palsy. In *Neurological Aspects of Plastic Surgery,* Volume 17, edited by S. Fredericks and G. S. Brady, pp. 133–137. St Louis: C. V. Mosby

HOFFER, M. M., PERRY, J. and MELKONIAN, G. J. (1979) Dynamic electromyography and decision-making for surgery in the upper extremity of patients with cerebral palsy. *Journal of Hand Surgery,* **4,** 424–431

HOFFER, M. M. (1982) Cerebral palsy and stroke: Part I. In *Operative Hand Surgery,* edited by D. P. Green, pp. 185–194. New York: Churchill Livingstone

HOUSE, J. H., GWATHMEY, F. W. and FIDLER, M. O. (1981) A dynamic approach to the thumb-in-palm deformity in cerebral palsy. *Journal of Bone and Joint Surgery,* **63A,** 216–225

INGLIS, A. E. and COOPER, W. (1966) Release of the flexor–pronator origin for flexion deformities of the hand and wrist in spastic paralysis. *Journal of Bone and Joint Surgery,* **48A,** 847–857

INGLIS, A. E., COOPER, W. and BURTON, W. (1970). Surgical correction of the thumb deformities in spastic paralysis. *Journal of Bone and Joint Surgery,* **52A,** 253–268

KEATS, S. (1965) Surgical treatment of the hand in cerebral palsy: correction of the thumb-in-palm and other deformities. Report of 14 cases. *Journal of Bone and Joint Surgery,* **47A,** 274–284

MATEV, I. (1963) Surgical treatment of spastic 'thumb-in-palm' deformity. *Journal of Bone and Joint Surgery,* **45B,** 703–708

MATEV, I. (1970) Surgical treatment of flexion–adduction contracture of the thumb in cerebral palsy. *Acta Orthopaedica Scandinavica,* **41,** 439–445

McCARROL, H. R. (1949) Surgical treatment of spastic paralysis. In *American Academy of Orthopaedic Surgery Instructional Course Lectures,* **6,** 134–151

McCUE, F. C., HONNER, R. and CHAPMAN, W. C. (1970) Transfer of the brachioradialis for hand deformed by cerebral palsy. *Journal of Bone and Joint Surgery,* **52A,** 1171–1180

MILNER-BROWN, H. S. and PENN, R. D. (1979) Pathophysiological mechanisms in cerebral palsy. *Journal of Neurology, Neurosurgery and Psychiatry,* **42,** 606–618

MITRAL, M. A. (1979) Lengthening of the elbow flexors in cerebral palsy. *Journal of Bone and Joint Surgery,* **61A,** 515–522

MOBERG, I. E. (1976) Reconstructive hand surgery in tetraplegia, stroke and cerebral palsy: some basic concepts in physiology and neurology. *Journal of Hand Surgery,* **1,** 29–34

MOWERY, C. A., GELBERMAN, R. H. and RHOADES, C. E. (in press). Upper extremity tendon transfers in cerebral palsy: electromyographic and functional analysis. *Journal of Pediatric Orthopaedics*

OMER, G. E. and CAPEN, D. A. (1976) Proximal row carpectomy with muscle transfers for spastic paralysis. *Journal of Hand Surgery,* **1,** 197–204

O'REILLY, D. E. and WALENTYNOWICZ, J. E. (1981) Etiology factors in cerebral palsy. *Developmental Medicine and Child Neurology,* **23,** 633–642

PAGE, C. M. (1923) An operation for the release of flexor contracture in the forearm. *Journal of Bone and Joint Surgery,* **5,** 233–234

PHELPS, W. M. (1957) Long-term results of orthopaedic surgery in cerebral palsy. *Journal of Bone and Joint Surgery,* **39A,** 53–59

POLLACK, G. A. (1982) Surgical treatment of cerebral palsy. *Journal of Bone and Joint Surgery,* **44B,** 68–81

SAKELLARIDES, H. T. and MITAL, M. (1976) Treatment of the pronator contracture of the forearm in cerebral palsy. *Journal of Hand Surgery,* **1,** 79–80

SAMILSON, R. L. and MORRIS, J. M. (1964) Surgical improvement of the cerebral palsied upper limb: electromyographic studies and results of 128 operations. *Journal of Bone and Joint Surgery,* **46A,** 1203–1216

SAMILSON, R. L. (1966) Principles of assessment of the upper limb in cerebral palsy. *Clinical Orthopaedics and Related Research,* **47,** 105–125

SARKIN, T. L. (1972) Surgery of the hand in infants with cerebral palsy. *South African Medical Journal,* **45,** 655–657

SHERK, H. H. (1977) Treatment of the severe rigid contractures in cerebral palsied upper limbs. *Clinical Orthopaedics and Related Research,* **125,** 151–155

SILVER, C. M., SIMON, S. D., LITCHMAN, H. M. and MEHRDAD, M. (1976) Surgical correction of spastic thumb-in-palm deformity. *Developmental Medicine and Child Neurology,* **18,** 632–639

SMITH, R. J. (1977) Surgery of the hand in cerebral palsy. *Operative Surgery,* R. G. Pulvertaft, consultant editor, pp. 215–230. London: Butterworths

SMITH, R. J. (1982) Flexor pollicis longus abductor-plasty for spastic thumb-in-palm deformity. *Journal of Hand Surgery,* **7,** 327–334

SWANSON, A. B. (1960) Surgery of the hand in cerebral palsy and the swan-neck deformity. *Journal of Bone and Joint Surgery,* **42A,** 951–964

SWANSON, A. B. (1968) Surgery of the hand in cerebral palsy and muscle origin release procedures. *Surgical Clinics of North America,* **48,** 1129–1138

TACHDIJIAN, M. O. and MINEAR, W. L. (1958) Sensory disturbances in the hands of children with cerebral palsy. *Journal of Bone and Joint Surgery,* **40A,** 85–90

TACHDIJIAN, M. O. (1972) *Pediatric Orthopaedics,* Volume II. Philadelphia: W. B. Saunders

WHITE, W. F. (1972) Flexor muscle slide in spastic hand. *Journal of Bone and Joint Surgery,* **54B,** 453–459

ZANCOLLI, E. A. and ZANCOLLI, E. R. (1981) Surgical management of the hemiplegic hand in cerebral palsy. *Surgical Clinics of North America,* **61,** 395–496

ZANCOLLI, E. A., GOLDNER, L. J. and SWANSON, A. B. (1983) Surgery of the spastic hand in cerebral palsy: report of the committee on spastic hand evaluation. *Journal of Hand Surgery,* **5,** 766–771

2
The rheumatoid hand

John Stanley

INTRODUCTION

The restoration and preservation of function to maintain an independent lifestyle remains the aim of treatment for the patient with rheumatoid arthritis. Patients who suffer from inflammatory and erosive polyarthropathy present complex interrelated problems. There are both medical and social aspects. In order to assess patients for treatment programmes a clear view of the aims and objectives of such treatment must be held by both the physician and surgeon. A proper understanding of the pathology, and how this is likely to affect a given individual in his or her daily life, will lead to rational and realistic surgical and medical management, increasing the likelihood of functional improvement. The aims of surgery in the rheumatoid patient are traditionally said to be the relief of pain and the improvement of function. It is clear from our own experience that, although patients commonly complain of pain, it is the loss of function following incomplete medical control of the disease that causes the patient and rheumatologist to seek a surgical opinion. Pain is a feature of both the acutely inflamed joint and the chronically destroyed joint. Surgery during the former stage is contraindicated, but during the latter stage is strongly indicated.

The term rheumatoid arthritis was first coined by Sir Alfred Garrod in 1850. It is a systemic disease, and systemic treatment is necessary to achieve control of the disease. The use of 'first-line' drugs, such as the non-steroidal anti-inflammatory preparations (NSAIDs) in addition to the 'second-line' management using gold salts, penicillamine and others, has reduced the prevalence of florid synovitis, and the incidence of joint damage associated with this. The introduction of antimetabolites has meant that a larger group of patients will come under partial or full control and total lymphoid irradiation (Calin, 1964) may improve this control still further in selected patients. This reinforces the position of rheumatologists as prime movers in the management of rheumatoid patients. It is essential that rheumatologists be fully aware of current surgical thinking, and especially aware of the surgical procedures that are available to the patient at local level. Whether the contact is through the joint consultative clinic, or informally, is a personal choice, but without understanding the role of the surgeon the rheumatologist cannot advise his patient fully and, of course, the surgeon must view the rheumatologist in the same light. Surgical procedures will not then be doomed to failure because of poor rheumatological control, nor will patients develop progressive functional loss due to worsening deformity and instability to a point when surgery is merely a 'salvage procedure' for the destroyed hand.

ASSESSMENT OF THE RHEUMATOID HAND

Control of the disease process is, unfortunately, rarely complete. Ageing and the inevitable progress of secondary degenerative changes usually means that some aspect of the patient's problems will require a surgical solution.

Within the context of hand surgery, assessment of the patient's difficulties commences with broad questions related to the upper limb; discussion between the patient and therapist regarding the social and financial aspects. From these rather formal beginnings a relationship is built up which allows the therapist to appreciate the context of the answers to the more detailed questioning, and practical assessment of the upper limbs. The involvement of the lower limbs is highly relevant. The amount of help needed for walking, and getting up out of a chair or a bed, provided by the upper limbs, must be identified in advance of any hand surgery programme. Rarely is a single disability identified as the sole problem and more often a list of stiff or unstable, deformed and painful joints will emerge, and it is in these circumstances that priority must be given to the many disabilities. Several views exist as to whether simple 'test' surgery should first be performed on the non-dominant side (Souter, 1979), or whether treatment should be restricted to one or two surgical procedures in one admission (Millender, Nalebuff and Feldon, 1982). Alternatively a list of problems can be seen as an overall surgical problem, and the maximum achievable under a single tourniquet as the limit to one 'session' (Strickland and LaSalle, 1982).

There is no doubt that several factors must be taken into account: the patient's wishes, the patient's surgical 'tolerance', the surgeon's operative experience, and the compatibility of the various surgical procedures. The patient may be reluctant to undergo any surgery and the decision to replace the wrist, fuse the interphalangeal joint of the thumb and replace all the finger metacarpophalangeal joints might deter them. If this be the case, an appreciation of the patient's views, through the therapist, will warn of such danger, and a non-dominant thumb–interphalangeal joint fusion would reassure the nervous patient and rheumatologist that surgery can be successful. However, with a variety of problems presenting, generally some form of multiple surgery is necessary if several admissions for hand surgery are not to be added to admissions for hip, knee and foot surgery. The activities of daily living, Fries assessment (Fries, 1983), practical tasks (such as the button test), range of movement, deformity and stability are the basis for our decision-making both with regard to the selection of patients for surgery and the choice of the surgical procedure.

It is useful to group patients into three broad bands, based upon a rough assessment of their upper limb disability. The first group is the '80 per cent' function group, the second is the '50 per cent' group and the third is the '5 per cent' group.

The '80 per cent hand' represents the patients with mild disease, limited deformity and good function. Within this group exists the patient with early disease, and often significant early synovitis. These patients are those for whom preventive surgery would be considered. Synovectomy and rebalancing of joints might form part of a surgical programme in the event of incomplete medical control of the disease. Dorsal tenosynovectomy, flexor tenosynovectomy and synovectomy of the proximal interphalangeal joint (PIP) are usually successful in this group with minimal loss of hand function after surgery. However, postoperative assessment shows little or no change in the overall picture; the main advantage of surgery has been the prevention of further disability, and the relief of pain.

The '50 per cent hand' is the situation where wrist surgery, joint replacement, tendon repairs and other procedures can improve function to 75–80 per cent of normal, an increase of up to 50 per cent. This is the most common group.

The '5 per cent hand' represents the group of patients who are dependent upon others for the basic activities of daily living, feeding, dressing and attending to personal hygiene. Apart from the patient with complete destruction of the wrist, with little or no hand disability, who can be improved by wrist fusion to 80 per cent function, the remainder of this group require simple surgery, and can achieve at best 25–30 per cent of hand function following thumb and wrist surgery, improving many of them to the position of independence.

The philosophy for each group is different, and regard to this overall view prevents over-ambitious surgical treatment causing disappointment to the patient, surgeon, therapist and rheumatologist.

When faced with multiple problems a 'priority' list is of value and our priorities are outlined in *Table 2.1*.

Table 2.1 The priority order for surgical treatment

(1) Nerves
(2) Flexor tendons
(3) Wrist joint
(4) Extensor tendons
(5) Thumb
(6) Metacarpophalangeal (MCP) joint
(7) Proximal interphalangeal (PIP) joint
(8) Distal interphalangeal (DIP) joint

Nerve compression syndromes

These are present in the majority of patients presenting with rheumatoid disease. In one series 69 per cent of patients had a carpal tunnel syndrome (Barnes and Curry, 1970). In addition to the more obvious median nerve compression, elbow joint synovitis with ulnar nerve compression within the cubital tunnel is often present, and easily overlooked. Patients suffering from multiple joint disease are reluctant to volunteer symptoms they regard as less important than hip, knee, shoulder, elbow and wrist pain. Long-standing nerve compression leads to progressive impairment of motor function. This adds to the overall effect of joint and tendon damage, and can prejudice the result of a surgical programme. The highest priority is given to this aspect of hand disability.

Flexor tendons

Synovitis associated with rheumatoid disease is present in almost half of patients (Brewerton, 1957), and, although remittent in many, may be chronic, and it is in this group that careful assessment is particularly warranted. It may present as diffuse proliferative synovitis or as discrete nodules. The discrete nodule occurs on or within the flexor digitorum sublimis (FDS), the flexor digitorum profundus (FDP), or the flexor pollicis longus (FPL), and can lie at the level of the A1 pulley, giving rise to 'triggering'; at the level of the C1/A2 pulley it causes restriction of flexion, since the nodule can often not escape from the fibrous flexor sheath, and when distal to the FDS decussation (Helal, 1970) it may prevent excursion of the flexor digitorum profundus. Thickening of the synovium alone is best treated by steroid injection, but failure to improve or early recurrence of symptoms must be treated surgically. Proliferative synovitis throughout the length of the fibrous sheath must be regarded with suspicion, since chronic synovitis in this situation may result in flexor tendon rupture of one or both tendons and, as the tendon ruptures within the thickened synovial sheath, healing can occur, but in a markedly lengthened state. This attenuation and lengthening weakens the action of the flexor muscles, weakens grasp and may give rise to swan-neck deformity of the proximal interphalangeal joint. Even if rupture of the tendons does not occur, resolution of the synovitis often leaves residual scarring and adhesions, impeding tendon gliding motion. These effects will compromise the results of metacarpophalangeal (MCP) joint replacement surgery, and more significantly proximal interphalangeal joint replacement surgery. A positive approach to proliferative synovitis of the flexor sheath is indicated. Flexor synovitis present after 3–4 months, despite adequate rheumatological care, should be explored, and a tenosynovectomy performed.

Proliferative synovitis within the radial bursa at the wrist level, apart from precipitating median nerve compression, can cause ischaemia and rupture of tendon in just the same way as occurs within the fibrous sheath; the time-scale is longer, the effect the same. We feel this results in 'rupture in continuity', markedly weakening the power of grasp and preventing the achievement of satisfactory joint replacement within the fingers. Triggering may also occur at the wrist. Hence our high priority within the list of problems to be treated.

Rupture of the flexor pollicis longus occurs in association with a spur arising from the scaphotrapezial joint which erodes through the volar radiocarpal ligament, and abrasion of the flexor pollicis longus against this spur causes attrition of the tendon (Mannerfelt and Norman, 1969). Delayed primary repair or grafting gives better results than are achieved with repair or graft of the finger flexors.

At the wrist, sharp dissection of the synovium from the three groups of tendons, flexor pollicis longus, flexor digitorum sublimis and flexor digitorum profundus is done first, checking the floor of the carpal tunnel for spurs, and ensuring that the transverse carpal ligament is divided, completes the surgical procedure. Unfortunately, a recurrence of the synovitis is seen in some patients, and this fact must be conveyed to the rheumatologist and patient alike, before surgery, lest they regard this as a surgical failure, and decline any further treatment. Therefore, careful therapy programmes with close supervision not only improve the results of the tenosynovectomy but also identify the recurrence early should it occur.

WRIST

The importance of the wrist joint cannot be overemphasized: pain and instability at this level has a profound effect upon the function of the hand. A number of mechanisms come into play, either singly or in combination: supination of the hand upon the forearm with rotary instability of the wrist; translocation of the carpus;

volar collapse; synovitis of the wrist joint and intercarpal arthritis. All significantly impair wrist function, and this adversely affects hand function.

A common presentation is the so-called caput ulnae syndrome, with limited supination of the forearm, loss of extension of the little finger and dorsal subluxation of the ulnar head, with the 'piano key' sign (Backdahl, 1963). The distortion of the extensor retinaculum is asymmetrical, and the ulnar side of the retinaculum is pulled towards the volar side by the triquetral attachment, giving rise to a sharp ridge under which the extensor digiti minimi is compressed (Abernethy and Dennyson, 1979). The common extensor tendons are affected to a lesser degree, but the extensor of the little finger is at high risk of rupture; the risk diminishes towards the radial side, probably related to the ischaemia resulting from the synovitis under the extensor retinaculum rather than attrition due to a Vaughan-Jackson lesion (Vaughan-Jackson, 1948). In our experience, only seven such lesions were associated with rupture in a series of 115 cases. Established supination of the wrist often worsens during attempts to grasp, as the extensor carpi ulnaris is always displaced to the volar side and acts as a flexor of the wrist, pulling the triquetrum under the volar aspect of the ulna. However, not all wrists exhibit this type of deformity. Relative overactivity of the radial wrist extensors due to synovitis of extensor carpi radialis leads to ulnar translocation and radiocarpal collapse, with rotational instability of the scaphoid. The natural axis of the hand which lies through the radius and the third metacarpal is disturbed, and a Z deformity, which collapses upon finger extension, gives rise to painful inhibition of power grasp (Volz, 1982). The appearance of the crypt or anterior synovial cyst is a prelude to volar collapse. The crypt described by Mannerfelt is an extension of synovium along the anterior marginal vessels, with the formation of an ever-increasing synovial cyst in the radius, with subsequent collapse. Over-lengthening of the flexor tendons to the fingers is the net result, and failure of axial compression stability.

Synovitis of the wrist joint gives rise to apparent stretching of all the ligaments, and instability, which tends to perpetuate the synovitis. Much more painful is the intercarpal synovitis, with characteristically haemorrhagic synovium. This often causes marked deterioration of hand function, but eventually this type appears to progress towards spontaneous intercarpal fusions.

Taking into account these mechanisms, it must be realized that any surgical intervention at the metacarpophalangeal joint level in the presence of significant wrist pain or instability will have limited success. The treatment options available for the wrist are dependent upon the bone stock. Gross destruction of the lower radius with proximal carpal loss will leave few options. However, good bone stock and stability of the joint allow all options to be considered. The options are as follows:
(1) Synovectomy – dorsal or volar with rebalancing of tendons.
(2) Excision lower ulna.
(3) Interpositional arthroplasty (silicone rubber).
(4) Limited wrist fusion (radiolunate).
(5) Wrist fusion (radiocarpal).
(6) Excisional arthroplasty.
(7) Excisional arthroplasty with Silastic spacer.
(8) Total wrist replacement.

All dorsal approaches to the wrist are performed through straight longitudinal incisions. Lazy S incisions may heal poorly with tip necrosis. A dorsal tenosynovectomy should be performed for all except the first compartment, and extensor retinaculum must be placed deep to the tendons, due care being taken to preserve the dorsal branches of the ulnar and radial nerves. This 'exteriorization' of the tendons protects them, and in Clayton's series (Clayton, 1982), only one tendon ruptured in 174 patients in a three-year follow-up.

Excision of 1 cm of the terminal branch of the posterior interosseous nerve lying in the loose areolar tissue deep to the common extensor tendons has become popular, and does denervate part of the joint. A capsular flap is based on the third metacarpo-capitate junction, reflected from the distal radius from the line of extensor carpi radialis longus to the radio-ulnar joint, provides adequate access to the joint. This access is greatly improved if the terminal 1–2 cm of ulna is excised through an incision in its capsule. Extraperiosteal excision reduces the incidence of regeneration of the ulna to form the 'carrot'-shaped stump (Swanson, 1972). After removal, access can be gained to the ulnar side of the radiocarpal joint.

Volar wrist synovectomy may be performed at the same time as flexor tenosynovectomy, but although some favour the approach (Taleisnik, 1979), the restriction of access and the inability to perform distal ulnar surgery or reconstruction of the wrist if necessary lowers the value of this approach.

Excision of the lower ulna described by Darrach (Darrach and Dwight, 1915), Smith-Peterson, Aufranc and Larson (1943) for rheumatoid arthritis, and as described above, can allow for correction of the supination of the carpus, the importance of which is widely recognized. Reconstruction of the ulnar structures is made easier by careful preservation of the collateral ligament, and splitting of the ulnar head. Removing it in two halves facilitates this (*Figure 2.1*). The use of a flap of volar capsule based distally, brought up over the stump of ulna, as described by

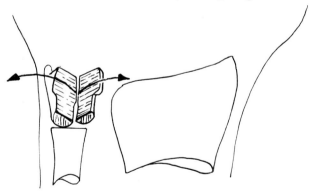

Figure 2.1 Longitudinal division of the ulnar head allows safer dissection of the two halves, each half being dissected away from the volar structures

Blatt (Blatt and Ashworth, 1979), stabilizes the lower ulna and restrains dorsal instability. At the Mayo Clinic (Lipscomb, 1967) half of the extensor carpi ulnaris is used, based distally as a reinforcement to the posterior capsule. Both these methods are static tethers of the ulna. The use of careful capsular repair over a silicone cap (Swanson, 1972), allowing repositioning of extensor carpi ulnaris (Hastings and Evans, 1975), creating a dynamic sling is, in our view, more likely to have a lasting effect.

The rebalancing of the wrist by relocation and centralization of extensor carpi ulnaris is but one technique for attempting to correct deformity, and transfer of extensor carpi radialis longus to the ulnar side, as described by Clayton (Clayton and Ferlic, 1974), is also useful. The scope for surgery such as described, in addition to dorsal tenosynovectomy and joint synovectomy, is limited (Millender, Nalebuff and Feldon, 1982), and reconstruction of the wrist joint is much more frequently required. The options are either fusion or arthroplasty. Arthroplasty in the form of proximal row carpectomy has been superseded by the use of an internal spacer (Swanson, 1973), or interposition, and in some centres, total joint replacement.

In the presence of reasonable joint alignment with minimal translocation and no volar subluxation, a Jackson interpositional arthroplasty of the wrist using 1 mm silicone elastomer sheeting cut to a teardrop shape and inserted through the ulnar side of the wrist joint after ulnar head excision, gives excellent pain relief (Souter, 1981). The range of movements is usually improved only if the major part of the preoperative restriction of range is due to pain. In our own series the best improvement in range is in extension, and improvements from 20° preoperatively to 70° postoperatively can be achieved within six weeks of surgery. Flexion usually improves from 10° to 45°. No special instruments are required, and the excision of the ulnar head can be accompanied by dorsal tenosynovectomy, and repair of tendons if necessary. The extensor carpi ulnaris is relocated over the head of the ulna, and the use of the silastic ulnar cap facilitates this manoeuvre, giving some bulk to the lower ulna to allow for improved action of the extensor carpi ulnaris in balancing the hand.

Limited wrist fusion, as advocated by Chamay (Chamay, Della Santa and Vilaseca, 1983), involves fusion of the lunate to the radius, and allows intercarpal movement to mimic radiocarpal movements. The results are good in selected cases; that is those wrists without significant intercarpal arthritis, with minimal or correctable translocation, good lunate stock, and no volar subluxation. The range to be expected is up to 50 per cent of normal range. The technique is simple, and the period of immobilization is six weeks. Fixation with Kirschner wires is unsatisfactory and the use of screws, plates and other methods of fixation appear bulky. However, the concept is sound, and the early reported results are encouraging.

Wrist arthrodesis using internal fixation has been described and well documented. Clayton's first use of a Steinman pin (Clayton, 1965), committed the fusion to the neutral position. Mannerfelt (Mannerfelt and Malmsten, 1972), using a Rush pin, achieved some dorsiflexion. Millender (Millender and Nalebuff, 1973), using a Steinman pin between the second and third metacarpals by a closed technique, allowed early mobilization to be contemplated. The third metacarpal provides excellent distal fixation; the radius excellent proximal fixation. The two links in between need to be stabilized. After a routine dorsal tenosynovectomy, the carpus is decorticated, using a bone rongeur for two-thirds of its depth. This preserves some length, and prevents bone chips bulging in the volar ligaments. The radius is likewise rongeured for two-thirds of its depth. The ulnar head is invariably removed in the rheumatoid patient. If cut correctly it provides an excellent corticocancellous graft (*Figure 2.2*), and can be held with the dorsal capsule and extensor retinaculum, remaining in position during healing. A plaster slab for two weeks, during which time finger exercises are insisted upon, and a work splint for four weeks, complete the postoperative programme.

In our series of 91 wrist fusions with a follow-up of six months to six years, the countersink pin of our design has been used in 72 wrists, and non-union of the

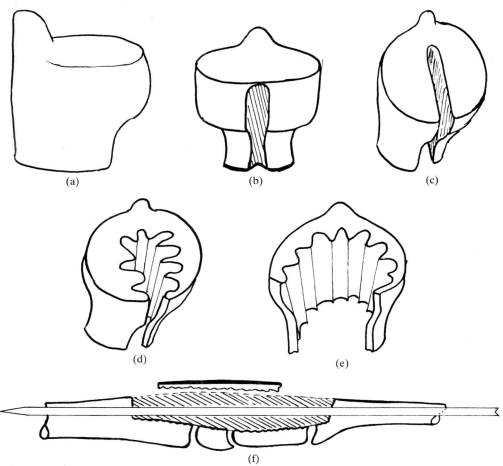

(a)　　　　　　(b)　　　　　　(c)

(d)　　　　　　(e)

(f)

Figure 2.2(a) The ulnar head is removed intact and excess synovium removed. (*b*) The use of sharp bone nibblers allows removal of a channel from the shaft and this channel is carried over (*c*) into the distal surface of the ulnar head. Crushing the remaining bone longitudinally (*d*) gradually opens out the ulnar head (*e*) into a flat graft which is corticocancellous and can be placed directly over the disintegrated carpus (*f*)

radiocarpal joint occurred in one patient, but painful movement of the third metacarpo-capitate joint in four patients. One patient had a fracture of the shaft of the third metacarpal at the tip of the pin in association with this movement; therefore fusion must include the third metacarpo-capitate joint. Countersinking to a depth of 15 mm from the metacarpal head allows a fibrous plug to form, preventing extrusion of the pin through the third metacarpal. Countersinking the pin to half the length of the shaft of the third metacarpal allows simultaneous replacement of the third metacarpophalangeal joint, providing 0.5 cm is trimmed from the stem of the Silastic implant.

The results of wrist fusion are well known, with marked pain relief, stability and improvement in hand function, but the grip that remains is simple power grasp, or baggage grip. However, sophisticated activity of the hand requires the ability to ulnar deviate the hand, and this movement is lost with fusion. Thus it is our practice, if the bone stock allows, to perform a radiocarpal wrist fusion of the non-dominant wrist, and a Swanson type replacement on the dominant side. The fusion is performed first as this provides the power grasp – the fixing, holding hand – and requires to be soundly fused. The replacement wrist ought not to perform power activity and thus the fusion must be achieved before commencing replacement of the dominant wrist, usually at a four-month interval.

The concept of fusion in some dorsiflexion, as described by Seddon (1952), has now been superseded by the view of neutral fusion to facilitate pesonal hygiene.

Wrist replacement is well documented (Swanson and Swanson, 1982) and our experience matches this and other reports (Beckenbaugh and Linscheid, 1982; Nalebuff and Garrod, 1984).

The indications for flexible hinge arthroplasty of the wrist in our Unit are as those described by Swanson and Nalebuff: stiffness, instability, pain and deformity affecting hand function. We prefer, in the presence of good bone stock, to replace the dominant wrist to preserve sophistication of grasp. Absence of the extensors of the wrist is a contraindication to replacement surgery. The stability of the implant, either Silastic or total joint replacement, is dependent upon adequate balance of the wrist prime movers, and imbalance due to rupture or weakness creates forces which prejudice the long-term survival of the implant.

It is clear from our own series of 97 wrist replacements of the Swanson type, in which we have four fractured implants, that two factors conspire to load the implant abnormally. The first is excessive movement. The early series of patients were encouraged to achieve up to 60° of extension, and 40° of flexion, with 20° of ulnar deviation, and 5–10° of radial deviation; this we feel now is over-ambitious, and to prevent this mechanism causing implant failure due to pinching of the implant and setting up tears we now aim for 30° of flexion and extension, and 10° of ulnar deviation, with a jog of radial deviation.

The second mechanism is failure of the extensor carpi ulnaris to 'balance' the ulnar side of the wrist; this failure causes supination of the hand, much magnified in the wrist with a large range, creating rotational stresses upon the implant, with resultant fracture. The surgical technique is well described by Swanson (Swanson and Swanson, 1982). There are, however, some difficulties encountered which can be minimized or avoided. There are four major problems.

(1) Having exposed the wrist from the dorsal aspect and having removed the ulnar head, preserved the extensor retinaculum and performed a dorsal teno-synovectomy if appropriate, the first problem is to decide upon the correct osteotomy cuts. With marked synovitis and volar collapse it is tempting to take too much from the radial side; the osteotomy cut must be at right angles to the shaft of the radius, both to the anteroposterior and longitudinal axis, and is cut as a compromise between the anterior and the posterior lips of the radius as assessed at the mid-part of the radiocarpal joint (*Figure 2.3a*). The second osteotomy cut is much easier and lies through the distal two-thirds of the lunate and through the waist of the scaphoid (*Figure 2.3b*). This removes the tip of the capitate and leaves a corona of lunate, which is removed piecemeal if necessary.

(2) The second problem is to achieve further enlargement of the newly created space without major bone resection, which will cause effective over-

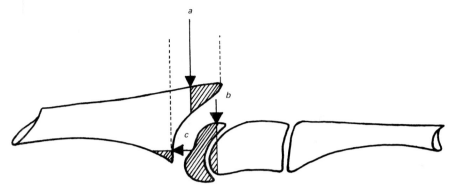

Figure 2.3 A lateral view of the wrist, with marked volar subluxation. The shaded areas represent bone to be excised. (*a*) The osteotomy here is at the compromise position between the dorsal and volar extremes of the radius. (*b*) The osteotomy here shows the need to leave some lunate bone to prevent excessive removal of the body of the capitate. (*c*) This represents the excision of the anterior osteophyte which is often small but significant (*see text*)

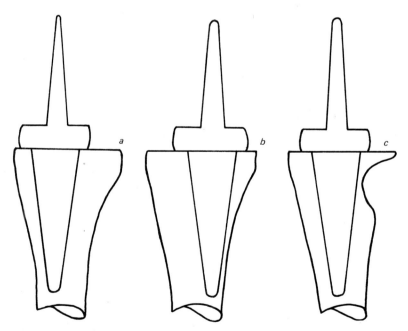

Figure 2.4(a) Reaming of the shaft of the radius in this position creates radial translocation which is cosmetically unsightly or creates a shear force across the distal stem of the implant. (*b*) Correct positioning of the implant allows the hand to be neutrally placed, and the axis of the third metacarpal is correctly aligned with the radius. (*c*) Excessive radio-ulnar erosion, due to proliferative synovitis, prevents adequate placing of the silicone implant and may be so severe as to preclude this procedure

lengthening of the finger flexors with increasing weakness of grasp. To achieve satisfactory lengthening, removal of the anterior osteophyte from the radius is essential, and the removal of 2 or 3 mm of bone will increase the joint space by up to 1 cm (*Figure 2.3c*). Any detachment of the volar ligament must be repaired.

(3) The third problem, of course, is reaming of the radius, and this must start from the ulnar side. Recognition of any erosion due to the radio-ulnar synovitis is taken into account (*Figure 2.4*). This minimizes ugly translocation.

(4) Finally, reaming of the capitate/third metacarpal must be angled dorsally to avoid entering the palm (*Figure 2.5*). Using both the standard and wide body series allows accurate choice of the implant to be made.

The long-term results are very acceptable. The choice appears to be between power from a fusion, or sophistication from the replacement, and one of each, we feel, is an excellent compromise. Although patients in our series with bilateral wrist surgery prefer replacement to wrist fusion, those patients with bilateral wrist replacements do have limitation of power, and those with bilateral fusions have limitation of sophisticated grasp.

Extensor tendons

Rupture of the extensor tendons occurs commonly from the ulnar side and results in the 'dropped' fingers so often seen in long-standing rheumatoid arthritis. The importance of not mistaking dislocated tendons which come to lie to the ulnar side

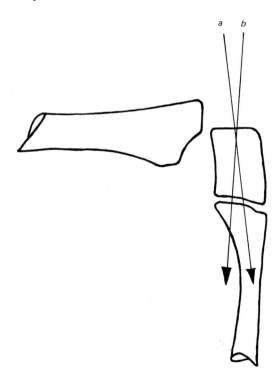

Figure 2.5(a) The direction for reaming of the capitate and third metacarpal must be angled. (*b*) The vertical approach leads to broaching of the cortex and injury to the structures in the palm of the hand

of the metacarpal heads, and lose the leverage necessary to extend the metacarpophalangeal joint for tendon ruptures, is clear. The diagnosis is also clear upon careful examination. Not so clear is the compression of the posterior interosseous nerve at the elbow (Chang *et al.*, 1972) causing weakness, and occasionally frank palsy of the common extensor tendons mimicking rupture. Single rupture of the little finger tendon is best treated by side-to-side suture to the tendon of the ring finger, utilizing a limited weave. Double ruptures and triple ruptures require tendon transfers, and extensor indicis proprius is the transfer of choice. Loss of independent index extension is not a problem, and adaptation occurs early in all age groups. Quadruple rupture of the finger extensors is uncommon and difficult to treat. No tendon is easily available for transfer. The wrist flexors and extensors are essential to wrist stability, and are not available unless the wrist is fused. The superficial tendon to the ring finger has been advocated for transfer, taken through the interosseous membrane or taken around the ulna. This can be successful in some patients, but a tenodesis effect appears to allow this transfer to work modestly (Nalebuff and Patel, 1973).

Extensor pollicis longus ruptures commonly, since it lies in a confined tunnel, and takes a sharp change of direction around the tubercle of Lister. The effect of this rupture is to prevent active movement of the thumb behind the plane of the hand; extension of the interphalangeal joint may be absent but not invariably so, and the only reliable test of this tendon is the ability to lift the thumb behind the plane of the palm. Disability is not invariably present, and many rheumatoid patients have little or no functional deficit. For those that do have a problem, extensor indicis proprius transfer to the long thumb extensor is very successful. Some would say use extensor pollicis brevis. If this transfer is unavailable, the next choice must be a graft. Despite poor results of grafting, this is preferable to transfer of the long radial wrist extensor, with consequent loss of balance of the wrist.

THUMB

The classification of deformities introduced by Nalebuff (Millender, Nalebuff and Feldon, 1982) remains useful by virtue of the implicit understanding of the mechanics of the deformity, essential in the process of selection of correct and effective surgical management.

The boutonnière deformity. flexion at the metacarpophalangeal joint and extension at the interphalangeal joint, he describes as type I. The deformity arises from two principal causes: failure of the extensor expansion secondary to a proliferative synovitis and rupture of the flexor pollicis longus tendon. When the deformity is correctable passively the problem is at the metacarpophalangeal level. The treatment must be directed towards synovectomy of the metacarpophalangeal joint and reconstruction of the retinaculum of the extensor hood. If joint destruction has occurred, replacement or fusion of the joints is indicated in addition to soft tissue surgery. Rupture of the flexor pollicis longus can be managed by repair, graft (usually one stage), or tenodesis of the distal joint of the thumb.

Type III or swan-neck deformity arises solely from the destruction of the carpometacarpal (CMC) joint. Treatment of this joint is indicated early in the development of the deformity. (Type II is a combination of I and III.)

Metacarpotrapezial disease can be managed by excision of the base of the metacarpal, and the insertion of a convex condylar silicone implant. The toe implant has been used on occasions (Swanson, 1981).

Erosion of the scaphoid, with or without translocation of the carpus, indicates that the above-described procedures are to be preferred to total trapezial replacement, which has an increased dislocation rate in poor tissues, commonly seen in rheumatoid disease.

The adduction deformity, Kessler (1973) pointed out, exists in the fascial covering of the intrinsic muscles, and our findings confirm those of Nalebuff (Millender, Nalebuff and Feldon, 1982), and Kessler (1973); correction of the deformity is achieved by releasing the fascia only.

Ulnar collateral rupture or attenuation (gamekeeper's thumb), and radial collateral ligament failure (reverse gamekeeper deformity) are considered as type IV. Treatment depends upon the quality of the metacarpophalangeal joint. Repair or reconstruction using a strip of extensor pollicis longus tendon is only valid when the joint is relatively undamaged or when joint replacement is performed. Fusion is the logical alternative, and if the metacarpophalangeal joint is the only joint affected, fusion is the treatment of choice, as the carpometacarpal and the interphalangeal joints have sufficient range to compensate. A previous fusion of the interphalangeal, or disease of the carpometacarpal joint, would favour replacement and reconstruction of the metacarpophalangeal joint. Fusions of this joint or interphalangeal joints of the thumb are generally straightforward. We have for some time favoured the technique described by Omer (1968), but have sometimes used Harrison-Nicolle polypropylene pegs (Harrison, 1974). Marked bone loss, as in the mutilans type of rheumatoid, requires a 'shish kebab' graft (Millender, Nalebuff and Feldon, 1982).

Reconstruction of the thumb can be the most rewarding surgical procedure a patient undergoes. In the great majority of cases that seem hopeless, stabilization of the thumb will give a functional improvement out of proportion to the surgical effort, to the delight of both patient and surgeon alike.

The restoration of thumb function, and the stabilization of the wrist, provide important improvements to the rheumatoid patient. The metacarpophalangeal joints of the finger are commonly affected in rheumatoid disease, and instability, stiffness, volar subluxation, ulnar drift, and pain may result in profound disability in spite of adequate wrist, thumb and flexor tendon surgery. The more proximal surgery is aimed at providing a pain-free, stable base for finger action, and thus the next logical step in the management of the rheumatoid hand is the metacarpophalangeal joint.

METACARPOPHALANGEAL JOINTS OF FINGERS

Synovitis at this level gives rise to stretching of tissues, progressive joint destruction and deformity. Surgery is indicated if medical control of the disease is incomplete or, as a result of the synovitis and its effects, a disability is present. Most authorities would regard synovectomy and soft tissue reconstruction as having a very limited application if performed at the metacarpophalangeal level alone. Recurrence of the synovitis within 1–3 years, the slow progression of deformity in some patients after surgery and the natural remission of the disease in others without surgery, has meant that the results of synovectomy are not predictable. There is a place for synovectomy when gross synovitis is unresponsive to splintage, intra-articular steroid injection and second-line therapy, and is accompanied by progressive deformity in the presence of good joints without significant subcollateral erosions, as seen on a radiograph taken in Brewerton's view (Brewerton, 1957). Beyond these criteria, the loss of advantage occasioned by the scarring, and the loss of confidence of the patient and rheumatologist, outweigh the possible benefits.

The understanding of the deforming forces is less than complete in the metacarpophalangeal joints of the hand. Some understanding is necessary if, at the time of surgery, rebalancing of the structures around the joint is to be successful. Three major deformities occur at the metacarpophalangeal joint: volar subluxation, ulnar deviation and pronation; flexion and extension deformities are less significant.

Volar subluxation

This is often seen early in the disease process, and can be recognized by testing the integrity of the dorsal capsule with the metacarpophalangeal joint held in 60° of flexion. The method is simply assessing the amount of displacement that can be produced at the joint by attempting to move the proximal phalanx into the palm; the normal hand has very little movement in this direction. The mechanisms of this deformity would seem to be three-fold: stretching of the dorsal capsule; failure of the accessory collateral ligament; loss of part of the metacarpal head on its volar surface (*Figure 2.6*), and the dorsal aspect of the proximal phalanx. Secondary

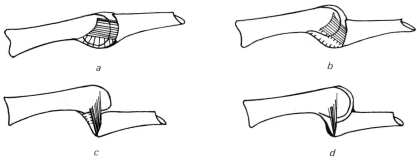

Figure 2.6 (*a*) The normal situation with intact suspensory ligament supporting the volar plate. (*b*) Early volar subluxation involves attenuation of the dorsal capsule and stretching of the suspensory ligament. (*c*) Erosion of the head of the metacarpal removes the normal restraint imposed by the ball and socket configuration of the joint. (*d*) Significant erosion of the dorsal aspect of the proximal phalanx also reduces the flexion range of the metacarpophalangeal joint and creates a difficult surgical problem

changes supervene to perpetuate and worsen the problem. Contracture of the volar plate, erosion and distortion of the transverse metacarpal ligament all result in a severe disturbance of adjacent metacarpophalangeal joints. Surgical correction of this deformity can be extremely difficult and, more importantly, it is difficult to maintain the correction following joint replacement.

Ulnar deviation

This is a common deformity, by itself not necessarily a cause of disability, but of considerable importance when joint replacement has been performed, since lateral instability, in concert with normal flexion and extension, places considerable shear, rotational and compression forces upon the implant, increasing the risk of its failure. Gross ulnar deviation is a cause of significant disability and arises as a result of many factors, only some of which may be relevant in a given individual case. Recognized elements in producing ulnar drift deformity are radial wrist collapse leading to radial deviation of the hand (Shapiro, 1968), synovitis of the subcollateral recess with collateral ligament failure (Flatt, 1966), extensor tendon displacement, flexor tendon displacement (Smith *et al.*, 1966), key grip pinch and intrinsic muscle imbalance (Boyes, 1969). In practical terms, surgical correction relies upon wrist surgery, relocation of the extensor tendons, and rebalancing the intrinsic muscles. Soft tissue surgery remains the keystone of arthroplasty of the metacarpophalangeal joints of the fingers.

Pronation

Pronation of the fingers prevents normal pulp to pulp pinch. Lateral pinch of the thumb to index finger hastens ulnar drift. The mechanism of pronation is not wholly clear. Failure of the normal supination action of the first dorsal interosseous muscle, coupled with failure of the radial accessory collateral ligament, allows ulnar displacement of the A2 pulley, prevents adequate supination, and the deformity results.

METACARPOPHALANGEAL JOINT ARTHROPLASTY

Many procedures have been described. Until the advent of implant surgery excisional arthroplasty was performed with variable results by, amongst others, Vainio (1974) and Fowler (1962) who used extensor tendon or volar plate respectively. The development of implant arthroplasty has occurred along two main paths: the metallic and the silicone elastomer.

Early experience with the metallic implants was encouraging (Flatt and Ellison, 1972), but the lack of tolerance of soft rheumatoid bone to the movement of metal within the medullary canal led to the development of cemented prostheses based upon the metal to high-density polyethylene implant (Steffee *et al.*, 1981), developed for the hip by Charnley. These in turn were less than satisfactory, due either to the occurrence of unexplained flexion deformity and poor range, or to loosening of the methylmethacrylate cement, again, in part, due to the poor quality of bone stock in the rheumatoid hand. The development of cementless prostheses, and those using dacron-coated stems, have reached clinical application.

The Silastic implants designed by Swanson have been the alternative to metal implants and, in the rheumatoid hand, have the advantage of being made of a material softer than the often very soft bone into which they are inserted. The use of other plastics (Nicolle and Calnan, 1972) has not met with the same long-term success as the silicone rubber and, overall, the Swanson flexible hinge remains, at this time, the most widely used. Niebauer (Niebauer, Shaw and Doren, 1968) developed a silicone implant with a dacron coating to stabilize the stems; the experience at the Mayo Clinic (Beckenbaugh and Linscheid, 1982) noted some problems of bone resorption, prosthetic buckling, and fracture with the early design of this implant.

Success of the Swanson implant is related to the principle that the implant provides an internal inert flexible splint which stabilizes the excisional arthroplasty and that meticulous rebalancing of soft tissues, with controlled early postoperative movements, protected by lively splintage, allows the formation of a capsule around the implant. This allows stable movement, with pain relief and improved function. The early Silastic material had poor tear resistance properties; the later material is much improved in this respect (Swanson and Swanson, 1982).

The surgical technique has been described by Swanson in detail (Swanson and Swanson, 1982). Certain minor alterations to the basic technique are helpful in difficult situations. The transverse incision, with preservation of the veins and nerves in the intermetacarpal groove, allows ease of access of all the joints, and allows them to be visualized at the same time without retraction of four incisions. The opening of the extensor expansion along the radial side of the extensor tendon allows for easier access in the patient with marked ulnar drift, and when closing, makes the decision to release the intrinsics more accurate. Additionally, advancement of the first dorsal interosseous tendon is made more easy when the fibres inserted into the extensor hood are seen directly. Advancement of the first dorsal interosseous tendon must not allow any correction of the pronation deformity to be lost. Dissection of the extensor tendon from the capsule of the joint must be done preserving this structure, the close of which, over the implant, recreates a smooth gliding surface. Minimal resection of bone from the metacarpal head, preserving the collateral ligaments, and the release of the volar plate from the proximal phalanx allows easy reaming of the medullary canals, ensuring that the index finger is in some supination. Marked volar subluxation with dorsal erosion of the proximal phalanx presents the most difficult dissection (*Figure 2.7*), and some excision of bone from the proximal phalanx is inevitable.

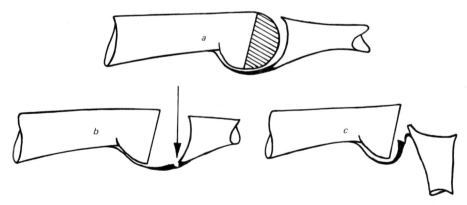

Figure 2.7 (*a*) Removal of the head of the proximal phalanx, preserving the collateral ligaments, facilitates partial incision of the volar plate at its insertion into the base of the middle phalanx. (*b*) The careful stripping of the soft tissues away from the volar aspect of the middle phalanx allows (*c*) dislocation of the whole of the base of the middle phalanx

Crossed intrinsic transfer is usually reserved for the simpler preventive surgery, and is usually unnecessary in metacarpophalangeal replacement. The first dorsal interosseous muscle is the first line of defence in the prevention of recurrent ulnar drift, and provides a dynamic correcting force. Therefore, having advanced its insertion, active index finger abduction exercises are commenced the day following surgery; this is in addition to the flexion and extension exercises normally performed.

Committed patients, lively splintage and close supervision by a hand therapist contribute to maximum improvement in a given patient (Swanson, Swanson and Leonard, 1978).

What constitutes a good result? The answer to this will vary according to whether the question is asked of the patient, the therapist, the rheumatologist, or the surgeon. The criteria for success must not be measured in range of movement, but in functional improvement, since the former is under the control of the patient, who will only achieve the range of movement that he or she requires. Any surplus range gained by therapy programmes is often lost over succeeding months.

PROXIMAL INTERPHALANGEAL JOINT

This joint responds much more reliably to synovectomy, and the indications are wider than those for the metacarpophalangeal joint or wrist. However, this joint, like the thumb, suffers from the effects of tendon imbalance, which act to produce two major deformities: the swan-neck deformity, and the boutonnière deformity. Both may coexist in the same hand. Nalebuff has described a classification of swan-neck deformity (Millender, Nalebuff and Feldon, 1982); that is, hyperextension of the proximal interphalangeal joint with flexion of the distal interphalangeal (DIP) joint, and he uses this classification as a basis for treatment.

Type I is mobile, correctable, with a good joint surface, and can be due to a longstanding mallet finger deformity, rupture of the superficial flexor tendon, or failure of the volar plate. The treatment of the first is to fuse the distal interphalangeal joint. The second and third require either a dermodesis (Millender, Nalebuff and Feldon, 1982), sublimis tenodesis (Curtis, 1980) (through bone or the flexor sheath), or reconstruction of the oblique ligament (Littler, 1969).

Type II swan-neck, stiff in metacarpophalangeal joint extension, and mobile with the metacarpophalangeal joint flexed, indicates intrinsic contracture, and release of the intrinsics is appropriate. Dermodesis or sublimis tenodesis may be performed. Metacarpophalangeal volar subluxation must be corrected prior to proximal interphalangeal joint surgery, as metacarpophalangeal joint disease is a common factor in the production of swan-neck deformity.

Type III presents with a stiff joint, good radiographs, and tight soft tissues, and probably represents a long-standing type I. Manipulation will only be successful if the flexor tendons have a good excursion; lateral band release is often necessary, and lengthening of the central strip may be needed (Nalebuff and Millender, 1975).

The presence of flexor tendon disease would require tenolysis; this also must be considered in type IV, with stiffness and joint destruction, where fusion of the index proximal interphalangeal joint, and Swanson silicone implant arthroplasty of the lesser finger proximal interphalangeal joints, restores grasp within the limits of the flexor tendon excursion.

Boutonnière deformity

This deformity consisting of flexion of the proximal interphalangeal joint, and extension of the distal interphalangeal joint, is less disabling than the swan-neck, since the pulps of the fingers reach the palm, and a closed grasp is possible. The mechanism is an attenuation, or rupture, of the central slip of the extensor mechanism, and, if no radiographic changes have occurred, synovectomy and repair of the central slip in the early case will be sufficient. However, the well-established deformity, with a good joint, requires advancement of the central slip, relocation of the lateral bands, and a Fowler extensor tenotomy over the middle phalanx. Joint destruction, with gross flexion can, with serial splintage, be improved to a point where consideration might be given to a proximal interphalangeal joint Swanson arthroplasty. In patients with correctable deformity, this procedure can stabilize and correct the major part of the deformity, and thence the disability.

The technique of flexible hinge arthroplasty of the proximal interphalangeal joint is well described (Swanson, 1981); particular care must be given to the preservation of the collateral ligaments, and to the adequate release of the volar plate. Release of the volar plate attachment from the anterior lip of the base of the middle phalanx allows excellent exposure of the middle phalanx, and removal of osteophytes and sharp bone spicules, often seen at this level (*see Figure 2.7*). The reattachment of the central slip, to be lengthened in swan-neck, and shortened in a boutonnière, to bone via drill holes, and the closure of the capsule as a separate layer, complete a procedure which requires very careful supervision, and the patient must be aware that 12 weeks after surgery, if an unsatisfactory range of movement is present, a manipulation might be required. Rupture of the radial collateral ligament of the proximal interphalangeal joint occurs spontaneously in the rheumatoid patient, and is usually associated with joint damage; this can be mistaken for collapse of the ulnar condyle. The former would require fusion, the latter a replacement.

Fusion of the proximal interphalangeal joint is indicated in the index finger, and also in the joints of the ulnar fingers, when replacement is inadvisable because of absent flexor tendons, collaterals, or previous failed arthroplasty. The use of two or

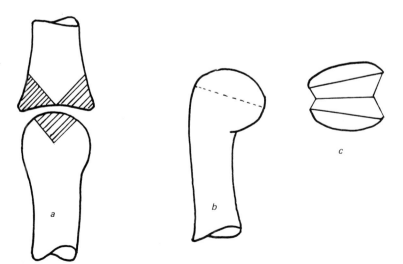

Figure 2.8 (*a*) The chevron excision of bone, if angled toward the volar aspect (*b*) gives control as to the final position of the joint with maximum bone contact. (*c*) This angulation is achieved by excising a wedge wider on the volar surface than the dorsal

three Kirschner wires, or Harrison–Nicolle polypropylene pegs, coupled with reversed chevron bone excision (Omer, 1968; *Figure 2.8*), (the 'V' cut from the head of the proximal phalanx, and the base of the middle phalanx shaped to fit), is followed by a high union rate, and allows removal of wires, if necessary, at 3–4 weeks. The position of fusion is different for each finger; 30° of flexion in the index, increasing to 45° or 50° in the little finger. This improves grasp.

Distal joint disease

This is associated with joint destruction in the arthritis mutilans type, or as a result of extensor tendon rupture, mallet deformity, or flexor tendon rupture, leading to hyperextension. Both these conditions respond well to fusion of the joint, the optimum position being in neutral for all the fingers (Millender, Nalebuff and Feldon, 1982).

CONCLUSION

The importance of a surgeon appreciating the rheumatological management is emphasized when faced with a patient taking antimetabolite drugs, or 'third-line' management, for their rheumatoid disease. Only a small proportion of patients have rheumatoid disease so severe that this method of management is necessary. However, it is clear from our own experience that these patients seem to mature the scar collagen, formed after surgery, extremely slowly, and it is our practice to splint these patients for considerably longer (up to double the time), than the patient who is on first and second-line therapy. Whether this formation of poor collagen is a reflection of the severity of the disease process, or whether it is a reflection of the effects of antimetabolite drugs, is uncertain. Patients who require surgery, and who have vasculitis, also fall into the category of patients in which surgery must be regarded with some caution. The use of plasmapheresis (Wilkinson, 1980), reported to improve vasculitis has, in our Unit, allowed for healing of vasculitic lesions, and the creation of a vasculitic free period, sometimes lasting many months, which allows for surgical correction of the joint and tendon disease, and satisfactory wound healing. These latter two examples highlight the close cooperation necessary between the disciplines of the management of patients with rheumatoid arthritis.

Concern has been expressed recently about the appearance of 'silicone synovitis'. This has been seen in situations where Silastic articulates under some pressure, in other words, the radial head and the small bones of the wrist. This appears as a marked inflammatory reaction with histological appearances of a synovitis containing fine Silastic particles. Cyst formation within adjacent bone in addition to the synovitis characterizes this uncommon occurrence. Removal of the implant with curettage, synovectomy and bone grafting may be necessary. The incidence of this particular complication is extremely low but has given rise to concern.

In our own experience of several thousands of implants, we have seen this condition once in association with a radial head implant, which when removed showed significant wear. It would seem clear that it is important that Silastic articulates with the pseudo-capsule rather than bone; however, we have not seen this silicone synovitis in trapezium implants nor in convex condylar replacement of the carpometacarpal joint of the thumb.

References

ABERNETHY, P. J. and DENNYSON, W. G. (1979) Decompression of extensor tendons in rheumatoid arthritis. *Journal of Bone and Joint Surgery*, **61B**, 64–68

BACKDAHL, M. (1963) The caput ulnae syndrome in rheumatoid arthritis. *Acta Rheumatologica Scandinavica*. Supplement, **5**, 1–75

BARNES, C. G. and CURRY, H. L. F. (1970) Carpal tunnel syndrome in rheumatoid arthritis. A clinical and electrodiagnostic survey. *Annals of the Rheumatic Diseases*, **26**, 226–233

BECKENBAUGH, R. D. and LINSCHEID, R. L. (1982) Arthroplasty. In *Operative Hand Surgery*, edited by David P. Green, pp. 153, 170–173. New York: Churchill Livingstone

BLATT, G. and ASHWORTH, C. R. (1979) Volar capsular transfer for stabilisation following resection of the distal end of the ulna. *Orthopaedic Transactions*, **3**, 13

BOYES, J. H. (1969) The role of the intrinsic muscles in rheumatoid deformities. In *La Main Rheumatoide (The Rheumatoid Hand)*, edited by R. Tubiana, pp. 63–64. Paris: Expansion Scientifique Française

BREWERTON, D. A. (1957) Hand deformities in rheumatoid disease. *Annals of the Rheumatic Diseases*, **16**, 183

CALIN, A. (1964) X-radiation in the management of rheumatoid disease. *British Journal of Hospital Medicine*, **33**, 261–265

CHAMAY, A., DELLA SANTA, D. and VILASECA, A. (1983) Radio-lunate arthrodesis, a factor of stability for the rheumatoid wrist. *Annales de Chirurgie de la Main*, **2**, 5–17

CHANG, L. W., GOWANS, J. D. C., GRANGER, C. V. and MILLENDER, L. H. (1972) Entrapment neuropathy of the posterior interosseous nerve. A complication of rheumatoid arthritis. *Arthritis and Rheumatism*, **15**, 350–352

CLAYTON, M. L. (1965) The surgical treatment of the wrist in rheumatoid arthritis. *Journal of Bone and Joint Surgery*, **47A**, 741–750

CLAYTON, M. L. (1982) The caput ulnae syndrome: update. In *Difficult Problems in Hand Surgery*, edited by J. W. Strickland and J. B. Steichen, pp. 199–202. St Louis: C. V. Mosby

CLAYTON, M. L. and FERLIC, D. C. (1974) Tendon transfer for radial rotation of the wrist in rheumatoid arthritis. *Clinical Orthopaedics*, **100**, 176–185

CURTIS, R. (1980) Sublimis tenodesis. In *Campbell's Operative Orthopaedics*, 6th edition, edited by A. S. Edmondson and A. H. Crenshaw. St Louis: C. V. Mosby

DARRACH, W. and DWIGHT, K. (1915) Derangement of the inferior radio-ulnar articulation. *Proceedings of the New York Academy of Medicine. Medical Record*, **87**, 708

FLATT, A. E. (1966) Some pathomechanics of ulnar drift. *Plastic and Reconstructive Surgery*, **37**, 295–303

FLATT, A. E. and ELLISON, M. R. (1972) Restoration of rheumatoid finger function. III. *Journal of Bone and Joint Surgery*, **54A**, 1317–1322

FOWLER, S. B. (1962) Arthroplasty of the metacarpophalangeal joints in rheumatoid arthritis. *Journal of Bone and Joint Surgery*, **44A**, 1037–1038

FRIES, J. F. (1983) Toward an understanding of patient outcome measurement. *Arthritis and Rheumatism*, **26**, 697–704

HARRISON, S. H. (1974) The Harrison–Nicolle intramedullary peg: follow-up study of 100 cases. *The Hand*, **6**, 304–307

HASTINGS, D. E. and EVANS, J. A. (1975) Rheumatoid wrist deformities and their relation to ulnar drift. *Journal of Bone and Joint Surgery*, **57A**, 930–934

HELAL, B. (1970) Distal profundus entrapment in rheumatoid disease. *The Hand*, **2**, 48–51

KESSLER, I. (1973) The aetiology and management of adduction contracture of the thumb in rheumatoid arthritis. *The Hand*, **5**, 170–174

LIPSCOMB, P. R. (1967) Synovectomy of the distal two joints of the thumb and fingers in rheumatoid arthritis. *Journal of Bone and Joint Surgery*, **49A**, 1135–1140

LITTLER, J. W. (1969) Restoration of the oblique retinacular ligament for correcting hyperextension deformity of the proximal interphalangeal joint. In *La Main Rheumatoide (The Rheumatoid Hand)*, edited by R. Tubiana, pp. 155–157 Paris: Expansion Scientifique Française

MANNERFELT, L. and NORMAN, O. (1969) Attrition rupture of flexor tendons in rheumatoid arthritis caused by bony spurs in the carpal tunnel. *Journal of Bone and Joint Surgery*, **51B**, 270–277

MANNERFELT, L. and MALMSTEN, M. (1972) Arthrodesis of the wrist in rheumatoid arthritis. *Scandinavian Journal of Plastic and Reconstructive Surgery*, **5**, 124–130

MILLENDER, L. H. and NALEBUFF, E. A. (1973) Arthrodesis of the rheumatoid wrist. *Journal of Bone and Joint Surgery*, **55A**, 1026–1034

MILLENDER, L. H., NALEBUFF, E. A. and FELDON, P. G. (1982) Rheumatoid arthritis. In *Operative Hand Surgery*, edited by David P. Green, pp. 1164, 1195, 1224–1233, 1241–1255. New York: Churchill Livingstone

NALEBUFF, E. A. and GARROD, K. J. (1984) Present approach to the severely involved rheumatoid wrist. *Orthopaedic Clinics of North America*, **15**, 369–380

NALEBUFF, E. A. and MILLENDER, L. H. (1975) Surgical treatment of the swan-neck deformity in rheumatoid arthritis. *Orthopaedic Clinics of North America*, **6**, 733–752

NALEBUFF, E. A. and PATEL, M. R. (1973) Flexor digitorum sublimis transfer for multiple extensor tendon ruptures in rheumatoid arthritis. *Plastic and Reconstructive Surgery*, **52**, 530–533

NICOLLE, F. V. and CALNAN, J. S. (1972) A new design of finger joint prosthesis for the rheumatoid hand. *The Hand*, **4**, 135–146

NIEBAUER, J. J., SHAW, J. L. and DOREN, W. W. (1968) The silicone–dacron hinge prosthesis. *Journal of Bone and Joint Surgery*, **50A**, 634

OMER, G. E. (1968) Evaluation and reconstruction of the forearm and hand after peripheral nerve injuries. *Journal of Bone and Joint Surgery*, **50A**, 1454–1478

SEDDON, H. J. (1952) Reconstructive surgery of the upper extremity. *Report of the Second Poliomyelitis Conference*. Philadelphia: Lippincott

SHAPIRO, J. S. (1968) The aetiology of ulnar drift: a new factor. *Journal of Bone and Joint Surgery*, **50A**, 634

SMITH, E. M., JUVINALL, R. C., BENDER, L. F. and PEARSON, J. R. (1966) Flexion forces and metacarpophalangeal deformities. *Journal of the American Medical Association*, **198**, 130–134

SMITH-PETERSON, M. N., AUFRANC, D. E. and LARSON, C. B. (1943) Useful surgical procedures for rheumatoid arthritis involving joints of the upper extremity. *Archives of Surgery*, **46**, 764–770

SOUTER, W. A. (1979) Planning treatment of the rheumatoid hand. *The Hand*, **11**, 3–16

SOUTER, W. A. (1981) The hand in rheumatoid disease. In *The Practice of Hand Surgery*, edited by D. W. Lamb and K. Kuczinski, p. 355. Oxford: Blackwell Scientific Publications

STEFFEE, A. D., BECKENBAUGH, R. D., LINSCHEID, R. L. and DOBYNS, J. H. (1981) The development, technique and early clinical results of a total joint replacement for the metacarpophalangeal joints of the fingers. *Orthopaedics*, **4**, 175

STRICKLAND, J. W. and LASALLE, W. B. (1982) The surgical management of multiple level deformities of the rheumatoid hand: a practical approach. In *Difficult Problems in Hand Surgery*, edited by J. W Strickland and J. B. Steichen, p. 224. St Louis: C. V. Mosby

SWANSON, A. B. (1972) The ulnar head syndrome and its treatment by implant resection arthroplasty. *Journal of Bone and Joint Surgery*, **54A**, 906

SWANSON, A. B. (1973) Flexible implant arthroplasty for arthritis disabilities of the radio-carpal joint. A silicone rubber intramedullary stemmed flexible hinge implant for the wrist joint. *Orthopaedic Clinics of North America*, **4**, 383–394

SWANSON, A. B. (1981) Arthroplasty in the rheumatoid hand. In *The Practice of Hand Surgery*, edited by D. W. Lamb and K. Kuczinski, pp. 379–388. Oxford: Blackwell Scientific Publications

SWANSON, A. B. and SWANSON, G. DEG. (1982) Flexible implant arthroplasty of the radio-carpal joint; surgical technique and long term results. In *American Academy of Orthopaedic Surgeons Symposium on Total Joint Replacement of the Upper Extremity*. St Louis: C. V. Mosby

SWANSON, A. B., SWANSON, G. DEG. and LEONARD, J. (1978) Postoperative rehabilitation programme in flexible implant arthroplasty of the digits. In *Rehabilitation of the Hand*, edited by J. M. Hunter, L. H. Schneider, E. J. Macklin and J. A. Bell, p. 477. St Louis: C. V. Mosby

TALEISNIK, J. (1979) Rheumatoid synovitis of the volar compartment of the wrist joint: its radiological signs and its contribution to wrist and hand deformity. *Journal of Hand Surgery*, **4**, 526–535

VAINIO, K. (1974) The surgery of rheumatoid arthritis. *Surgical Annals*, **6**, 309–335

VAUGHAN-JACKSON, O. (1948) Rupture of extensor tendons by attrition at the inferior radio-ulnar joint. A report of two cases. *Journal of Bone and Joint Surgery*, **30B**, 528–530

VOLZ, R. G. (1982) Total wrist arthroplasty: a clinical and biomechanical analysis. In *American Academy of Orthopaedic Surgeons Symposium on Total Joint Replacement of the Upper Extremity*, edited by A. E. Inglis, p. 273. St Louis: C. V. Mosby

WILKINSON, D. S. (1980) Rheumatoid vasculitis. In *Vasculitis*, edited by K. Wolff and R. K. Winkleman, p. 201. London: Lloyd Luke

3
Osteoarthritis of the hand
Clayton A. Peimer

INTRODUCTION

Osteoarthritis is one of the oldest known diseases affecting all races of man and his vertebrate predecessors, and all species of mammals regardless of climate. It is only in this century, however, that inflammatory connective tissue arthritis was first differentiated from osteoarthritis (OA) (Goldthwait, 1904). Although virtually universal by the sixth and seventh decades of life, ageing and the development of osteoarthritis are not synonymous: osteoarthritis is not entirely a 'wearing out' of joints with concomitant cartilaginous degeneration (Lawrence, Bremner and Bier, 1966). Osteoarthritis is probably not one specific disorder, but a complex of disease groups with similar clinical and pathological findings. Probably the single, most frequent cause of rheumatological symptoms in individuals over the age of 50 (Wood, 1971), osteoarthritis constitutes a major economic problem.

In 1802 the English physician, William Heberden, asked 'What (are) those little hard knobs about the size of a pea, which are frequently seen on the tops of fingers, a little below the tip, near the joint?' Haygarth proposed a polyarticular form of osteoarthritis in 1805, and in 1857 such a syndrome was first described in detail (Adams, 1857). In the early part of the twentieth century nodular deformities of the hand were often thought to be relatively painless and to occur predominantly without associated involvement of other joints.

CLASSIFICATIONS OF OSTEOARTHRITIS

Osteoarthritis is usually described either as primary (idiopathic) or as secondary. It is primary when it occurs in the absence of exogenous predisposing factors. (Heredity is excluded as a predisposing factor for purposes of this definition.) It is secondary when an important and recognizable underlying condition contributes to its onset and pathogenesis. Although osteoarthritis is typically classified as a 'non-inflammatory' type of arthritis, the various subgroups of osteoarthritis may be more properly viewed as a continuum including end-stage wearing out, extending into the inflammatory rheumatoid-like conditions, as well as primary generalized osteoarthritis, erosive inflammatory osteoarthritis, and diffuse idiopathic skeletal hyperostosis (Kellgren and Moore, 1952; Crain, 1961; Peter, Pearson and Marmor, 1966; Ehrlich, 1972; Tillman, 1977; Resnick *et al.*, 1978; Gardner, 1983; Pinals, 1983). Whether these various symptoms and stages of disease represent subgroups of osteoarthritic diseases or merely reflect the severity and expression of osteoarthritis in particular individuals is presently unknown. It is now recognized that generalized (polyarticular) osteoarthritis is probably two syndromes, the primary type associated with little pain and the erosive-inflammatory group presenting with a significant resemblance to other inflammatory polyarticular arthropathies (Crain, 1961; Ehrlich, 1972). The abrupt onset of pain, swelling, erythema and the increased joint temperature associated with limited function at the interphalangeal joints, for example, characterize the inflammatory syndrome associated with nodular deformities.

PATHOLOGICAL PROCESS

To understand osteoarthritis one must appreciate normal joint anatomy and histochemistry. Hyaline cartilage is composed mostly of water (up to 80 per cent). Its water content accounts for much of its mechanical resilience. By dry weight, type 2 collagen represents about 50 per cent and proteoglycans about 20 per cent of cartilage substance. Proteoglycans (formerly referred to as protein-polysaccharides or chondromucoproteins) are complex macromolecules that consist of a linear protein core to which long-chain polysaccharides (glycoseaminoglycans) are linked. (The term for glycoseaminoglycans was originally mucopolysaccharides.) The ability of the proteoglycans to hold water gives cartilage its shock-absorbing properties. Both the collagen matrix and proteoglycans are formed by chondrocytes, which have no direct blood supply in adults, but gain nourishment by diffusion from the synovial fluid. Cartilage is therefore considered 'isolated' from the blood system. In the early stages of osteoarthritis cartilage water decreases, proteoglycans decrease, and eventually the collagen disrupts.

A number of theories suggest that various events may underlie the pathological process. It has been suggested that the initial lesion is an abnormally wide separation of collagen fibres. The mechanical strength of the matrix deteriorates, leading to secondary structural damage during joint loading (Meachim *et al.*, 1974; Freeman and Meachim, 1979). Because a reduction in the quantity or quality of the matrix proteoglycans may harm the collagen framework, it has been further theorized that alteration in chondrocyte proteoglycan synthesis leads to an early lesion (McDevitt and Muir, 1976). An alternative explanation is that increased enzymatic degradation from synovial cells, chondrocytes, or other factors could lead to loss of cartilage matrix or proteoglycans and water (Bentley, 1971). Increased deposition of crystallines within joints (in certain diseases) has been associated with increased incidence and severity of symptoms (Gardner, 1983). Radin, Paul and Rose (1972) and Townsend *et al.* (1977) have suggested that mechanical changes, primarily due to ageing and cyclic loads on bone, reduce bone resilience, increase cartilage wear, and lead to destructive change. Primary or secondary alteration in the quantity or quality of synovial fluid would potentially diminish joint lubrication, increase friction, and hasten wear-induced mechanical destruction.

Probably several of these events interact. Functionally, there is a significant interplay among subchondral bone, articular cartilage, synovial lubrication, chondrocytes, and proteoglycans. We still need to know more about the interaction of biological and mechanical factors that lead to the progression from cartilage pathology to the development of symptomatic and dysfunctional disease. It is interesting to note that although osteoarthritis of the hip is common, osteoarthritis of the ankle is not, and that the hand and wrist are two of the most frequently affected and disabling sites of this condition. At this time we do not yet know why this is true.

In the later stages of primary and secondary osteoarthritis, cartilage and bone changes both in weight-bearing and non-weight-bearing joints are essentially similar. In moderate cases, cartilage shows fibrillation througout the collagen framework, still continues to produce proteoglycans, and contains increased water. There is necrosis of chondrocytes and some increased mitoses, perhaps reflecting (frustrated) attempts at healing. A horizontal separation at the interface of uncalcified and calcified cartilage is often assumed to be the result of shearing. Thinning of the cartilage surface, presumably from abrasion, is also found. Late stage osteoarthritis is defined as the point at which the joint lesions have progressed to cartilage loss with exposure of bone tissue to the joint surface. The bone shows increased osteoblastic and osteoclastic activity, resulting in the radiographic appearance of sclerosis intermingled with osteolytic zones or 'cysts', which are typically filled with fluid or debris and surrounded by dead bone. In joints with extensive chronic change, tracks or grooves can develop on the exposed bone surfaces (*Figure 3.1a*). In general, osteophytic lipping can occur throughout the spectrum of osteoarthritic grades. Osteophytes may result from stimulation by synovial debris, altered surface contours, or their appearance may be an attempt at new bone formation for the purpose of remodelling. The joint capsule may fibrose, adhering and trapping the joint debris, and an acute or chronic secondary inflammatory response will result.

Frequency of occurrence in various joints of the hand

The distal interphalangeal (DIP) joints of the index and middle fingers are more commonly affected than the distal interphalangeal joints of the ring and little fingers. The distal joint of the thumb is about as commonly involved as the distal joint of the index. The proximal interphalangeal (PIP) joints are affected only about two-thirds as often as the distal interphalangeal joints. Although symmetrical involvement is common, osteoarthritis occurs slightly more frequently in the dominant than in the non-dominant hand. The metacarpophalangeal (MCP) joints are rarely involved. The basalar joint of the thumb (first carpometacarpal) is the joint affected in at least one-third of the patients (Crain, 1961; Balbosa, Cirillo and Malara, 1968; McEwen, 1968; Ehrlich, 1972). Symptoms and changes at the radiocarpal and radio-ulnar joints are most uncommon, but simultaneous involvement of large joints and of the spine may be found. In the non-inflammatory syndrome both distal interphalangeal and proximal interphalangeal joints are involved; degeneration at the base of the thumb is common. It is the severity, rather than the number of joints involved, that accounts for most of the disability associated with osteoarthritic hand dysfunction (Labi, Gresham and Rathev, 1982).

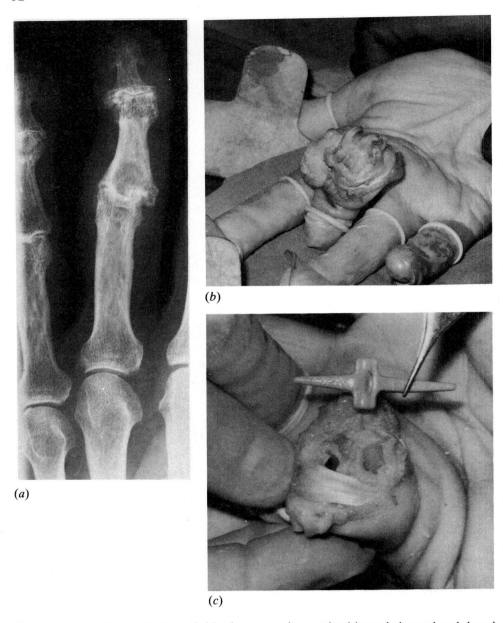

(a)

(b)

(c)

Figure 3.1 (*a*) Advanced osteoarthritic changes at the proximal interphalangeal and dorsal interphalangeal joints with spurring (Bouchard's and Heberden's nodes, respectively) are seen in this middle finger. Note the marked grooving (tracking) in the middle phalanx. Only the proximal interphalangeal joint was symptomatic. (*b*) A modified Bruner incision, division of both collateral ligaments, and sharp release of the palmar plate proximal to its middle phalangeal insertion allowed the proximal interphalangeal joint to be hyperextended like the breech of a shotgun. (The flexor tendons are retracted ulnarward.) (*c*) The medullary canals are easily prepared for insertion of the Swanson Silastic HP prosthesis

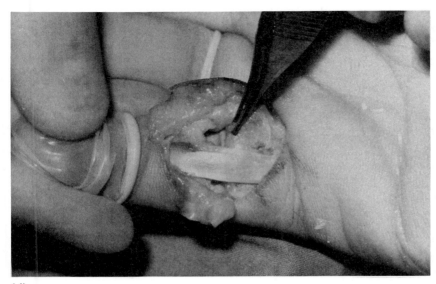

(*d*)

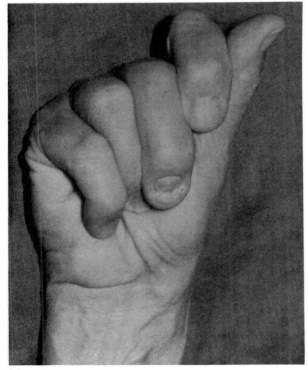

(*e*)

Figure 3.1 (*d* and *e*) After prosthetic insertion the ligaments are repaired and flexor sheath closed if possible. The joint is splinted in mild flexion for 10–14 days, then therapy is begun

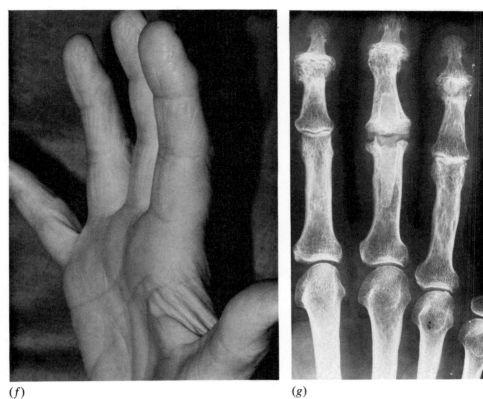

(*f*)   (*g*)

Figure 3.1 (*f* and *g*) Radiograph and clinical results of this middle finger Swanson proximal interphalangeal arthroplasty nine months following surgery. The palmar incision is virtually invisible. Our average active arc of motion is 45–50°

Grades of disease

Although radiographs have been employed for grading and diagnosing osteo-arthritis only during the last three decades, they have revealed that there is little correlation among symptoms, clinical findings, and X-ray changes with respect to the severity of disease. The presence of clinical signs has relatively little predictive value for radiological changes and, conversely, radiological changes are not indicative of exacerbation of symptoms (Valkenburg, 1981; *Figure 3.2*). A uniform radiographic grading system has been developed to classify affected joints into four relatively distinct groups (*Table 3.1*) (*Atlas of Standard Radiographs*, 1963).

Table 3.1 Radiographic grading of osteoarthritis

Grade I	Small osteophytes
Grade II	Osteophytes without joint space impairment
Grade III	Osteophytes with moderate loss of normal joint space
Grade IV	Osteophytes with significant loss of joint space and sclerosis of subchondral bone
Grade V	Grade IV with subluxation

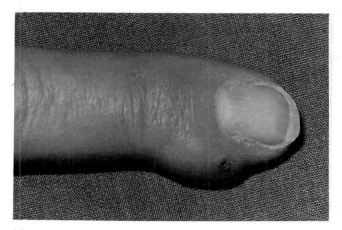

(a)

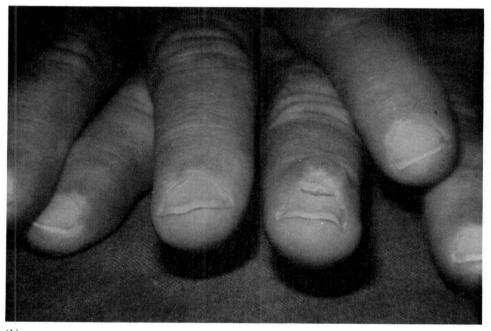

(b)

Figure 3.2 (*a*) Mucous cyst from the radial aspect of the left index in a painless dorsal interphalangeal joint which showed grade I–II changes on X-ray. The overlying skin is quite thin and had drained spontaneously in the past. The cyst and joint were injected with cortisone after aspiration. About a year later excision required removal of the contiguous skin but allowed direct closure. (*b*) Grooving of the fingernails is seen when mucous cysts arise near the germinal matrix. Grooving appears in both middle fingernails; a large cyst is visible in the lower hand

Incidence

It is estimated that 30 per cent of adults are affected. For some there may be an occupational predisposition (Bard, Sylvestre and Dussault, 1984). Population studies note the essential exponential age-related increase in frequency and severity of osteoarthritis after the age of 50. Vazici *et al.* (1975) describe only a 30 per cent incidence of Heberden's nodes in the sixth decade compared to a 69 per cent incidence in the age group over 75 years. Whether the age-specific incidence of osteoarthritis reflects the effects of increasing incongruity and mechanical wear or of secondary autoimmune reaction to cartilage debris remains in dispute (Burch, 1977).

Cartilaginous degeneration and wear, extremely common in asymptomatic adult synovial joints, increases with age but varies with symptomatic expression. Since asymptomatic joints in the early pathological stages of human osteoarthritis are not routinely available for histological examination, not a great deal is known about the initial changes in man. Overall, the incidence of osteoarthritis of the hand is higher in men under 45 than in those older. Conversely, it occurs more frequently in women over 45. There is no difference by sex if all ages are considered. Stecher notes in 1955 the strong hereditary association of Mendelian dominance in women for Heberden's nodes. Kellgren and Moore (1963) described the disease as often oligoarticular, but characterized by a generalized, frequently systemic and inflammatory presentation, predominantly in middle-aged women but also as a recessive trait in men.

TREATMENT

Drugs

Medication for osteoarthritis depends on patient cooperation and the appropriate use of additional supportive measures. The patient must understand the nature of his or her disease and that the goal of all therapies is preservation of maximal function. Because it is easier to prevent deformity and loss of function than to correct or restore them, the management of the patient with osteoarthritis has both short-term and long-term objectives beginning with relief of pain and progressing to correction of deformity. The patient's best friend is his or her rheumatologist, but he or she may gain significantly from assistance by a qualified hand therapist. Often the elderly patient has other medical problems which will influence the decision as to which and how much of the drug(s) should be used. Altered metabolic function in the liver and kidneys, reduced cardiac output, gastrointestinal problems, and intolerence for certain drugs significantly influence the choice and use of medication. Although analgesics and non-steroidal anti-inflammatory drugs (NSAIDs) are excreted renally, hepatic function affects their half-life and detoxification. All patients should be given the least toxic medication at the lowest effective dose. This is especially important in treating the elderly patient who is more susceptible than a younger person to hypersensitivity, drug idiosyncrasy, overdose, interactions with other medication, and side-effects.

Salicylate preparations, in low doses, are the most reasonable first choice because they offer both analgesic and anti-inflammatory effects. A proliferation of other prescription NSAIDs has occurred in the last three decades. The dozen or so

NSAIDs now available in the United States have small differences in indication, efficacy, safety, and pharmacokinetics (Calabro, 1984). Whatever drug is prescribed, its potential benefits and both the common and serious side-effects should be explained in detail to the patient and reviewed at frequent follow-up visits.

Therapy

Physical and occupational therapy may considerably benefit the patient with osteoarthritis. Local heat, paraffin, and regular exercises to prevent stiffness and to strengthen the hand have a significant place in the treatment routine. Custom-made and commercial splints will often support or unload (partially immobilize) a symptomatic or unstable joint and improve function (*Figure 3.3*). Hand therapists with backgrounds in physical and occupational therapy advise patients regarding assistive devices and modification of the activitities of daily living, which can improve their functional capacity and comfort.

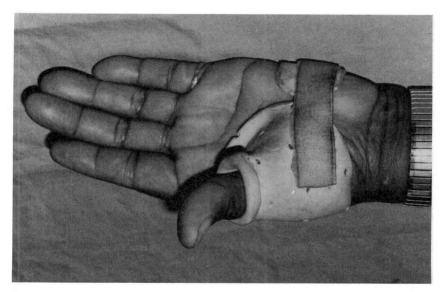

Figure 3.3 Custom 'short opponens' splint which supports and partially immobilizes the thumb carpometacarpal joint but leaves the interphalangeal joint free. In addition to this well-worn splint the patient had received a local steroid injection and NSAIDs orally

Intra-articular steroids can be considered an important and useful adjunctive measure in the presence of acute inflammation. Usually local steroids are considered when systemic medication, physical modalities, and splinting have failed to control symptoms adequately, or, in the presence of a painful effusion, to relieve discomfort and allow preservation or restoration of mobility. Installation of an insoluble steroid (acetate) is frequently helpful. The duration of benefit varies, and there is some controversy regarding complications of repeated, frequent administration of intra-articular steroids (Sweetnam, 1969; Gibson *et al.*, 1976).

Systemic effects are rare, as is iatrogenic infection. However, some patients may experience post-injection pain or inflammation 'flare'. Localized subcutaneous or cutaneous atrophy and hypopigmentation (especially in black people) are usually transient but can persist (Gray, Tenenbaum and Gottlieb, 1981). In general, a 22-gauge needle is used for injection without aspiration for the wrist and elbow, and a 25-gauge or 26-gauge needle is used for the smaller joints. Aspiration of an effusion or of a ganglion cyst often requires a larger needle and syringe first. A local anaesthetic, such as carbocaine, is mixed with the steroid that is instilled.

Surgery

A specific surgical treatment is determined by the clinical course of the disease. As patients present complaining of problems at given joints, it is most reasonable to approach the discussion of active and operative treatment organizationally on an anatomical basis.

Distal interphalangeal (DIP) joints

The distal interphalangeal joint is a common site of involvement not only in osteoarthritis but also in several other arthritides. It is useful for diagnostic purposes to consider other common problems which produce a destructive distal interphalangeal joint arthritis, such as psoriasis (Behrens, Shepherd and Mitchel, 1976; Pinals, 1983). Pitting and discoloration of the fingernails and the presence of a rash suggest this diagnosis. Chronic ulcerative colitis and Reiter's syndrome may also present with distal interphalangeal joint involvement (Pinals, 1983). Patients with rheumatoid arthritis may have distal interphalangeal joint involvement occasionally, whereas those with polyarticular juvenile rheumatoid arthritis may show inflamed distal interphalangeal joints somewhat frequently. Secondary or post-traumatic distal joint involvement is seen in younger adults, but rarely affecting more than one finger. In such cases the anteroposterior or lateral radiograph will disclose the localized, healed fracture.

In primary osteoarthritis Heberden's nodes may appear gradually, often first noticed as a painless enlargement in one or more fingers or a non-tender cystic swelling proximal to the nail, generally without a traumatic history (*see Figure 3.1*). In some patients these cysts may be rather large and associated with a history of spontaneous drainage of 'clear liquid'. The skin is often thin and virtually transparent (*see Figure 3.2*). The cyst is usually associated with an asymptomatic osteophyte, and the fluid, when aspirated, is identical to that in a ganglion cyst. These osteoarthritic mucous cysts may cause nail deformity by bringing pressure on the germinal matrix but, more often, the patient complains of the ugly appearance of the finger. It is reasonable to aspirate the cyst contents and inject the joint with steroids on one or two occasions. If it recurs, the cyst and the atrophic skin should be excised, and the osteophyte should be removed. The osteophyte is best exposed after the cyst has been removed. Retraction or longitudinal splitting of the terminal extensor tendon may be required to permit adequate exposure. Following the excision, the joints should be immobilized in extension for 7–10 days. The patient should understand before agreeing to the procedure that a permanent cure may require arthrodesis.

Excision of a Heberden's node (the osteophyte), in the absence of a mucous cyst, is a reasonable cosmetic request if the joint is relatively asymptomatic and, except for the lipping, radiographically benign. Under such circumstances, the patient should understand that the disease process will not be altered, that the osteophytes may recur, and that cysts may later develop anyway.

The symptomatic, dysfunctional, subluxated joint may be treated by arthroplasty or arthrodesis. We consider arthroplasty at this joint merely theoretical, neither to be recommended nor performed because of the nature of stresses to which the distal interphalangeal joint is subject and the properties and complications of wear of available materials (Smith, Atkinson and Jupiter, 1985; Peimer *et al.*, 1985). Arthrodesis is the best way to correct distal interphalangeal joint instability, deformity, and discomfort. Distal joint fusion results in excellent function, and the major morbidity is the risk of non-union. The candidate for distal interphalangeal arthrodesis typically has a painful, stiff joint and appreciates being pain-free and able to perform both fine and heavy motor activities. The exact position of arthrodesis varies with the surgeon's preference. We generally fuse the thumb interphalangeal joint at 5–15° of flexion and the digital distal interphalangeal joints at about 20° of flexion. We use a dorsal H-incision and divide the terminal tendon, avoiding power tools (and the concomitant risk of thermal osteonecrosis). We prefer fixation with the combination of longitudinal K-wires and intraosseous wires for compression (Lister *et al.*, 1977).

Proximal interphalangeal (PIP) joints

Primary osteoarthritis, more common at the proximal interphalangeal joints than generally appreciated, is rarely present in the absence of distal interphalangeal joint involvement. Unfortunately, the disease is often inflammatory at the proximal interphalangeal joints, which tend to develop erosive changes, making it necessary to consider the possibility of an inflammatory polyarthritis such as rheumatoid arthritis. Bouchard's nodes may be a prominent feature of proximal interphalangeal joint osteoarthritis and, as at the distal interphalangeal joints, early in the disease process more deforming than painful. Usually, a gradual loss of joint motion, often with the joint tending to stiffness in mild to moderate flexion, occurs without significant malangulation (*see Figure 3.1*). When symptomatic, the joints are usually stiffer after activity. Although radiographic findings may be impressive, clinical signs are typically limited. Post-traumatic or secondary osteoarthritis at the proximal interphalangeal joint is usually easily distinguishable historically and radiographically.

Functional impairment, which may be due to pain, decreased mobility, or malposition can produce impingement on adjacent digits or interference with hand function. Surgical treatment may include excision of osteophytes for cosmetic reasons or for correction of bony impingment with any motion. Arthrodesis or arthroplasty are employed to relieve intractable symptoms.

In our experience, requests are rather uncommon for osteophytic removal at the proximal interphalangeal joint as an isolated procedure. If the areas of bony enlargement are not dysfunctional, patients are rarely willing to undergo surgery requiring two incisions on each of several digits merely to achieve a moderate reduction in the size of their knuckles. Rarely, a palmar osteophyte may prevent flexion, but in such instances examination will reveal a passive flexion block in the presence of a bony prominence which is radiographically identifiable. To gain access to that bony prominence (spur) in order to excise it will generally require a lateral or palmar approach and dissection of the palmar plate and accessory colateral ligament. These important soft tissue structures are repaired and motion started within a few days of surgery, usually utilizing an extension block splint during the first 2–3 postoperative weeks.

Most patients who require surgical treatment desire to retain small joint mobility, typically for light activities such as cooking, handling playing cards or mah-jong tiles, and playing golf. Only arthroplasty will afford sufficient mobility to perform these activities. The choices of procedure include fascial interposition and silicone or cemented prostheses. Fascial arthroplasties require resection of less bone than cemented prostheses so that alteration of digital length is minimal. The complications of implant breakage or wear and secondary synovitis are avoided; an unsuccessful procedure may be salvaged by performing implant arthroplasty or arthrodesis. However, fascial arthroplasty is definitely not indicated unless the joint surface is essentially well preserved and digital malposition is limited. If involvement of one of the joint surfaces is not significant, techniques such as Eaton's volar plate arthroplasty may be successful (Eaton and Malerich, 1980).

Prosthetic arthroplasty at the proximal interphalangeal joint has a checkered history. The original, hinged prostheses developed numerous problems (Ellison, Flatt and Henard, 1973). In recent years, silicone implants have been the most popular and successful of those available in the United States (Swanson, 1972b; Swanson, Maupin and Gajjor, 1983). The joints modified with silicone implants are typically pain-free. The average active range of motion is about 45°. Not more than 80 per cent of prostheses survive five years. Joint stability is dependent on soft tissue support (reconstruction) rather than on the prosthesis, which is only a bone spacer. A dorsal or palmar approach may be appropriate for the surgery, depending on the particular patient and deformity. In general, we prefer the more aesthetic palmar approach whenever possible, in the manner described by Eaton and Malerich (1980) for the volar plate arthroplasty, which also 'spares' both the flexor and extensor tendons and permits earlier mobilization of the joint under the guidance of a hand therapist (*see Figure 3.1b–d*). When the Eaton approach is used the finger is splinted for about 5–7 days before an active therapy program with an extension block splint (to protect the repaired palmar ligaments) is started. Since many complications of implant arthroplasty may not appear until after the second or third postoperative year, it is essential that the patient understands such risks and the need for continuing follow-up at regular intervals by both X-ray and clinical examination.

We find limited indication for proximal interphalangeal arthrodesis unless there is marked malposition, instability, and disabling pain or in the face of a failed prosthesis, infectious process, or heavy manual demands. A fused proximal interphalangeal joint is awkward regardless of the position of the arthrodesis even for a young patient with an otherwise normal hand and a secondary osteoarthritic deformity. Although the finger may be stable and durable, it may be so awkward that the subject may not be able to perform heavy work or use machinery. When a question exists, we sometimes find it helpful to 'arthrodese the joint temporarily' by immobilizing it with a percutaneous K-wire for 2–3 weeks. We are more likely to arthrodese an index proximal interphalangeal joint than the three ulnar digits since the index is subjected to frequent lateral stress in pinch.

Metacarpophalangeal (MP) joints

Although primary osteoarthritis affecting the metacarpophalangeal joints is very uncommon, secondary osteoarthritis following the trauma of articular fractures and open joint injuries is common. The choice of treatment depends on the joint involved and the patient's functional needs. Because the thumb metacarpal phalangeal joint is required for so many vigorous activities, an arthrodesis is generally preferred. Following even the most successful prosthetic arthroplasty in a finger metacarpophalangeal joint, restored mobility does not compare with that of the unaffected joints. However, moderate digital metacarpophalangeal mobility is generally preferable to arthrodesis. Because the metacarpophalangeal joint implants can be larger and are surrounded by more robust soft tissues, including adjacent digits and intrinsic muscles, they have been more satisfactory than implants for other joints of the hand. Again, the patient must be aware that implant fracture or gradual wear may occur long after the implant arthroplasty is performed. Should the joint become recurrently symptomatic, these two possibilities should be considered in making a diagnosis (Beckenbaugh *et al.*, 1976; Ferlic and Clayton, 1981).

A thumb metacarpophalangeal joint arthrodesis is approached from the dorsum. The joint is fused at about 20° of flexion, slight abduction, and mild pronation. Typically, we use intraosseous wires and K-wire technique for arthrodeses. Rarely do we find that autogenous grafting is required. Finger metacarpophalangeal fusions are generally fixed at about 50° of flexion. The finger metacarpophalangeal joints are approached from the dorsum for both arthroplasty and arthrodesis.

Carpometacarpal (CMC) joints

The basilar joint of the thumb is a frequent site of dysfunction. Patients with inflammatory polyarthritis may be symptomatic. Pain and swelling in this region of the hand must be differentiated from inflammation emanating from the first dorsal compartment. Osteoarthritis as the origin of these symptoms must also be differentiated from other chronic inflammatory diseases. In addition, acute trauma or the secondary effects of chronic injury must be considered. It is not clear whether the carpometacarpal 'boss', which may be found at the dorsal base of the second and third carpometacarpal joints, is necessarily an expression of osteoarthritic disease and not a secondary ossification center or a chronic tendon injury (Artz and Posch, 1973). Osteoarthrosis at the fifth carpometacarpal (metacarpohamate) joint is more likely to be post-traumatic than osteoarthritis at the other carpometacarpal joints.

The carpometacarpal boss may require only diagnosis, injection, or, on occasion, excision. Post-traumatic osteoarthritis of the metacarpohamate joint may become symptomatic after the hand has undergone vigorous activity involving forced or prolonged grasping (fifth carpometacarpal flexion). Patients who fail to respond to conservative treatment may require surgery. We strongly prefer arthrodesis because this joint is highly subject to stress. The carpometacarpal joint is fixed in mild flexion in order to preserve the transverse arch of the hand (Clendenin and Smith, 1984). Typically we add autogenous radial bone graft and immobilize the joint with crossed K-wires.

Among the most common indications for treatment of osteoarthritis in the hand are symptoms at the thumb carpometacarpal joint. Upon longitudinal loading of the first ray (in pinch and grasp), patients experience pain and a concomitant decrease in their pinch strength. The carpometacarpal joint is often prominent and the first metacarpal subluxated radially and dorsally, producing a functional adduction contracture, which limits grasp further and places secondary stresses on the metacarpal phalangeal joint and its collateral ligaments. As the carpometacarpal joint space narrows and subluxation progresses a large osteophyte typically develops about the ulnar condyle of the trapezium (*Figure 3.4a*). Depending on whether the assessment is made by X-ray (Swanson, 1972a) or anatomic dissection (North and Eaton, 1983), the incidence of generalized peritrapezial osteoarthritis varies, but may be as high as 50 per cent of symptomatic cases. At presentation in the office, patients are generally quite uncomfortable. We agree with Dell, Brushart and Smith (1978) that the combination of local steroid injection, oral NSAIDs, and a custom short opponens (thumb post) splint should be used to position the thumb in opposition and partially to immobilize the painful joint without interfering with the distal joints of the thumb and index (*see Figure 3.3*). Patients are instructed to use the splint to perform activities for which they perceive it to be helpful (it is somewhat awkward). Although everyone responds at least initially, many patients eventually return for further treatment because of recurrent symptoms or dissatisfaction with the inconvenience of depending on a splint to prevent symptoms. If pain and/or malposition are disabling, we recommend surgical treatment.

Arthrodesis of the trapeziometacarpal joint will relieve the symptoms of carpometacarpal joint arthritis but because other peritrapezial joints are affected in patients with osteoarthritis, some pain may persist (Eaton and Littler, 1969; Stark *et al.*, 1977; Crosby, Linsheid and Dobyns, 1978). In addition, a carpometacarpal fusion prevents full opposition and extension of the thumb beyond the plane of the palm. A fusion may be the most appropriate alternative for patients who have a particular need for strength and durability of the joint. An example of such a patient might be a young person with post-traumatic carpometacarpal arthrosis.

We know of at least eight prostheses available in the United States for insertion as implants at this joint by trapezial resection or hemiarthroplasty technique (Swanson, 1972b; Ashworth *et al.*, 1977; Ferlic, Busbee and Clayton, 1977; Haffajee, 1977; Swanson, Swanson and Watermeier, 1981; Braun, 1982; Engel *et al.*, 1982; Smith and Amadio, 1982). Other authors have advocated a resection with soft tissue interposition (Froimson, 1970; Weibly, 1971; Carroll and Hill, 1973; Lucht, Vang and Munck, 1980; Amadio, Millender and Smith, 1982). There is also support for extra-articular basilar metacarpal osteotomy to produce predictable improvement in patients with adduction contracture (Wilson and Bossey, 1983).

When a silicone implant is used its stem is placed in the metacarpal or trapezium if the resection is limited, but the implant must be seated very carefully and stabilized by meticulous, often complex, ligament reconstructions. The technique of silicone implant arthroplasty with total trapezial resection has been serially revised as the problems of implant subluxation, dislocation, and instability became evident. The recommended technique now includes, additionally, a partial resection of the trapezoid, K-wire or suture fixation of the implant, and transposition of half of one or more tendons to enhance the ligaments and pseudocapsule further. When results are good, mobility and pain relief are reportedly excellent. Studies which carefully compared the results of soft tissue and silicone arthroplasty for the basilar joint of the thumb reveal that soft tissue technique is as effective or more effective than silicone implant arthroplasty (Amadio, Millender and Smith, 1982; Pellegrini and Burton, 1985). Furthermore, the soft tissue technique avoids the frequent early complications with the implant. In long-term follow-up studies it becomes clear that survival of silicone implants, which are cyclically loaded axially, decreases significantly over time (Smith and Amadio, 1982; Pellegrini and Burton, 1985). Our own studies of the effects of axial load and abrasion of Silastic implants and the resultant microparticulate-induced synovitis in many patients make it impossible for us to recommend this material as a prosthesis for this joint. In short, we believe that resection arthroplasty offers the best result for osteoarthritis deformity at this joint. Our technique is to maintain the 'resected space' by non-parallel, smooth K-wires for a period of 6–8 weeks postoperatively (*Figure 3.4b–e*). We insert no material or tendon graft, but allow the body to fill the space by natural means over the 6–8 weeks. The abductor

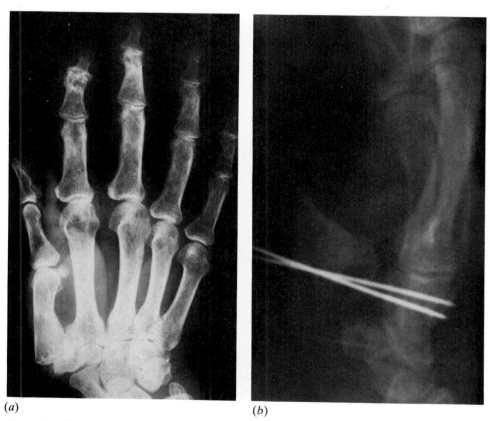

(a)   *(b)*

Figure 3.4 (*a*) Radiograph showing advanced trapeziometacarpal arthritis and subluxation in a symptomatic patient who had only transient relief from conservative measures. (*b*) Trapezial resection was performed and the joint space maintained by distraction-fixation using non-parallel, smooth K-wires, which hold the first metacarpal in wide palmar abduction and pronation. The wires and postoperative splint are removed about six weeks following surgery

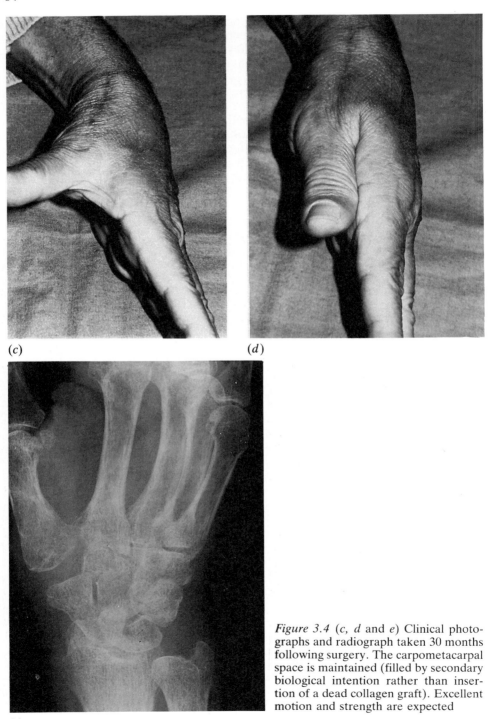

(c)

(d)

(e)

Figure 3.4 (*c*, *d* and *e*) Clinical photographs and radiograph taken 30 months following surgery. The carpometacarpal space is maintained (filled by secondary biological intention rather than insertion of a dead collagen graft). Excellent motion and strength are expected

pollicis longis is advanced about 1.5 cm. and the first compartment retinaculum is released. In our patients with carpometacarpal and pantrapezial disease, this method of resection arthroplasty has afforded very satisfactory, predictable, and reproducible results.

Wrist joints

Primary osteoarthritis at the radiocarpal and intercarpal joints is uncommon, as is ulnocarpal impingement. On the other hand, secondary involvement due to idiopathic aseptic necrosis of the scaphoid (Preiser's), to lunate (Kienbock's), or to chronic (undiagnosed) scaphoid non-unions and intercarpal ligament instabilities is common (Mack *et al.*, 1984; Watson and Baltel, 1984; Watson and Ryu, 1984). It is important to differentiate early intracarpal pathology from tendinitis about the second, third, and fourth dorsal compartments. The disease process seems to involve the periscaphoid joints primarily. The scaphotrapezial and scapho-trapezoidal articulations are most frequently involved in the presence of primary disease (Bertheussen, 1981). Radioscaphoid disease may be more typically a secondary phenomenon. Proximal carpal migration and ulnar translocation occur late in the disease process. Both may occur at approximately the same time, and in addition ulnocarpal disease may be present. The patient's symptoms depend on which joint is involved and the progress of the disease. Initially, conservative treatment should be considered for all patients. Those who fail to respond to the combination of oral medication, symptomatic splinting, and local steroid injection may need to be treated surgically.

We have found that arthrodesis for scaphotrapeziotrapezoidal (STT) disease can be quite helpful (Watson and Hempton, 1980; Bertheussen, 1981). We prefer a dorsoradial approach, autogenous radial bone graft, internal fixation with multiple crossed smooth K-wires, and thumb gauntlet-type immobilization. The major disadvantage is the length of immobilization, which can be as much as 12 weeks or more, until radiographic union is evident. In addition to relief of pain, the arthrodesis eliminates most active wrist radial deviation and 25 per cent or more of dorsiflexion. Patients should be informed of this outcome before surgery is undertaken.

In patients with more advanced collapse involving diffuse intercarpal or radiocarpal disease, the choice may be limited to a (generic) radiocarpal arthroplasty or arthrodesis. Because of the complications of silicone carpal implants (Peimer *et al.*, 1985; Smith, Atkinson and Jupiter, 1985) we cannot recommend them, even in association with a limited arthrodesis (*Figure 3.5*). Patients with limited but significant symptomatic disease may be candidates for single bone carpectomies and appropriate intercarpal arthrodeses to prevent secondary collapse. It has been our experience that a proximal row carpectomy has been generally predictable and satisfactory for patients with diffuse wrist osteoarthritis, for whom it is important to preserve some wrist mobility. Although we would be unlikely to recommend a proximal row carpectomy for someone whose career required heavy, repetitive use of the hand and wrist (Neviaser, 1983), we have found it very useful for patients who are draftsmen, engineers, and machinists. Generally, these are not individuals for whom a silicone or cemented total wrist is appropriate (Cooney, Beckenbaugh and Linscheid, 1984).

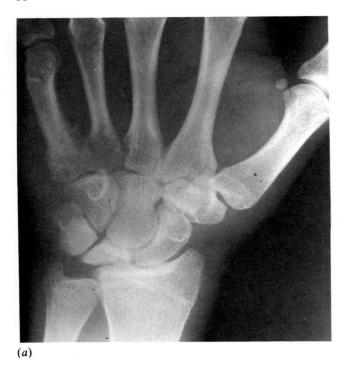

(*a*)

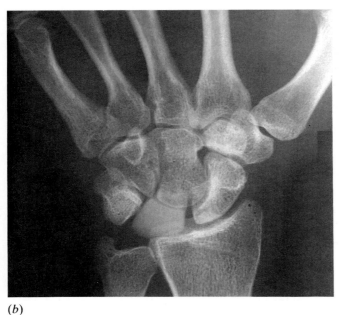

(*b*)

Figure 3.5 (*a* and *b*) Radiographs show results of Silastic HP carpal lunate replacement for symptomatic Kienbock's disease in this 31-year-old labourer who had excellent relief of symptoms and postoperative motion, and was able to return to regular employment

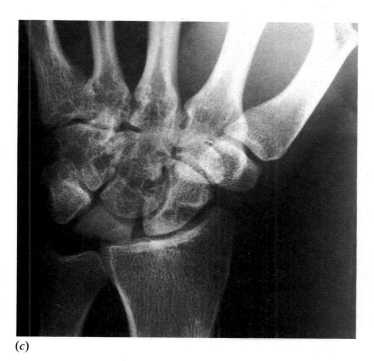

(*c*)

Figure 3.5 (*c*) Patient returned 49 months following surgery complaining of 3–6 months of increasing swelling and discomfort. Radiographs revealed these multiple, diffuse, lytic defects, loss of implant volume and contour, and carpal height. Such radiographs are typical of destructive silicone-induced microparticulate synovitis

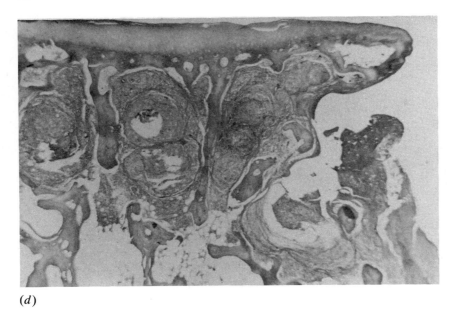

(*d*)

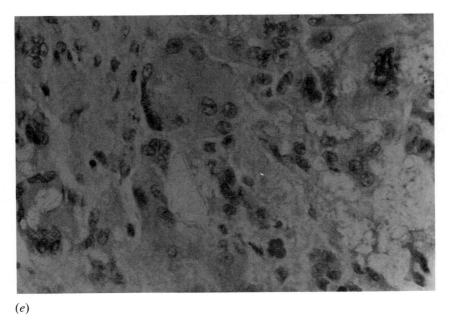

(*e*)

Figure 3.5 (*d* and *e*) Histologic sections showing inflammatory synovitis invading and destroying subchondral bone and producing the lytic defects (which are *not cysts* but tissue-filled spaces). Giant cells and numerous weak refractile foreign bodies, some within giant cells, are seen. On X-ray spectrography the tissue was shown to contain large quantities of silicon. (H & E × 43 and × 100)

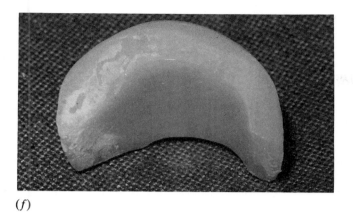

(f)

(g)

Figure 3.5 (*f*) The excised implant shows loss of normal contours from abrasive wear. Fatigue loading of dorsal and palmar poles is seen as 'powdery deposits' which are free silicone microparticles on SEM inspection. The 'fixation stem' sheared long ago and the site of origin is polished smooth. (*g*) Proximal row carpectomy, aggressive synovectomy, and curettage of the multiple lytic defects were performed with successful symptomatic relief

Radiocarpal arthrodesis in neutral position or slight dorsiflexion can offer someone engaged in heavy labor a functional wrist, which is generally durable, predictable, and typically pain-free. There are obvious disadvantages to the loss of all wrist mobility, and these must be discussed in detail with the patient undergoing the surgery. Although each of the many available techniques has its advocates, our own best results have been obtained with a modification of the Mannerfelt and Smith-Petersen technique (Smith-Petersen, 1940; *Figure 3.6*). We approach the wrist by a straight mid-line dorsal incision, exposing the fourth and fifth compartments and retracting the tendons. The dorsal half of the proximal and distal carpal row is decorticated, and the dorsal half of the mid-portion of the radial metaphysis is moved distally as a corticocancellous graft. The distal 2–3 cm of ulna is excised and morcellized for additional autogenous graft. Stability is achieved with the use of a large, smooth Steinmann pin drilled through the fourth web space into the medullary canal of the radius and then tapped up the medullary canal. The radial graft may require stabilization by one or two additional smooth K-wires, which are subsequently removed. A short arm splint is replaced by a short arm cast

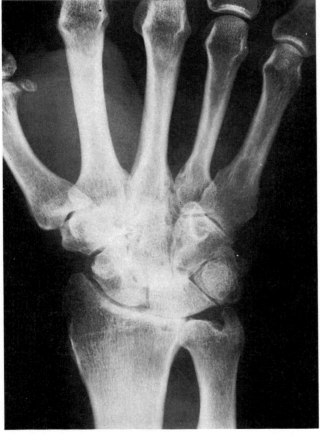

(a)

Figure 3.6 (a) Diffuse, symptomatic osteoarthritis in a 56-year-old truck driver unresponsive to conservative care

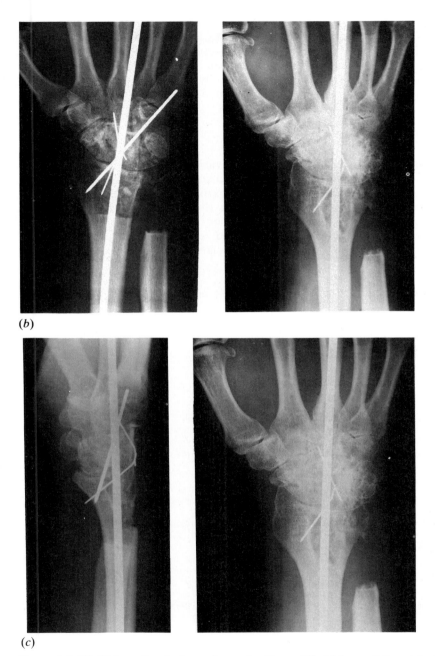

(b)

(c)

Figure 3.6 (b) Wrist arthrodesis, performed with modified Mannerfelt and Smith-Petersen techniques, utilized the dorsal half of the radius as a sliding graft into a trough made in the dorsal half of the continguous carpals and supplemented with morcellized bone graft from a generous ulnar resection. (c) Radiographic results at 4 months. Patient returned to work at 10 weeks; he has excellent fixation, no restrictions in forearm rotation, and no complaints about the distal ulna

after swelling subsides, about two weeks postoperatively. All external immobilization can generally be removed within 6–8 weeks, and the patient can return to
unrestricted activities after 12–16 weeks. The morbidity of prolonged immobilization, loss of forearm rotation, and an iliac graft donor site is avoided by this
procedure. The technique is simple, and we rarely encounter patients who later
request removal of the buried longitudinal Steinman pin.

CONCLUSION

The expressions of osteoarthritis in the hand are varied. Symptoms and dysfunction
can cause significant impairment, deformity, and economic loss. Based on current
theories of pathogenesis, our approach remains conservative, and we try to work
closely with our hand therapists and referring rheumatologists. Surgery, when
indicated, may afford significant improvement, but each procedure carries
important limitations, restrictions, and potential complications which the patient
should understand and the surgeon should appreciate.

Acknowledgements

The assistance of Frances S. Sherwin, MA, in the preparation of this manuscript is
gratefully acknowledged.

References

ADAMS, R. (1857) *A Treatise on Rheumatic Gout.* London: Churchill
AMADIO, P. C., MILLENDER, L. H. and SMITH, R. J. (1982) Silicone spacer or tendon spacer for trapezium
    resection arthroplasty – comparison of results. *Journal of Hand Surgery*, **7**, 237–244
ARTZ, T. D. and POSCH, J. L. (1973) The carpometacarpal boss. *Journal of Bone and Joint Surgery*, **55A**,
    747–752
ASHWORTH, C. R., BLATT, G., CHUINARD, R. D. and STARK, H. H. (1977) Silicone rubber interposition
    arthroplasty of the carpometacarpal joint of the thumb. *Journal of Hand Surgery*, **2**, 345–357
Atlas of Standard Radiographs (1963) Volume 2. The epidemiology of chronic rheumatism. Oxford:
    Blackwell Scientific Publications
BALBOSO, B., CIRILLO, R. and MALARA, B. (1968) La rizartrosi del pollice. *Rheumatilismo*, **20**, 195–208
BARD, C. C., SYLVESTRE, J. J. and DUSSAULT, R. G. (1984) Hand osteoarthropathy in pianists. *Journal of the
    Association of Canadian Radiologists*, **35**, 154–158
BECKENBAUGH, R. D., DOBYNS, J. H., LINSCHEID, R. L. and BRYAN, R. S. (1976) Review and analysis of
    silicone-rubber metacarpophalangeal implants. *Journal of Bone and Joint Surgery*, **58A**, 483–487
BEHRENS, F., SHEPHERD, N. and MITCHEL, N. (1976) Alterations of rabbit articular cartilage by
    intra-articular injection of glucocorticoids. *Journal of Bone and Joint Surgery*, **57A**, 1157–1160
BENTLEY, G. (1971) Papain-induced degenerative arthritis of the hip in rabbits. *Journal of Bone and Joint
    Surgery*, **53B**, 324–337
BERTHEUSSEN, K. (1981) Partial carpal arthrodesis as treatment of local degenerative changes in the wrist
    joints. *Acta Orthopaedica Scandinavica*, **52**, 629–631
BRAUN, R. M. (1982) Total joint replacement at the base of the thumb – preliminary report. *Journal of
    Hand Surgery*, **7**, 245–251
BURCH, T. A. (1977) Cited in Lawrence, J. S.: *Rheumatism in Populations*, p. 112. London: William
    Heinemann Medical Books
CALABRO, J. J. (1984) Principles of drug therapy. In *Osteoarthritis: Diagnosis and Treatment*, edited by
    R. W. Moskowitz, D. S. Howell, V. M. Goldberg and H. S. Manken. Philadelphia: H. B. Saunders
    Company

CARROLL, R. E. and HILL, N. A. (1973) Arthrodesis of the carpometacarpal joint of the thumb. *Journal of Bone and Joint Surgery*, **55B**, 292–294

CLENDENIN, M. B. and SMITH, R. J. (1984) Fifth metacarpohamate arthrodesis for post-traumatic osteoarthritis. *Journal of Hand Surgery*, **9A**, 374–378

COONEY, W. P., BECKENBAUGH, R. D. and LINSCHEID, R. S. (1984) Total wrist arthroplasty. *Clinical Orthopaedics and Related Research*, **187**, 121–128

CRAIN, D. C. (1961) Interphalangeal osteoarthritis. *Journal of the American Medical Association*, **175**, 1049–1053; 1949–1953

CROSBY, E. B., LINSCHEID, R. L. and DOBYNS, J. H. (1978) Scaphotrapezial trapezoidal arthrosis. *Journal of Hand Surgery*, **3**, 223–234

DELL, P. C., BRUSHART, T. M. and SMITH, R. J. (1978) Treatment of trapeziometacarpal arthritis: results of resection arthroplasty. *Journal of Hand Surgery*, **3**, 243–249

EATON, R. G. and LITTLER, J. W. (1969) A study of the basal joint of the thumb. The treatment of its disabilities by fusion. *Journal of Bone and Joint Surgery*, **51A**, 661–668

EATON, R. G. and MALERICH, M. M. (1980) Volar plate arthroplasty of the proximal interphalangeal joint: a review of ten years' experience: *Journal of Hand Surgery*, **5**, 260–268

EHRLICH, G. E. (1972) Inflammatory osteoarthritis: I. The clinical syndrome. *Journal of Chronic Diseases*, **25**, 317–328

ELLISON, M. R., FLATT, A. E. and HENARD, D. (1973) Finger joint replacement in the rheumatoid hand. A comparison of 525 implants of varying design and material. *Journal of Bone and Joint Surgery*, **55A**, 880

ENGEL, J., GANEL, A., PATISH, H. and KAMHIN, M. (1982) Osteoarthritis of the trapeziometacarpal joint. *Acta Orthopaedica Scandinavica*, **53**, 219–223

FERLIC, D. C., BUSBEE, G. A. and CLAYTON, M. L. (1977) Degenerative arthritis of the carpometacarpal joint of the thumb: a clinical follow-up of eleven Niebauer prostheses. *Journal of Hand Surgery*, **2**, 212–215

FERLIC, D. C. and CLAYTON, M. L. (1981) Total joint arthroplasty of the large joints of the upper extremities. *Colorado Medicine*, **78**, 262–265

FREEMAN, M. A. R. and MEACHIM, G. (1979) In *Adult Articular Cartilage*, 2nd edition, edited by M. A. R. Freeman, pp. 487–543. Tunbridge Wells: Pitman Medical Publishing

FROIMSON, A. (1970) Tendon arthroplasty of the trapeziometacarpal joint. *Clinical Orthopaedics*, **70**, 191–199

GARDNER, D. L. (1983) The nature and causes of osteoarthritis. *British Medical Journal*, **286**, 419–424

GIBSON, T., BURRY, H. C., POSWILLO, D. and GLASS, J. (1977) Effect of intra-articular corticosteroid injections in primate cartilage. *Annals of the Rheumatic Diseases*, **36**, 74–79

GOLDTHWAIT, J. E. (1904) The differential diagnosis and treatment of the so-called rheumatoid diseases. *Boston Medical Surgery Journal*, **151**, 529–534

GRAY, R. G., TENENBAUM, J. and GOTTLIEB, N. L. (1981) Local corticosteroid injection treatment in rheumatic disorders. *Seminar of Arthritis and Rheumatism*, **10**, 231–254

HAFFAJEE, D. (1977) Endoprosthetic replacement of the trapezium for arthrosis in the carpometacarpal joint of the thumb. *Journal of Hand Surgery*, **2**, 141–148

HAYGARTH, J. (1805) *Clinical History of Diseases*. London: Gadell and Davies

HEBERDEN, W. (1802) *Commentaries on History and Cure of Diseases*, pp. 148–149. London: T. Payne

KELLGREN, J. H., LAWRENCE, J. S. and BIER, F. (1963) Genetic factors in generalized osteoarthrosis. *Annals of the Rheumatic Diseases*, **22**, 237–255

KELLGREN, J. H. and MOORE, R. (1952) Generalized osteoarthritis and Heberden's nodes. *British Medical Journal*, **1**, 181–187

LABI, M. L. C., GRESHAM, G. E. and RATHEY, U. K. (1982) Hand function in osteoarthritis. *Archives of Physical Medicine and Rehabilitation*, **63**, 438–440

LAWRENCE, J. S., BREMNER, J. M. and BIER, F. (1966) Osteoarthrosis. Prevalence in the population and relationship between symptoms and X-ray changes. *Annals of the Rheumatic Diseases*, **25**, 1–24

LISTER, G. D., KLEINERT, H. E., KUTZ, J. E. and ATASOY, E. (1977) Arthritis of the trapezial articulations treated by prosthetic replacement. *Hand*, **9**, 117–129

LUCHT, U., VANG, P. S. and MUNCK, J. (1980) Soft tissue interposition arthroplasty for osteoarthritis of the carpometacarpal joint of the thumb. *Acta Orthopaedica Scandinavica*, **51**, 767–771

MACK, G. R., BOSSE, M. J., GELBERMAN, R. H. and YU, E. (1984) The natural history of scaphoid non-union. *Journal of Bone and Joint Surgery*, **66**, 504–509

MEACHIM, G., DENHAM, D., EMERY, I. H. and WILKINSON, P. H. (1974) Collagen alignments and artificial splits at the surface of human articular cartilage. *Journal of Anatomy*, **118**, 101–118

McDEVITT, C. A. and MUIR, H. (1976) Biochemical changes in the cartilage of the knees in experimental and natural osteoarthritis in the dog. *Journal of Bone and Joint Surgery*, **58B**, 94–101

McEWEN, C. (1968) Osteoarthritis of the fingers with ankylosis. *Arthritis and Rheumatism*, **11**, 734–743

NEVIASER, R. J. (1983) Proximal row carpectomy for post-traumatic disorders of the carpus. *Journal of Hand Surgery*, **8**, 301–305

NORTH, E. R. and EATON, R. C. (1983) Degenerative joint disease of the trapezium: a comparative radiographic and anatomic study. *Journal of Hand Surgery*, **8**, 160–166

PEIMER, C. A., MEDIGE, J., ECKERT, B. S., WRIGHT, J. R. and HOWARD, C. S. (1985) Destructive synovitis following silastic arthroplasty. *Journal of Hand Surgery*, (in press)

PELLEGRINI, V. D. and BURTON, R. I. (1985) Surgical management of basal joint arthritis of the thumb. *Journal of Hand Surgery*, (in press)

PETER, J. B., PEARSON, C. M. and MARMOR, L. (1966) Erosive osteoarthritis of the hands. *Arthritis and Rheumatism*, **9**, 365–388

PINALS, R. S. (1983) Approaches to rheumatoid arthritis and osteoarthritis: an overview. *American Journal of Medicine*, Suppl.: Arthritis Symposium, p. 2–9

RADIN, E. L., PAUL, I. L. and ROSE, R. M. (1972) Role of mechanical factors in the pathogenesis of primary osteoarthritis. *Lancet*, **1**, 519–522

RESNICK, D., SHAPIRO, R. F., WIESNER, K. B., NIWAYAMA, G., UTSINGER, P. D. and SHAUL, S. R. (1978) Diffuse idiopathic skeletal hyperostosis (DISH) (ankylosing hyperostosis of Forestier and Rotes-Querol). *Seminars in Arthritis and Rheumatism*, **7**, 153–187

SMITH, R. J. and AMADIO, P. C. (1982) Controversies in hand surgery: resection arthroplasty versus silicone replacement arthroplasty for trapeziometacarpal osteoarthritis. In *Difficult Problems in Hand Surgery*, edited by J. W. Strickland and J. B. Steichen, pp. 21, 183. St Louis: C. V. Mosby Co.

SMITH, R. J., ATKINSON, R. E. and JUPITER, J. B. (1985) Silicone synovitis of the wrist. *Journal of Hand Surgery*, **10A**, 47–61

SMITH-PETERSEN, M. N. (1940) A new approach to the wrist joint. *Journal of Bone and Joint Surgery*, **22**, 122–124

STARK, H. H., MOORE, J. F., ASHWORTH, C. R. and BOYES, J. H. (1977) Fusion of the first metacarpotrapezial joint for degenerative arthritis. *Journal of Bone and Joint Surgery*, **59A**, 22–26

STECHER, R. M. (1955) Heberden's nodes. A clinical description of osteoarthritis in the finger joint. *Annals of the Rheumatic Diseases*, **14**, 1–10

SWANSON, A. B. (1972a) Disabling arthritis of the base of the thumb. *Journal of Bone and Joint Surgery*, **54A**, 456–471

SWANSON, A. B. (1972b) Flexible implant arthroplasty for arthritic finger joints. *Journal of Bone and Joint Surgery*, **54A**, 435–455

SWANSON, A. B., MAUPIN, B. K. and GAJJOR, N. V. (1983) Long-term review of flexible implant arthroplasties in the proximal interphalangeal joint of the hand. *Journal of Hand Surgery*, **8**, 620

SWANSON, A. B., SWANSON, G. DE G. and WATERMEIER, J. J. (1981) Trapezium implant arthroplasty. *Journal of Hand Surgery*, **6**, 125–141

SWEETNAM, R. (1969) Corticosteroid arthropathy and tendon rupture (editorial). *Journal of Bone and Joint Surgery*, **51B**, 397–398

TILLMANN, K. (1977) Pathological aspects of osteoarthritis related to surgery. *Inflammation. Vol. 2*, Suppl. S57–S74

TOWNSEND, P. R., ROSE, R. M., RADIN, E. L. and RAUX, P. (1977) The biomechanics of the human patella and its implications for chondromalacia. *Journal of Biomechanics*, **10**, 403–407

VALKENBURG, H. A. (1981) Clinical versus radiological osteoarthrosis in the general population. In *Epidemiology of Osteoarthritis*, edited by J. G. Peyron, pp. 53–58. Paris: Geigy

WATSON, H. K. and BALTEL, F. L. (1984) The SLAC wrist: Scapholunate advanced collapsed pattern of degenerative arthritis. *Journal of Hand Surgery*, **9**, 358–365

WATSON, H. K. and HEMPTON, R. F. (1980) Limited wrist arthrodesis. Part I: The triscaphoid joint. *Journal of Hand Surgery*, **5**, 320–327

WATSON, H. K. and RYU, J. (1984) Degenerative disorders of the carpus. *Orthopaedic Clinics of North America*, **15**, 337–353

WEIBLY, A. (1971) Surgical treatment of osteoarthritis of the carpometacarpal joint of the thumb: indications for arthrodesis, excision of the trapezium, and alloplasty. *Scandinavian Journal of Plastic and Reconstructive Surgery*, **5**, 136–141

WILSON, J. N. and BOSSLEY, C. J. (1983) Osteotomy in the treatment of osteoarthritis of the first carpometacarpal joint. *Journal of Bone and Joint Surgery*, **65**, 179–181

WOOD, P. H. N. (1971) Rheumatic complaints. *British Medical Bulletin*, **27**, 82–88

YAZICI, H., SAVILLE, P. D., SALVATI, E. A., BOHNE, W. H. and WILSON, JR., P. D. (1975) Primary osteoarthrosis of the knee or hip: prevalence of Heberden's nodes in relation to age and sex. *Journal of the American Medical Association*, **231**, 1256–1260

4
Dupuytren's disease

D. A. McGrouther

INTRODUCTION

The curious condition of retraction of the fingers described by Baron Gauillaume Dupuytren (1832) remains an enigma, but there has been considerable progress towards an understanding of the biological processes responsible. Epidemiological evidence is presently being expanded (McFarlane, 1983) and the relationship to associated diseases clarified. The basic cellular processes are under intense investigation in relation to the cells, collagen fibres and ground substance of the normal and Dupuytren's tissue.

Knowledge of the anatomy of the palmar fascial ligamentous systems has been rationalized and expanded so that the lesions of Dupuytren's disease (nodules, pits, distortion of palmar creases, joint contractures) can be explained in mechanical terms (McFarlane, 1974; McGrouther, 1982).

A better understanding of the nature of the disease allows us to analyze the widely varying surgical treatments available. The role of surgery in release, excision of fibroblastic foci or prophylaxis can be understood and common principles of surgical management defined.

La maladie de Dupuytren has for many years been termed Dupuytren's contracture in the English literature. As the affliction may present without finger contracture, simply as skin nodules or pits, the use of the term Dupuytren's disease has become accepted. There is no positive evidence, however, of a single disease process; the clinical features may reflect a number of different conditions which disrupt the fine internal anatomical structures of the hands. Tightness of the palmar fascial ligaments may not be a more specific clinical sign than joint stiffness. The clinical picture is, however, currently designated Dupuytren's disease.

INCIDENCE

Determining the true prevalence of Dupuytren's disease is very difficult. Early (1962) has described the problem that population surveys may refer only to flexion deformity but not include the earlier manifestations. Heathcote, Cohen and Noble (1981) showed that whereas in a group of diabetic patients 19% were considered to have Dupuytren's disease on examination by a physician, this figure rose to 42% when examined by an orthopaedic surgeon. Certainly Mikkelsen (1976) has emphasized that the patients presenting for surgery are a highly selected group; of the patients in his study who had contractions of such an extent that surgery was advisable, less than one in four had been operated upon.

Mikkelson's (1972, 1977) routine examination of 15 950 persons of the town of Haugesund, Norway, remains the most comprehensive population study; 901 were found to have Dupuytren's disease. Early (1962) reviewed different populations in the north-west of England and recorded a rising incidence with age, reaching 18.1% in men aged 75 and over. Among women the corresponding figure was 9%. Dupuytren's disease is extremely rare in patients before the age of 20, and it seems to be a more severe and progressive condition when it occurs before the age of 40.

There seem to be widely differing incidences from country to country and this has been suggested to be principally due to racial differences, although sociological factors, such as longevity, and the incidence of associated conditions, may to some extent explain apparent regional variations. The disease is commonly seen in all northern European countries, in Scandinavia and in Russia. Hueston (1982) has suggested a relation to racial groups who arose from northern Europe and Scandinavia, but the evidence for this is indirect (Early, 1962). As the disease was not recorded before the Napoleonic Wars, with one exception (Plater, 1641), it is difficult to relate its present distribution to past racial migrations throughout the old world. Certainly the inhabitants of the new world who have migrated from northern Europe do have a high incidence of the condition (Hueston, 1982). The condition is uncommon in Japan (Ushijima, Tsuneyoshi and Enjoji, 1984) and very rare in China (Chow, Luk and Kung, 1984) or south-east Asia. Within India the condition is rarely seen in the south but may occur infrequently in the north. In negroes the condition is so rare as to justify single case reports (Zaworski and Mann, 1979). When it occurs it has been attributed to genetic admixture but Plasse (1979) and Furnas (1979) have suggested a small but definite incidence in blacks. Mennen (1986) has described a number of cases and by genotyping has excluded Caucasian genes. Although these tests are not quite specific they are highly suggestive of pure negro ancestry. The incidence in the Middle East is largely unknown. It must be emphasized, however, that much of the evidence of geographical distribution is based on anecdotal accounts of the practices of hand surgeons in these areas rather than on true scientific population study. There are also differences in the suppleness of connective tissues in peoples who have different racial backgrounds and there are certainly differences in wound healing and scar forming properties. Dupuytren's disease is rare in the racial groups prone to keloid scars. Basic knowledge on collagen metabolism in different racial groups is, however, lacking.

HEREDITY AND DUPUYTREN'S DISEASE

Heredity plays a strong part. The family trees of Dupuytren's patients have been studied by Ling (1963) who examined patients and relatives and proposed an autosomal inheritance, Dupuytren's contracture being the result of a single dominant gene. Hueston (1963) feels that a more complex genetic system may be involved. Matthews (1979) has described a family pedigree in which a strong Dupuytren's trait is manifest predominantly on the female side, and it seems that the degree of penetrance of the gene is at least as important as its transmission. Chromosomal abnormalities (mosaicism) have been noted in the palmar fascial fibroblasts by Bowser-Riley *et al.* (1975) and Sergovich *et al.* (1983) but their significance is uncertain. HLA typing (Tait and MacKay, 1982) has shown no difference in antigens between Dupuytren's contracture and normal subjects.

OTHER CONDITIONS AND DUPUYTREN'S DISEASE

Diabetes

Certain conditions have been reported as occurring in association with Dupuytren's disease. A relationship with diabetes seems certain. Noble, Heathcote and Cohen (1984) have reported Dupuytren's disease in 42% of adult diabetics. They noted that the disease was of benign prognosis, rarely needing operation. In a separate study they noted that 13% of patients with Dupuytren's disease had a raised blood glucose level. They raised the question as to whether the biochemical disturbance causes Dupuytren's disease or whether the pattern of inheritance predisposed to both conditions.

Epilepsy

Lund (1941) found a high incidence of Dupuytren's disease among epileptic patients. Early (1962) and Critchley *et al.* (1976) observed that epilepsy and Dupuytren's disease were commonly associated with knuckle pads and plantar nodules. Dupuytren's disease in epileptics also tended to be bilateral and symmetrical. James (1974) has reviewed the genetic patterns of idiopathic epilepsy and Dupuytren's disease and found no evidence of linked inheritance. Critchley *et al.* (1976), however, have compared the high incidence of the condition in modern series with earlier literature and conclude that Dupuytren's disease is due to the prolonged administration of anticonvulsants, especially phenobarbitone. Noble (personal communication, 1985) has noted differing incidences of Dupuytren's disease in different epilepsy populations in the United Kingdom despite similar medication and other, as yet undefined, factors therefore appear to apply in this relationship.

Alcohol

Alcohol and Dupuytren's disease are closely linked in the minds of medical students. A study by Graubard (1954) in New York brewery workers displayed a high incidence which he thought was due to occupation; however, the contracture probably was attributable to alcoholic history or other factors. Wolfe *et al.* (1956) have shown a relationship with alcoholism and hepatic cirrhosis but there is no relationship to bilharzial cirrhosis. This association therefore requires further clarification.

Other conditions

Other medical conditions which have been linked to Dupuytren's disease are chronic pulmonary disease and gout.

Vascular changes have been implicated by Wilflingseder, Bauer and Iannovich (1971) and Bauer (1976), who demonstrated by plethysmography that there was diminished blood flow in the digit.

Bocanegra *et al.* (1981) have compared black and caucasoid groups for Dupuytren's contracture and found that despite the presence in black patients of diabetes mellitus, epilepsy and alcoholism, Dupuytren's contracture is extremely rare. There therefore seems to be a multifactorial aetiology.

A reduced incidence of Dupuytren's disease has been suggested in patient's with rheumatoid arthritis by Arafa, Steingold and Noble (1984).

USE OF THE HAND

That the disease may appear in some individuals after a single injury is generally agreed (Hueston, 1968). It may also follow operation. Palmar nodules are not infrequent as part of the dystrophic process which may follow Colles fractures and other limb injuries. These nodules rarely progress to a full-blown contracture (Stewart, Innes and Burke, 1985). Dupuytren (1832) believed that chronic work related trauma may be responsible but Early (1962) found no difference in incidence in manual workers and clerks at Crewe locomotive works. Mikkelsen (1978), by contrast, found the prevalence to be higher and the contracture more severe in people doing hard manual work than in people doing light or non-manual work. When certain employments are scrutinized the incidence may be even higher. Bennett (1982) noted double the expected incidence in men doing a particular type of hard manual work. Roberts (1981) described two cases where transmitted hand-to-arm vibration may have been a contributing factor. Because of the medicolegal significance of work-related trauma it is difficult to derive conclusions from individual case histories. At the present time it seems likely that the role of work is a triggering factor in a genetically predisposed individual. Bell and Furness (1977) have expressed the opinion that some patients who have developed Dupuytren's contracture would not have done so until later had they been engaged in a lighter occupation.

Summary

Most cases of Dupuytren's disease present without any obvious cause. How, therefore, can one correlate the known associations? Firstly, a genetic predisposition, or diathesis (Hueston, 1963), must be present *if* the person is to develop the disease. *When* the disease develops it may be triggered by systemic disease or possibly by mechanical influences. *Where* the disease develops depends on hand anatomy and biomechanics, together with the influence of external forces or injury. *The rate of progression* of contracture is influenced by age, collagen metabolism, 'neurovascular' factors, use of the hand and psychological make-up.

THE ANATOMY

There are two reasons for the surgeon to study the anatomy of the normal palmar fascia: firstly, the evolution of the lesions of Dupuytren's disease is related to the anatomy; secondly, the distribution is not random and a working knowledge of certain anatomical relationships will facilitate the operative dissection.

Dupuytren's contracture follows anatomical pathways but McFarlane (personal communication, 1984) has emphasized that only certain anatomical fascial pathways are involved. The fascia within the palm and the digits is a precise three-dimensional system of ligaments (Stack, 1973; McFarlane, 1974; McGrouther, 1982) orientated transversely, longitudinally or vertically. Each of these three fibre systems has a separate function. The transverse fibres contribute to retinacular restraint for tendons, prevent bowstringing of neurovascular bundles and the most superficial limit skin tension in the webs. The longitudinal fibres act as

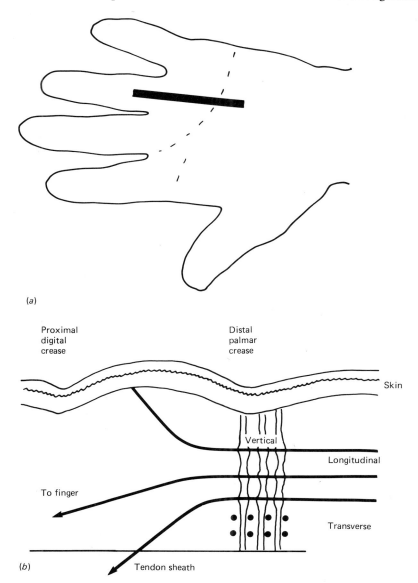

Figure 4.1 (*a and b*) Sagittal section of the distal palm. This shows the three distal insertions of the longitudinal fibres of the palmar fascia

skin anchors, resisting a tendency to longitudinal slip of the skin during gripping (that is, they balance shearing forces). The vertical fibres anchor specific zones to the underlying base to form skin joints. The palmar skin has no elasticity and the complex anchorage and draping of the skin of the hand to allow motion are controlled by the palmar fascial ligaments. Without these ligamentous systems the skin would slide off the hand like a glove.

The longitudinal fibres in the palm are those principally involved in Dupuytren's contracture. They arise proximally from the palmaris longus tendon. If this is absent they merge with the flexor retinaculum. These well-defined bundles of fibres are best developed in the palmar pretendinous area of each finger ray and on the radial aspect of the thumb. The distal insertions in three layers are best appreciated by reference to a sagittal section of the distal palm (*Figure 4.1*).

The first layer

The most superficial fibres insert into the dermis of the distal palm midway between the distal palmar crease and the proximal digital crease. The reader may appreciate an indentation in his own palm in this area on flexing the palm, especially in the ring finger. Involvement of this layer in Dupuytren's disease may cause a number of different clinical features. The simplest of these is an indentation at the site of skin insertion which is gradually pulled towards the distal palmar crease. As it does so the skin distally becomes tight and may blanch on full extension (the blanching sign) (*Figure 4.2a*). The skin between the attachment point and the distal palmar crease is heaped up to form a clinical nodule (*Figure 4.2b*). Nodules do not occur at random sites but overlie contracted fibres. Histologically the dermis thickens, the band (normal ligamentous structures are bands, when involved they become cords) becomes hypertrophic and the intervening fat is displaced or replaced by immature fibroblastic tissue such that dermis, fibroblastic tissue and band all form one mass. The palmar creases will distort, a sign that the underlying fascia is contracted. Distortion of the creases may be horizontal, such that they are bowed proximally or distally or vertical, such that the creases persist on full extension of the hand. There may be no joint contracture at this stage. As the disease progresses the contracture may propagate distally through the dermis (*Figure 4.2c*), or fascial fibres just deep to the dermis, to give clinical skin involvement at the base of the digit. In the finger this becomes a central cord (McFarlane, 1974) (*Figure 4.3a and b*), and the metacarpophalangeal (MCP) or interphalangeal (IP) joints commence to flex.

The second layer

The second layer of longitudinal pretendinous fibres comprises deeper bands which pass in bundles on either side of the flexor sheath. They pass around the neurovascular bundles in their course to the finger (spiral band of Gosset, 1974) (*Figure 4.4*). Contracture developing along these bands is likely to displace the neurovascular bundles. The bands, which originally spiral around the nerves, contract and straighten and the nerves come to spiral around the cords of diseased tissue. Contraction of these fibres may flex either the metacarpophalangeal (MCP) or proximal interphalangeal (PIP) joints.

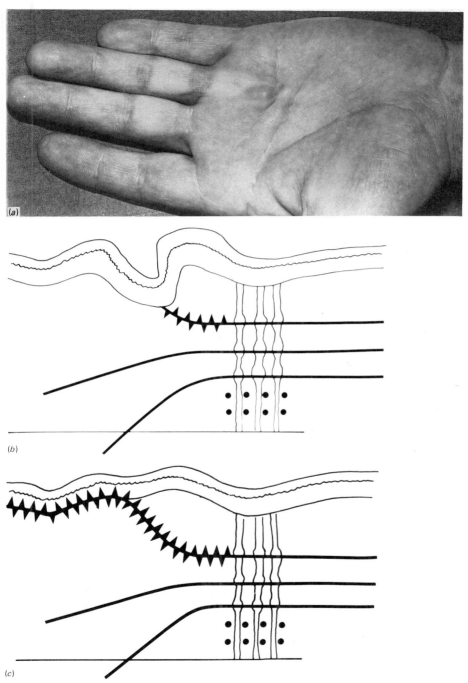

Figure 4.2 (*a*) The blanching sign. This is an early sign of Dupuytren's contracture. (*b*) A Dupuytren's contracture developing distal to the palmar crease. The skin is bunched up to produce a nodule. (*c*) Distal propagation through the dermis

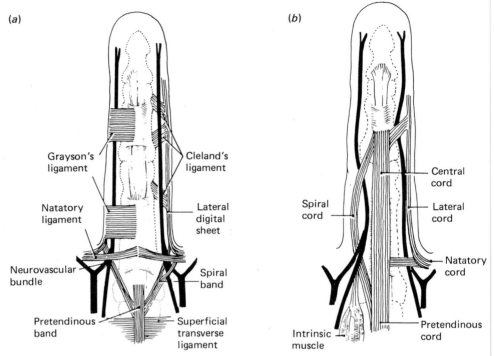

Figure 4.3 (*a*) The arrangement of the normal structures of the digital fascia. (After McFarlane, 1974) (*b*) The disease cords that cause contracture. (From Chui and McFarlane, 1978)

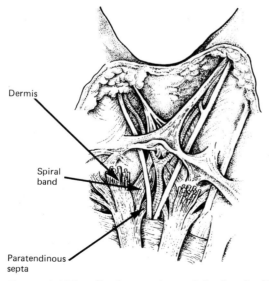

Figure 4.4 The distal extensions of the longitudinal fibres of the palmar fascia and their communications with the distal fascia. (Modified after Gosset, 1974)

The third layer

The deepest layer of longitudinal pretendinous fibres passes around the flexor sheaths to deep insertions either proximal or distal to the metacarpophalangeal joints. Contracture of these fibres will flex the metacarpophalangeal joint and not be amenable to correction by fasciotomy.

Transverse fibres exist in several layers and anatomical nomenclature is confusing. Skoog (1967) described a well-defined transverse fibre layer, the most distal edge of which lies beneath the distal palmar crease. The significance of this structure is that it is possible to use the transverse fibres as a safe surgical landmark. If these are preserved intact during fasciectomy the nerves and vessels lie safely beneath them. These transverse fibres never contract in the palm although a continuation across the thumb web as the proximal commissural ligament may do so (Tubiana, Simmons and De Frenne, 1982).

A separate system of transverse fibres exists on a much more superficial plane around the bases of the finger webs and across the palm just proximal to the webs (natatory ligaments). Involvement of these fibres in the contraction process will adduct adjacent fingers, giving rise to a tight web. This system may also be used as a safe surgical landmark as the neurovascular bundles are never superficial to this layer.

The vertical fibres have little surgical significance, but are the fibres which can be felt 'scratching' against the blade of the knife as the skin is dissected from the fascial plane of the longitudinal fibres. They are particularly condensed for a few millimetres on either side of the palmar creases rather than underlying the creases *per se*. Vertical contracture gives rise to skin pits which may subsequently be pulled by adjacent longitudinal cords such that they become quite deep and concave proximally. A deep pit is often an indication that a contracture cord is expending its tension on the skin surface rather than producing a finger contracture.

The fascial structures on the radial side of the hand have been well described by Tubiana, Simmons and De Frenne (1982). In the first web space there are two transverse ligamentous bands. The more distal of these lies at the free margin of the web (distal commissural ligament) and corresponds to the digital natatory system. Proximal to this is another transverse system, the proximal commissural ligament (continuous with the transverse palmar fibres of Skoog). Contracture of either gives rise to an adduction contracture of the first web space. The longitudinal band of fibres is situated towards the radial side of the thumb and contracture of this may give rise to flexion of either the metacarpophalangeal or interphalangeal joint when involved in Dupuytren's disease. The thumb therefore differs from the digits in that both transverse and longitudinal contractures are possible.

The fascial structures on the ulnar side of the hand have been dissected by White (1984). Fascial extensions of the abductor digiti minimi pass in four major directions – to the natatory ligament, Grayson's ligaments, the lateral digital sheath and the extensor expansion. Barton (1984) has described Dupuytren's contracture arising from the abductor digiti minimi and following these pathways. The cord originates from the muscle or overlying fascia and generally passes superficial to the neurovascular bundle which may be displaced radially. Contracture of this fibre bundle flexes the digit at the metacarpophalangeal and interphalangeal joints and forms a spiral cord with a strong tendency to displace the neurovascular bundle.

The normal fascial structures within the fingers have been beautifully described by McFarlane (1974) and can be conveniently described by classification, as in the palm, into longitudinal, transverse (and oblique) or vertical fibres. The major longitudinal system is laterally placed, the lateral digital sheet.

The second palmar layer (spiral band of Gosset, 1974) provides a normal fascial continuity between palm and digit by passing to the lateral digital sheet (McFarlane, 1974). The anterior edge of this collagenous sheet seems to be the structure described by Thomine (1974) as the retrovascular band. Proximally, fibres of the natatory system run into the lateral digital sheet. Distally, Law and McGrouther (1984) have defined a system of fibres which pass from the lateral digital sheet to the dorsal wrinkle skin over the proximal interphalangeal joint.

Cleland (1867) (quoted by Stack, 1973) described obliquely transverse fibres running from skin to bone and joint. His original description was imprecise and it has been left to later authors (Milford, 1968; McFarlane, 1974) to give precise definition to these fibres which lie posterior to the neurovascular bundles. Grayson's ligament is a transverse system of fibres lying anterior to the neurovascular bundle running from skin to tendon sheath.

In Dupuytren's contracture certain definable anatomical pathways are involved. McFarlane (1974) has classified digital contractures as being due to a central (or pretendinous) cord, a spiral cord or a lateral cord.

The central cord is a midline structure which has no anatomical counterpart and may possibly arise from the dermis. It forms in Dupuytren's disease as a continuation of the pretendinous fibres.

The spiral cord originates from a contracture which follows the normal pathway from the second palmar layer to the lateral digital sheet by way of the spiral band of Gosset. In the finger the contracture passes through Grayson's ligament to the tendon sheath and middle phalanx. It is this cord which is most likely to displace the neurovascular bundle.

The lateral cord follows the lateral digital sheet and neurovascular bundle displacement is less common.

Distally all finger cords may terminate in bone, tendon sheath or skin.

Strickland and Bassett (1985) have described cords which are confined to the fingers arising from the base of the proximal phalanx. These cords were either single or double, running superficial to the neurovascular bundles in the proximal digit and associated with displacement of the bundles.

Summary

The lesions of Dupuytren's disease arise by a cord-like contracture which follows the corresponding line of the anatomical band. Masses of new fibrous tissue arise in the subcutaneous spaces surrounding the thickened fibre bundles, thereby tethering them and the fat is displaced or replaced. As the disease progresses identification of the individual cords becomes difficult.

Dupuytren's contracture follows certain selected anatomical pathways to produce the characteristic clinical course commencing with the 'blanching sign', and leading to nodules and pits which have defined positioning, distortion of the palmar creases, cords and joint contractures.

PATHOLOGY

The longitudinal bands in the normal hand appear as discrete parallel glistening tendon-like structures with cross striations. When involved in the disease the cords, macroscopically, become white and opaque, and even quite gelatinous in the more advanced case. Microscopically, the initial change is a thickening of the bands (Millesi, 1959; Martini and Puhl, 1980). In the surrounding vessels there is proliferation of perivascular cells (Larsen and Posch, 1958). Kischer and Speer (1984) have described vascular occlusion within the bands and at the periphery but this may be a later reactive change.

Aggregations of cellular tissue form subcutaneous nodules extending outwith the cords enveloping them in such a way as to anchor them. Surrounding fat and connective tissues are displaced (Martini and Puhl, 1980). The skin may be heaped up by underlying cellular fibrous tissue or bunched up by tethering of thickened longitudinal ligamentous cords (see section on anatomy, pp. 78–84) to form clinical nodules.

Microscopic 'nodules' (different from clinical nodules) appear to arise within the bundles as areas of increased cellularity, and within these areas there is a corresponding reduction of fibres and apparent fibre discontinuity. These appearances have been interpreted by Skoog (1948) and Flint (personal communication; Colloquium on Dupuytren's disease, London, Ontario, October 1985) as evidence of microruptures and repair. They may, however, represent a reaction to stress without actual rupture.

The cells in the new fibroblastic tissue, presumably derived from perivascular cells, are myofibroblasts as described by Gabbiani and Majno (1972). These cells are recognized in many pathological states including granulation tissue, and have morphological features akin to smooth muscle cells; they have accordion-like folds of the nucleus and microfilaments in the cytoplasm. The microfilaments contain the polypeptides actin, desmin and vimentin and are thought to provide a mechanism enabling cell contraction.

The means by which myofibroblast contraction is conveyed to the cellular environment is unknown. Cell-to-cell contact by desmosomes (Gabbiani and Majno, 1972) or cell-to-fibrous stroma contact through a plexus of fibres are possibilities.

The collagen of the normal palmar fascia is type I, with a thin sheath of endotendineum around the individual bands of type III (this type is widely present in the fetus) (Bailey *et al.*, 1977). In Dupuytren's disease there is a marked increase in type III collagen (Bailey *et al.*, 1977; Bazin *et al.*, 1980; Brickley-Parsons *et al.*, 1981) and this can be demonstrated on immunofluorescence to be scattered throughout the nodules, the collagen being disrupted into microbundles.

Hunter, Ogden and Norris (1975) showed no primary chemical abnormality of the collagen. Brickley-Parsons *et al.* (1981) showed an increase in collagen and hexosamine with galactosamine in the most severely involved tissue. Delbruck, Reimers and Schonborn (1981) have shown no qualitative changes in enzyme activity and no increases of enzyme activity per cell (DNA).

There is general disorientation of the collagen fibres and elastic fibres may be present in excess (Millesi, 1974). These changes are most apparent in the nodules. Brickley-Parsons *et al.* (1981) showed progressive involvement in minimally involved fascia, longitudinal cords and nodules.

The collagen has multidirectional fibre orientation and the matrix shows an increase in glycosaminoglycan (GAG) content which is not uniformly spread amongst the three main GAG fractions (Flint, Gillard and Reilly, 1982). These macromolecules play an important role in determining the physical and functional characteristics of connective tissues. Dupuytren's cells have been grown in culture (Slack, Flint and Thompson, 1982) and the levels of GAG were not found to be elevated, suggesting that local mechanical conditions within the palm were responsible for the elevated GAG production. Chondroitin sulphate and dermatan sulphate were elevated but hyaluronate was not. Flint considered this to be a biological adaptation to decreased uniaxial tensional forces or to increased intermittent pressure forces.

In the late stages mature collagen bundles are seen with a gross and microscopic appearance similar to tendon (Hunter and Ogden, 1975). These bands are not vascular.

The question of biochemical changes in apparently uninvolved fascia is of considerable aetiological significance. Brickley-Parsons *et al.* (1981) noted biochemical changes before cell changes. Delbruck, Reimers and Schonborn (1981) have also shown that DNA synthesis is increased in apparently normal fascia.

Various attempts have been made to relate pathological and biochemical features to prognosis. Tyrkko and Viljanto (1975) correlated the appearance of several active nodules with a high frequency of postoperative recurrence. Gelberman *et al.* (1980) have related recurrence to the finding of myofibroblasts in the nodules.

The exact mechanism by which Dupuytren's contracture produces a contracture is not known. Contraction is not the same process as contracture (Smith, 1982), and some means of retaining the contracted position must be postulated. Brickley-Parsons *et al.* (1981) have suggested resorption and remodelling of the collagen rather than coiling or crimping.

All of the cellular and biochemical changes are not clearly distinguishable from those that occur during the active stages of connective-tissue wound repair. Dupuytren's contracture does not therefore appear to be a unique pathological process.

PRINCIPLES OF OPERATION

There is no single operative procedure which is universally applicable for Dupuytren's contracture (Luck, 1959; McFarlane, 1983) and the surgeon should make a choice from a range of available alternatives.

The many different surgical approaches all have features in common.

The aim of surgery is to restore to the digits the ability to extend fully, without creating the surgical complications of haematoma, wound scar contracture, damage to nerves or vessels, or joint stiffness.

A return to the normal anatomical arrangement is never possible. However, the aim is to revert to a normal biomechanical state whereby the skin and flexor sheath are separated by a sandwich of fat and there is a discontinuity in the tight fascia.

Views on the amount of tissue, involved or uninvolved, which must be removed vary widely, but it should be appreciated that it is release rather than removal of tissue which contributes to straightening of the digit.

It is known that after simple division (McGregor, McGrouther and Phillips, 1986) or even traumatic rupture of the contracture (Grace, McGrouther and Phillips, 1984), cords and nodules may apparently resolve, leading to a lasting release.

What therefore is the mechanism of operation?

The aim of surgery is to break up the line of contracture rather than to excise pathological tissue. The fascia which the surgeon will encounter will be of three types; visibly involved, not apparently involved but tight, or apparently normal. Most operations comprise a combination of release and excision but it is rarely possible to remove all of the pathological tissue and the concept of excision with a margin of clearance does not apply. The first step in all fasciectomy operations is a proximal 'fasciotomy' or release of the contracted tissues, whereupon by gentle manipulation there will be a considerable separation of the contracted fascial tissue. Thereafter a variable amount of fascia is removed, the wound is closed by reapplication of the original skin, taking steps to avoid longitudinal contracture. Alternatively the skin may be replaced if it is grossly involved with Dupuytren's disease.

Release of a single restraining cord (fasciotomy) will successfully restore function and the effect will be lasting if the cord does not reform. If the surrounding tissues are uninvolved simple release allows the cut ends of the cord to 'retreat' into normal fat. If, however, the state of scarring of the tissues prevents retraction, the continuity of the contracture cord will be restored by the hand flexing or by the short bridge segment healing by scar tissue.

The removal of tissue does virtually nothing to release the contracture. However, by following the band distally the identification of anatomical structures at risk is facilitated. Indirectly, therefore, removal of cords is justified on the basis of finding anatomy. Principally, however, it is done to prevent recurrence by ensuring a separation of the involved fascia.

There is no evidence that the removal of Dupuytren's tissue is removing a 'neoplastic' cell mass with a potential to recur.

Case selection and timing of surgery

The indication for operation is progressive contracture as judged from the history or repeated examination over a period of time. Proximal interphalangeal joint contracture of more than 30° is a strong indication for intervention as severe or long standing proximal interphalangeal joint contracture is extremely difficult to correct. McFarlane (1983) advises intervention as soon as the proximal interphalangeal joint begins to flex. There seems to be a critical angle of proximal interphalangeal contraction beyond which the condition will rapidly progress, perhaps because of the poor mechanical advantage of the extensor tendon or because the patient develops a habit of flexing the digit into the palm to keep it out of the way. The need to relieve proximal interphalangeal joint contracture at an early stage is not specific to Dupuytren's contracture but is related to anatomical features of the joint whereby prolonged immobilization in a flexed position is difficult to reverse.

Contracture of the metacarpophalangeal joint is a less urgent indication since this is always reversible.

Indications

Clinical impressions are an invaluable part of the assessment. The younger patient tends to develop a more aggressive contracture with nodules and more rapid progression. An assessment should be made of the type of hand involved by the contracture. The skin and subcutaneous tissues may be soft and supple and readily mobile over the deep contracted fascia or they may be tense and indurated. The moist sweaty hand is generally considered a bad prognostic sign, as is the thickened workman's hand. Such impressions are difficult to quantify but it is worth-while trying to identify patients likely to require additional postoperative supervision.

Operative procedures

The operative procedures for Dupuytren's contracture are:

(1) Fasciotomy.
(2) Limited fasciectomy.
(3) Radical fasciectomy.
(4) Digital fasciectomy.
(5) Procedures on the contracted proximal interphalangeal joint.

Fasciotomy

Fasciotomy or simple release was the technique advocated by Baron Dupuytren (1832). Colville (1983) has defined the role of closed fasciotomy, and in particular the precise indications for this selective procedure. It is an operation for the older patient. The band should be cord-like and an absence of bow-stringing is a contraindication. Ideally the overlying skin should be separated from the band by uninvolved subcutaneous fat. It may be considered as a preliminary to fasciectomy in the severely contracted hand.

Colville's technique employs a specially prepared no. 11 blade in which all of the cutting surface has been removed with the exception of the tip. This is inserted transcutaneously under limited local anaesthesia. The skin is freed distally, the band is placed under tension and gently cut. As the procedure is performed blind there is the risk of cutting a digital nerve. This risk is reduced to a minimum by attention to the above selection criteria and by undertaking the fasciotomy at the level of the distal palmar crease. The neurovascular bundles are deep to the transverse fibres at this level and therefore well away from the field of dissection.

Colville has also suggested fasciotomy proximal to the web crease and proximal to the proximal interphalangeal joint, but the danager of damaging digital nerves is greater in the finger. This technique is therefore for use on rare occasions. An alternative limited operation is open fasciotomy in which a small transverse or longitudinal incision may be used to allow visualization of the nerves. A longitudinal incision will have a tendency to remain closed after release of the contracture but a transverse incision will gape and require to heal by secondary intention. Alternatively, a small Z-plasty may be fashioned on top of the band. Watson (1984) has described the use of fasciotomy and Z-plasty in which the fascia is incorporated in the Z-plasty skin flap so that as the skin is transposed the direction of longitudinal tension in the fascia is also transposed and the tension line broken. This technique has been used throughout a wider age range than that in which closed fasciotomy would be applicable. It is, however, a judicious operation for the highly selected individual with a mature band. Fasciotomy and Z-plasty have a useful role in relieving contracture bands in the thumb.

Gonzales (1974) has used a full thickness skin graft as a means of maintaining separation between the ends of the divided cords after fasciotomy or fasciectomy. He feels that by treating Dupuytren's disease like any other scar contracture the morbidity of operation can be reduced. This technique therefore has a wider application than is the case with simple closed fasciotomy.

McGregor (1986) has developed the operation of fasciotomy and split skin grafting, using split skin interpositioning to separate cords and release tension. It is necessary to divide the palm from radial to ulnar borders and the digits from neutral line to neutral line to obtain a lasting result. All fascial fibres must be released and separation assured. This operation is particularly valuable in the hand where skin flap elevation is difficult; for example, the thick oedematous hand with multiple cords or nodules or in the case of recurrent contracture.

Limited fasciectomy

Fasciectomy operations have been described in various ways. Hueston (1961) described limited fasciectomy in which 'the apparently involved fascia is removed with a margin of clearance'. More recently, Hueston (1982) has applied the term regional fasciectomy and defined this as 'removal of the fascia within the area'. The actual amount of fascia removed has probably not changed but it is difficult to describe precisely which fascial structures are removed at operation and the extent of dissection that is necessary.

Skoog (1967) has described a much more specific anatomical dissection. He believes that the transverse palmar fibres are never involved and advises their preservation. In his operative description he expressed the desire that his method of fasciectomy would not be characterized simply as a particular skin incision pattern but rather that the focus of attention should be on the specific approach to the removal of the involved fascia. Regrettably, his wishes have not been observed. The Skoog technique specifically comprises:

(1) Preservation of the deep transverse palmar fibres.
(2) The excision of the involved longitudinal tissue (*Figure 4.5*).
(3) The neurovascular bundles are not uncovered proximal to the distal palmar crease but left undisturbed beneath the deep transverse fibres where they are safe. They are only sought distal to the distal palmar crease and uncovered only as necessary to ensure their preservation. This practice of limited exposure of the neurovascular bundles advocated by Skoog has been justified by the anatomical studies of McFarlane (1974) and McGrouther (1982) who have shown that the neurovascular bundles are not displaced in the proximal palm.
(4) Only the involved fascia should be removed and fat should be preserved.

This selective fasciectomy takes account of the fascial anatomy rather than treating the disease as an amorphous mass.

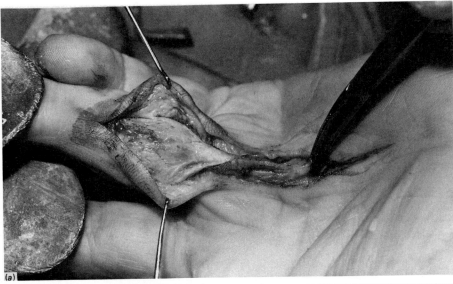

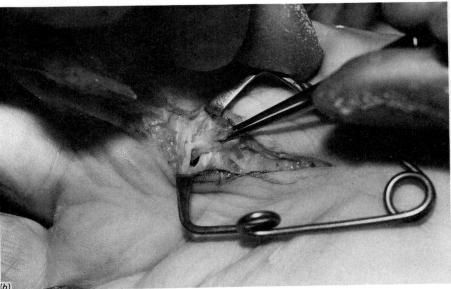

Figure 4.5 (*a*) A clinical example of a central Dupuytren's cord. (*b*) The same patient. At a deeper level a spiral cord is shown

Dermofasciectomy

Hueston (1962) has advised *en bloc* excision of the fascia and overlying skin in recurrences of Dupuytren's contracture. It has also been suggested that the procedure should be considered as a first operation in the young patient with skin involvement.

The procedure requires excision of all of the skin and fascia of the involved ray from the distal palmar crease of the proximal interphalangeal joint crease from neutral line to neutral line. The area is resurfaced by full thickness or thick split skin graft.

The operation is a radical procedure but Hueston believes that recurrence does not occur under a skin graft. Graft take can be difficult if the tendon sheath has been opened to permit proximal interphalangeal joint release.

A prolonged absence from work may be necessary to allow the skin to stabilize but the results are justified where there is considerable visible skin involvement.

Radical fasciectomy

Radical fasciectomy was formerly a popular operation in the United Kingdom and remains popular in central Europe. The part of the fasciectomy which is radical is within the palm and only involved digits are dissected. The extent of the operation is to remove the entire 'triangular palmar fascia' (that is, the longitudinal fibres to all four rays together with the transverse fibres). This concept does not take account of the various layers and individual ligamentous structures within the palmar fascia. Specific steps must be taken to preserve the skin blood supply. It is a time-consuming operation which in inexperienced hands carries a high risk of skin necrosis and haematoma resulting in subsequent stiffness. There is no evidence that a radical excision of the palmar tissue prevents the subsequent development of contracture in the fingers which have not been dissected, nor is there evidence that it reduces recurrence in the digits which have been operated upon. Recurrence of contracted tissues within the palm is not a problem to deal with and a radical operation to try to prevent this does not seem justified. The real therapeutic problems in Dupuytren's disease are of recurrence of contracture within the digit or the development of a severe contracture within an additional digit and a radical approach to the palm seems to have no role in preventing these problems.

Digital fasciectomy

The management of Dupuytren's disease in the digits can be discussed by considering each tissue separately. The skin is reflected to expose underlying cords and nodules using a non-linear incision. Different patterns of zigzag incision, such as that described by Bruner (1951), prevent later linear scar contracture. A straight line incision may be made with the formation of Z-plasties at the end of the dissection. Z-plasties have been deferred to a second operation (Robbins, 1981). Baker and Watson (1980) have advocated a series of triangular flaps to provide additional skin. Involved skin which is adherent to cords and nodules is deprived of its normal subcutaneous fat layer. It may be replaced by skin grafting as described above. Skin grafting may also be necessary to compensate for skin shortage. Skin flaps are an alternative means of making good skin shortage, particularly where the flexor tendon sheath has been opened. Harrison and Morris (1975) have described a dorsal transposition flap. Cross-finger flaps may be used as an alternative. Where the flexor sheath is opened the proximally based sliding volar flap has been suggested by Lane (1981), which leaves the subsequent skin defect for grafting over the middle phalanx.

Subcutaneous layers comprise fat and ligamentous bands, involved cords and nodules. Surgical approaches vary. It seems wise to conserve fat. Most surgeons remove involved fascia only as far as its distal insertion on the middle phalanx or tendon sheath. Central, spiral or lateral cords can generally be identified. McFarlane (1984) performs a radical fasciectomy in the digits, removing prophylactically all potentially involved anatomical structures.

The contracted proximal interphalangeal joint

The techniques of dealing with the contracted proximal interphalangeal joint have been reviewed by Tonkin *et al.* (1985) and Geldmacher (1985). If joint release is incomplete following fascial removal release of the flexor tendon sheath may be required. If this does not allow full digital extension, division of the check rein ligaments of the volar plates can be considered (Watson, Light and Johnson, 1979). These ligaments are fascial structures which appear in the digit with a contracted joint on the volar ridges of the proximal phalanx. Curtis (1970) has advised volar capsulectomy in selected cases where amputation may be entertained as an alternative. It is the author's experience that only a minority of patients benefit from such radical release.

Haemostasis

The prevention of haematoma is a vital part of all Dupuytren's operations. Surgeons vary in their approach to this problem. Hueston (1982) suggests a pressure dressing which may require release within 12 hours of operation and emphasizes the need for prolonged and careful haemostasis. Formal drainage has been suggested. The technique of McCash (1974), which provides open wound drainage, has received much attention in the literature and is generally a safe approach to prevent haematoma. The open palmar wound heals by secondary intention and leaves an excellent final scar. It does, however, take several weeks to heal and during this time the patient requires frequent dressings and encouragement to use the hand.

Salvage procedures in Dupuytren's disease

Arthrodesis of the proximal interphalangeal joint should be considered if the joint cannot be adequately straightened at operation. A proximal interphalangeal joint which can not be straightened beyond 45° on the table is likely to be stiff and the stiff proximal interphalangeal joint will creep down into greater flexion due to the strong flexor tendon action. Where extensive capsular release is therefore necessary it may be better in selected patients to undertake an elective proximal interphalangeal joint arthrodesis. The arthodesis is performed using intraosseous wires. In the severely contracted case where a preoperative decision for arthrodesis is made it is possible to approach the joint through a dorsal mid-line incision without opening the palmar tissues. Bone shortening can be achieved by a wedge excision in the region of the joint. An alternative to arthrodesis is amputation of the digit but the cosmetic result is less satisfactory. A fixed flexed digit may, however, be dangerous in certain occupations and pursuits; a fisherman can catch such a digit in a net and be pulled over the side of the boat. If amputation is undertaken through the metacarpal neck, scar tissue adjacent to the intrinsic muscles of the adjacent digit may be involved in later recurrences of Dupuytren's disease, making dissection extremely difficult. Alternatively, amputation may be undertaken at proximal interphalangeal joint level but the disadvantages are that the volar skin may be extremely scarred. A simple technique is to use the dorsal skin of the digit as a flap to resurface any scarred areas of the palm. Arthroplasty using a Swanson's prosthesis is an alternative means of avoiding amputation in elderly patients. Many patients given the choice between amputation and alternative salvage procedures, such as arthodesis or arthroplasty, will opt to keep the digit.

Results

It must be appreciated that Dupuytren's disease is a generalized condition. Surgical release is therefore no guarantee that the patient will be free of future trouble. Hueston (1982) has pointed out that after ten years only 20% of patients in Melbourne remained free of recurrence or extension.

References

ARAFA, M., STEINGOLD, R. F. and NOBLE, J. (1984) The incidence of Dupuytren's disease in patient's with rheumatoid arthritis. *Journal of Hand Surgery*, **9B**, 165–166

BAILEY, A. J., SIMS, T. J., GABBIANI, G., BAZIN, S. and LE LOUS, M. (1977) Collagen of Dupuytren's disease. *Clinical Science and Molecular Medicine*, **53(5)**, 499–502

BAKER, G. C. and WATSON, H. K. (1980) Relieving the skin shortage in Dupuytren's disease by advancing a series of triangular flaps: how to design and use them. *British Journal of Plastic Surgery*, **33(1)**, 1–3

BARTON, N. J. (1984) Dupuytren's disease arising from the abductor digiti minimi. *Journal of Hand Surgery (British)*, **9(3)**, 265–270

BAUER, M. (1976) Angiospasm and lesion of the ulnar nerve in Dupuytren's contracture. *Wien Klinische Wochenschrift*, Suppl. 88, 23, Suppl. 62, 1–18

BAZIN, S., LE LOUS, M., DUANCE, V. C., SIMS, T. J., BAILEY, A. J., GABBIANI, G. D., ANDIRAN, G., PIZZOLATO, G., BROWSKI, A., NICOLETIS, C. and DELAUNAY, A. (1980) Biochemistry and histology of the connective tissue of Dupuytren's disease lesions. *European Journal of Clinical Investigation*, **10(1)**, 9–16

BELL, R. C. and FURNESS, J. A. (1977) A study of the effect of recurrent trauma on the development of Dupuytren's contracture. *British Journal of Plastic Surgery*, **30(2)**, 149–150

BENNETT, B. (1982) Dupuytren's contracture in manual workers. *British Journal of Indian Medicine*, **39**, 98–100

BOCANEGRA, T. S., KING, P., VASEY, F. B., GERMAIN, F. B. and ESPINOZA, L. R. (1981) Dupuytren's contracture: a genetically predisposed disorder? (letter). *Journal of Rheumatology*, **8(6)**, 1026–1027

BOWSER-RILEY, S., BAIN, A. D., NOBLE, J. and LAMB, D. W. (1975) Chromosome abnormalities in Dupuytren's disease. *Lancet*, **2(7948)**, 1282–1283

BRICKLEY-PARSONS, D., GLIMCHER, M. J., SMITH, R. J., ALBIN, R. and ADAMS, J. P. (1981) Biochemical changes in the collagen of the palmar fascia in patients with Dupuytren's disease. *Journal of Bone and Joint Surgery (American)*, **63A(5)**, 787–797

BRUNER, J. M. (1951) Incisions for plastic and reconstructive (non-septic) surgery of the hand. *British Journal of Plastic Surgery*, **4**, 48

CHOW, S. P., LUK, K. D. and KUNG, T. M. (1984) Dupuytren's contracture in Chinese. A report of three cases. *Journal of the Royal College of Surgeons (Edinburgh)*, **29(1)**, 49–51

CHUI, H. F. and McFARLANE, R. M. (1978) Pathogenesis of Dupuytren's contracture: a correlative clinical pathological study. *Journal of Hand Surgery*, **3**, 1–10

COLVILLE, J. (1983) Dupuytren's contracture – the role of fascioctomy. *The Hand*, **15(2)**, 162–166

CRITCHLEY, E. M. R., VAKIL, S. D., HAYWARD, H. W. and OWEN, V. M. H. (1976) Dupuytren's disease in epilepsy: result of prolonged administration of anticonvulsants. *Journal of Neurology, Neurosurgery and Psychiatry*, **39**, 498–503

CURTIS, R. M. (1970) Surgical restoration of motion in the stiff interphalangeal joints of the hand. *Bulletin of the Hospital for Joint Diseases,* **31,** 1–6

DELBRUCK, A., REIMERS, E. and SCHONBORN, I. (1981) A comparative study of the activity of lysosomal and main metabolic pathway enzymes in tissue biopsies and cultured fibroblasts from Dupuytren's disease and palmar fascia. *Journal of Clinical Chemistry and Clinical Biochemistry,* **19,** 931–941

DUPUYTREN, G. (1832) *Lecons orales de clinique chirurgicale faites à l' Hotel Dieu de Paris,* Vol. 1, p.1. Paris: Baillière

EARLY, P. F. (1962) Population studies in Dupuytren's contracture. *Journal of Bone and Joint Surgery,* **44,** 602–613

FLINT, M. H., GILLARD, G. C. and REILLY, H. C. (1982) The glycosaminoglycans of Dupuytren's disease. *Connective Tissue Research,* **9(3),** 173–179

FURNAS, D. W. (1979) Dupuytren's contractures in a black patient in East Africa (letter). *Plastic and Reconstructive Surgery,* **64(2),** 250–251

GABBIANI, G. and MAJNO, G. (1972) Dupuytren's contractures: fibroblast contraction? *American Journal of Pathology,* **66,** 131

GELBERMAN, R. H., AMIEL, D., RUDOLPH, R. M. and VANCE, R. M. (1980) Dupuytren's contracture. An electronmicroscopic, biochemical and clinical correlative study. *Journal of Bone and Joint Surgery (America),* **62A(3)** 425–432

GELDMACHER, J. and KOCHERLING, F. (1985) Flexion contracture of the proximal interphalangeal joint in Dupuytren's disease. Anatomic and clinical observations. *Handchirurgie, Mikrochirurgie und Plastische Chirurgie,* **17(1),** 4–7

GONZALES, R. (1974) *Dupuytren's Disease,* edited by J. T. Hueston and R. Tubiana, pp. 123–127 London: Churchill Livingstone

GOSSETT, J. (1974) *Dupuytren's Disease and the Anatomy of the Palmodigital Aponeuroses in Dupuytren's Disease,* edited by J. T. Hueston and R. Tubiana. London: Churchill Livingstone

GRAUBARD, D. (1954) Dupuytren's contracture. An etiologic study. *Journal of the International College of Surgeons,* **21,** 15

GRACE, D. L., McGROUTHER, D. A. and PHILLIPS, H. (1984) Traumatic correction of Dupuytren's contracture. *Journal of Hand Surgery,* **9B, (1),** 59–60

HARRISON, S. H. and MORRIS, A. (1975) Dupuytren's contracture: the dorsal transposition flap. *The Hand,* **7(2),** 145–149

HEATHCOTE, J. G., COHEN, H. and NOBLE, J. (1981) Dupuytren's disease and diabetes mellitus (letter). *Lancet,* **27:1(8235),** 145–149

HUESTON, J. T. (1961) Limited fasciectomy. *Plastic and Reconstructive Surgery,* **27,** 569

HUESTON, J. T. (1962) Digital Wolfe grafts in recurrent Dupuytren's contracture. *Plastic and Reconstructive Surgery,* **29,** 342

HUESTON, J. T. (1962) *Dupuytren's Contracture.* Edinburgh: Livingstone

HUESTON, J. T. (1968) Dupuytren's contracture and specific injury. *Medical Journal of Australia,* **1,** 1084

HUESTON, J. T. (1982) In *Dupuytren's Disease in Hand Surgery,* edited by J. E. Flynn. pp. 797–822. Baltimore: Williams and Wilkins

HUNTER, J. A. A. and OGDEN, C. (1975) Dupuytren's contracture No. 2 – scanning electron microscope observations. *British Journal of Plastic Surgery,* **28,** 19–25

HUNTER, J. A. A., OGDEN, C. and NORRIS, M. G. (1975) Dupuytren's contracture No. 1 – chemical pathology. *British Journal of Plastic Surgery,* **28,** 10–18

JAMES, J. I. P. (1974) The genetic pattern of Dupuytren's contracture and idiopathic epilepsy. In *Dupuytren's Disease,* edited by J. T. Hueston and R. Tubiana, pp. 37–42. London: Churchill Livingstone

KISCHER, C. W. and SPEER, D. P. Microvascular changes in Dupuytren's contracture. *Journal of Hand Surgery (American),* **9A(1),** 58–62

LANE, L. S. (1981) The treatment of Dupuytren's contracture with flexor tendon sheath involvement – the sliding volar flap. *Annals of Plastic Surgery,* **6(1),** 20–23

LARSEN, R. and POSCH, J. (1958) Dupuytren's contracture; with specific reference to pathology. *Journal of Bone and Joint Surgery,* **40A,** 773

LAW, P. and McGROUTHER, D. A. (1984) The dorsal wrinkle ligaments of the proximal interphalangeal joint. *Journal of Hand Surgery,* **(3)**

LING, R. S. M. (1963) The genetic factor in Dupuytren's disease. *Journal of Bone and Joint Surgery,* **45B,** 709

LUCK, J. V. (1959) Dupuytren's contracture: a new concept of the pathogenesis correlated with surgical management. *'Journal of Bone and Joint Surgery,* **41A,** 635

LUND, M. (1941) Dupuytren's contracture and epilepsy. *Acta Psychiatrica Scandinavica,* **16,** 465

McCASH, C. R. (1974) The open palm technique in Dupuytren's contracture. In *Dupuytren's Disease*, edited by J. T. Hueston and R. Tubiana, p. 129. London: Churchill Livingstone

McFARLANE, R. M. (1974) Patterns of the diseased fascia in the fingers in Dupuytren's contracture. displacement of the neurovascular bundle. *Plastic and Reconstructive Surgery*, **54**, 31–44

McFARLANE, R. M. (1983) The current status of Dupuytren's disease. *Journal of Hand Surgery (American)*, **8(5 Pt 2)**, 703–708

McGREGOR, I. A. (1986) *Fasciotomy and Split Skin Grafting in Dupuytren's Disease*, 2nd edition, edited by J. T. Hueston and R. Tubiana. London: Churchill Livingstone

McGROUTHER, D. A. (1982) The microanatomy of Dupuytren's contracture. *The Hand*, **14(3)**, 215–236

MARTINI, A. K. and PUHL, W. (1980) Micromorphological studies in Dupuytren's disease. *Zeitschrift für Orthopaedie*, **118(3)**, 291–299. (English abstract) (German)

MATTHEWS, P. (1979) Familial Dupuytren's contracture with predominantly female expression. *British Journal of Plastic Surgery*, **32(2)**, 120–123

MENNEN, U, and GRABE, R. P. (1979) Dupuytren's contracture in a Negro: a case report. *Journal of Hand Surgery*, **4(5)**, 451–453

MENNEN, U. (1986) Dupuytren's contracture in the Negro. *Journal of Hand Surgery*, **11B**, 61–64

MIKKELSEN, O. A. (1972) The prevalence of Dupuytren's disease in Norway. A study in a representative population sample of the municipality of Haugesund. *Acta Chirurgie Scandinavica*, **138**, 695–700

MIKKELSEN, O. A. (1976) Dupuytren's disease – a study of the pattern of distribution and stage of contracture in the hand. *The Hand*, **8(3)**, 265–271

MIKKELSEN, O. A. (1977) Dupuytren's disease – initial symptoms, age of onset and spontaneous course. *The Hand*, **9(1)**, 11–15

MIKKELSEN, O. A. (1978) Dupuytren's disease – the influence of occupation and previous hand injuries. *The Hand*, **10(1)**, 1–8

MILFORD, L. W. (1968) *Retaining Ligaments of the Digits of the Hand*. Philadelphia: Saunders

MILLESI, H. (1959) Neue Gesichtspunkte in der Pathogenese der Dupuytrenschen Kontraktur. *Brunschweig Beitrage der Klinische Chirurgie*, 198–201

MILLESI, H. (1974) The clinical and morphological course of Dupuytren's disease. In *Dupuytren's Disease*, edited by J. T. Hueston and R. Tubiana. London: Churchill Livingstone

NOBLE, J., HEATHCOTE, J. G. and COHEN, H. (1984) Diabetes mellitus in the aetiology of Dupuytren's disease. *Journal of Bone and Joint Surgery*, **66-B(3)**, 322–325

PLASSE, J. S. (1979) Dupuytren's contracture in a black patient (letter). *Plastic and Reconstructive Surgery*, **64(2)**, 250

PLATER, F. (1641) *Observationum*, Volume 1, p. 150. Basel: Ludovici Konig

ROBBINS, T. H. (1981) Dupuytren's contracture: the defined Z-plasty. *Annals of the Royal College of Surgeons of England*, **63**, 357–358

ROBERTS, F. P. (1981) A vibration injury: Dupuytren's contracture. *Journal of the Society of Occupational Medicine*, **31(4)**, 148–150

SERGOVICH, F. R., BOTZ, J. S. and McFARLANE, R. M. (1983) Non-random cytogenetic abnormalities in Dupuytren's disease. *New England Journal of Medicine*, **308(3)**, 162–163

SKOOG, T. (1948) Dupuytren's contracture. *Acta Chirgurgie Scandinavica*, **96**(Suppl 139), 1

SKOOG, T. (1967) The superficial transverse fibers of the palmar aponeurosis and their significance in Dupuytren's contracture. *Surgical Clinics of North America*, **47**, 433

SLACK, C., FLINT, M. H. and THOMPSON, B. M. (1982) Glycosaminoglycan synthesis by Dupuytren's cells in culture. *Connective Tissue Research*, **9(4)**, 263–269

SMITH, R. J. (1982) A study of Dupuytren's tissue with the scanning electron microscope (letter). *Journal of Hand Surgery*, **7(2)**, 208

STACK, H. G. (1973) *The Palmar Fascia*. London: Churchill Livingstone

STEWART, H. D., INNES, A. R. and BURKE, F. D. (1985) The hand complications of Colles fráctures. *Journal of Hand Surgery*, **10B**, 103–106

STRICKLAND, J. W. and BASSETT, R. L. (1985) The isolated digital cord in Dupuytren's contracture: anatomy and clinical significance. *Journal of Hand Surgery (American)*, **10(1)**, 118–124

TAIT, B. D. and MACKAY, I. R. (1982) HLA phenotypes in Dupuytren's contracture. *Tissue Antigens*, **19(3)**, 240–241

THOMINE, J. M. (1974) *The Development and Anatomy of the Digital Fascia in Dupuytren's Disease*, edited by J. T. Hueston and R. Tubiana. London: Churchill Livingstone

TONKIN, M. A., BURKE, F. D. and VARIAN, J. P. W. (1985) The proximal interphalangeal joint in Dupuytren's disease. *Journal of Hand Surgery*, **10B**, 358–364

TYRKKO, J. and VILJANTO, J. (1975) Significance of histopathological findings in Dupuytren's contracture. *Annales Chirurgiae et Gynaecologiae Fenniae*, **64(5)**, 288–291

TUBIANA, R., SIMMONS, B. P. and DE FRENNE, H. A. (1982) Location of Dupuytren's disease on the radial aspect of the hand. *Clinical Orthopaedics,* **(168),** 222–229

USHIJIMA, M., TSUNEYOSHI, M. and ENJOJI, M. (1984) Dupuytren's type fibromatoses. A clinicopathologic study of 62 cases. *Acta Pathologica,* **34(5),** 991–1001

WATSON, H. K., LIGHT, T. R. and JOHNSON, T. R. (1979) Check rein resection for flexion contracture of the middle joint. *Journal of Hand Surgery,* **4,** 67

WATSON, J. D. (1984) Fasciotomy and Z-plasty in the management of Dupuytren's contracture. *British Journal of Plastic Surgery,* **37,** 27–30

WHITE, S. H. (1984) Anatomy of the palmar fascia on the ulnar border of the hand. *Journal of Hand Surgery,* **9B,** 50–56

WILFLINGSEDER, P., BAUER, M. and IANNOVICH, I. (1971) Venous-occlusion plethysmography in Dupuytren's contracture. *Fifth World Congress of Plastic and Reconstructive Surgery,* London: Butterworths, 599–605

WOLFE, S. J., WILLIAM, H. J., SUMMERSKILL, D. M. and DAVIDSON, C. S. (1956) Thickening and contraction of the palmar fascia (Dupuytren's contracture) associated with alcoholism and hepatic cirrhosis. *New England Journal of Medicine,* **255,** 559

ZAWORKSI, R. E. and MANN, R. J. (1979) Dupuytren's contractures in a black patient. *Plastic and Reconstructive Surgery,* **63(1),** 122–124

5
Infections of the hand

Neil Watson

INTRODUCTION

Meetings of hand societies seldom include papers about infections of the hand and indeed a search of the literature for the last ten years has revealed only a small number of publications. This might suggest that hand infections are both less common and less troublesome than previously. There would not appear to be any evidence to support that they are less numerous, though the patterns of infection have changed a bit. Some infections are undoubtedly rarer (for example, palmar space infection), whilst new ones are increasing (for example, genital herpes). If they are less troublesome that could reflect an improving standard of primary care. If so that is good news. For there seems little doubt that the final outcome of a hand infection is directly related to the primary treatment. That treatment cannot be correct unless the diagnosis is also correct. But unfortunately there are still many patients who are left with significant and disabling problems following infection of the hand, mostly because the primary treatment was inappropriate or inadequate.

Those of us who are regularly involved in the primary care of the injured or infected hand spend much time preaching this piece of gospel, believing that many difficult and often less than satisfactory retrieval procedures are avoidable if primary treatment is of a high quality. It is clearly and regrettably not logistically possible that all patients with a hand infection can be so treated. Hand surgeons collectively have a major educational responsibility to ensure that those doctors who are entrusted with such primary care are not only well instructed but also well supervised. Those doctors must of course also be acquainted with the conditions whose treatment is wholly inappropriate in a casualty or accident and emergency department and with those methods of treatment that are wrong, dangerous or ineffectual. Help and advice must be readily available. Sadly such assistance is often not to hand, leaving the primary care doctor to soldier on, referring the patient only when it becomes patently obvious that all is not well, by which time irreversible local complications are likely to have occurred. For there is no more such an entity as a minor hand infection than there is a minor hand injury. Those of you that have experienced either will testify to that notion.

Infections of the hand have obviously occurred throughout man's existence. The nature and extent of the problem has not featured prominently in the surgical literature. Kanavel (1905, 1933) seems to have been the earliest author in this century to collate information on the subject, and continued to do so over a long period. Pilcher *et al.* (1949), Bingham (1960), Rhode (1961), Entin (1964), Lowden (1964), Lindscheid and Dobyns (1975), amongst others, have produced reviews. Robins (1952), Scott and Jones (1952), and McConnell and Neale (1979) have reported on the outcome of large series of patients with hand infections. As well as sections in standard texts, monographs have also appeared, such as those by Bailey (1963), Sneddon (1970) and Carter (1983).

TAKING A HISTORY

It might seem unnecessary to even mention such a basic consideration as taking a proper history. But it must be done. Why? Because not only may there be particular and unusual organisms involved in certain infections, but there may also be general and local factors predisposing both to the initiation of a hand infection and to its failure to respond to conventional treatment. It is a good idea to spot these in advance.

General factors

These may be listed as follows:

(1) Diabetes.
(2) Anaemia.
(3) Conditions or drugs affecting immunological status.
(4) Hypoproteinaemia.
(5) Deficiency states.
(6) Existing infection at other sites.
(7) Skin conditions, such as eczema and psoriasis.
(8) Present medication.
(9) Drug sensitivities.

Local factors

These may be listed as follows:

(1) Unusual organisms, such as erisypeloid in butchers.
(2) Peripheral vascular disease.
(3) Occupational problems, such as regular maceration of hand skin.
(4) Chronic lymphoedema.
(5) Previous local radiotherapy.
(6) Undetected foreign body.

The lists are obviously not comprehensive. But it only takes a short time to make such enquiries and, almost as importantly, to record them. Such knowledge may well influence both treatment and outcome significantly. The hand has been described as the 'mirror of systemic disease'. It is clearly impossible to list all the conditions that may affect the hand here. However, a number of diseases may be complicated secondarily by hand infection or even masquerade as infection in the hand. Notable examples are mentioned.

DRESSINGS

The keratinized nature of hand skin renders it particularly susceptible to maceration from exudation. Absorbent dressings need to be changed at least daily. Sneddon (1970) thought many patients were able to cope with their own dressings but most hand surgeons prefer to see the patients themselves regularly.

SPLINTAGE

The requirement for splintage as part of the treatment both for the early resolution of infection, injury and inflammation of the hand and for the relief of pain has been recognized for centuries. Koch (1946) jogged failing memories about this. Younger surgeons, reared in the post-antibiotic era, tend to forget its importance. We should not allow ourselves and our trainees to forget it and should use it properly and effectively. Lamb and Kuczynski (1981) have popularized the term 'position of safe splintage', which has much to commend it. For it eliminates confusion and misunderstanding inherent in the terms 'position of rest' and 'position of function' which, when translated into a position of splintage, can and does result in some truly bizarre postures, not in the best interests of recovery.

ELEVATION

To splintage must be added elevation. The more swelling and inflammation the more is this so, to the extent that rest and elevation of the hand in hospital form vital adjuvants to the definitive surgical and/or antibiotic treatment, particularly when home circumstances are unsatisfactory.

ANTIBIOTICS

The inappropriate use of antibiotics in hand infections is to be deprecated (Watson, 1985 a and b; 1986). They have been responsible for many infections resulting in wholly avoidable morbidity. Antibiotics are not required for many of the hand infections which may properly be treated on an outpatient basis.

ANAESTHESIA

There can be no place for local infiltration techniques when dealing with hand infections surgically. Such manoeuvres flaunt accepted practice since uninvolved tissues are likely to be exposed to, or actually inoculated with, those organisms responsible for the infection. Local blocks are appropriate for infections in the distal part of the digit. A metacarpal block is to be preferred to the more traditional ring block which has the unwanted effect of increasing tissue tension within the digit. This is likely to hamper venous return and impede lymphatic drainage, both important for the early resolution of infection. As a general rule any infection occurring at or proximal to the proximal interphalangeal (PIP) joint of a finger, or the interphalangeal (IP) joint of the thumb would best be dealt with by axillary or supraclavicular regional block or general anaesthesia. The presence of ascending lymphangitis or axillary lymphadenopathy render regional blocks potentially hazardous. Winding an exsanguinating bandage over involved skin is clearly not sensible so that its application should be well proximal, or its use abandoned, with simple elevation being used prior to the application of the tourniquet, when that is indicated.

ACUTE PARONYCHIA

Commoner in women and nail biters this condition is often poorly treated. The reason is one of widespread misunderstanding, or ignorance, both of the normal anatomy of the nail and of the pathology of infection around it.

Anatomy

The nail is formed from cells in the nail germinal matrix which is closely applied to the proximal metaphysis of the distal phalanx (*Figures 5.1 and 5.2*). It merges proximally into the insertion of the extensor tendon and distally into the pink fleshy nail bed. The distal crescentic portion of the germinal matrix is visible through the nail as the lunula. The surrounding skin is reflected to cover the margins of the nail, the cuticle. The nail has a tendency to split at its lateral margins, producing hangnails.

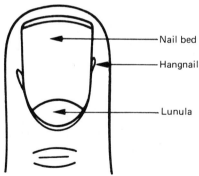

Figure 5.1 Anatomy of the nail (front view)

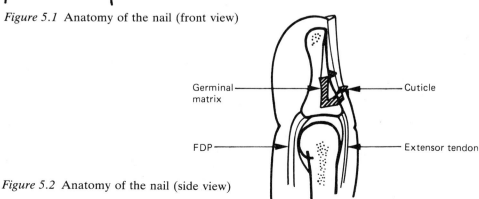

Figure 5.2 Anatomy of the nail (side view)

Pathology

The majority are due to *Staphylococcus aureus*, some to coliforms and a few to mixed organisms. Herpes simplex can sometimes be involved as can genital herpes. The portal for entry of the organisms is usually the base of the hangnail.

Stage 1

A bleb of pus forms at the margin of the hangnail (*Figure 5.3*). Traditionally incision has been practised. This is both unnecessary and inappropriate, for the pus is located between the margin of the nail and the overlying cuticle. Merely paring

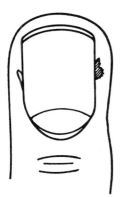

Figure 5.3 Acute paronychia, stage 1

back the cuticle will release it. Incising the skin exposes uninvolved tissues to infection. A dry dressing and a finger splint complete the treatment, as antibiotics are not required.

Stage 2

Now the pus has insinuated itself under the lateral margin of the nail so that simply paring back the cuticle will not provide adequate drainage (*Figure 5.4*). That part of the nail overlying the pus must therefore be removed, with great care. The

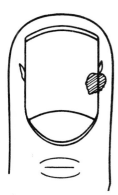

Figure 5.4 Acute paronychia, stage 2

removed portion should be distal to the lunula for the germinal matrix may be permanently damaged if a more proximal excision of the nail is attempted. Dressings and splintage complete the treatment.

Stage 3

This, the so called horseshoe paronychia (*Figure 5.5*), occurs when a more widespread proximal extension of the pus actually lifts the proximal part of the nail away from the germinal matrix, though the distal part of the nail may still be closely applied to the nail bed. Again, traditional treatment has frequently involved two

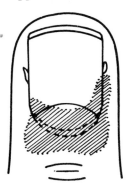

Figure 5.5 Acute paronychia, stage 3

linear incisions, allowing the proximal cuticle to be reflected. This would appear wholly unnecessary. It is a simple matter to 'flip out' the proximal part of the nail. (It has already been separated from the germinal matrix as the result of the infection.) The proximal part of the nail then lies on top of the proximal cuticle and may then be cut transversely at a point distal to the lunula, leaving the distal nail still on the nail bed. Obviously, in more advanced examples, the whole nail may need removal if all of it has been lifted up. Dead keratin should be excised. Similar aftercare is appropriate, though time to resolution will necessarily be longer than with earlier stages.

Herpetic whitlow

This is an infection of childhood. The physical signs consist of redness and swelling around the cuticle. There may be evidence of regional lymphadenitis and sometimes fever. Spontaneous resolution over a week or two is the rule. Surgical intervention is not normally appropriate. This condition seems to be regularly reported. Jarris and Kirkwood (1984) have provided a recent review and the place for the administration of acyclovir in recurrent cases has been discussed by Laskin (1985).

CHRONIC PARONYCHIA

Several digits, both of the hand and of the feet, may be affected by this condition which is fungal in origin. The characteristic red hypertrophic cuticles are associated with scaling and pitting of the nails. Pus is not formed and there is rarely a place for surgery in the management of this troublesome condition (Baran and Bureau, 1981). Its successful eradication requires often prolonged treatment with the appropriate antifungal agents.

OTHER FUNGAL CONDITIONS IN THE HAND

Tinea has a different presentation in the hand. Whereas the feet are involved with interdigital infection, the changes in the hand are those of pitting of the palmar skin and dry accentuation of the palmar creases. Interdigital infection can result from candida, the condition being called erosio blastomycetica interdigitalis. Onychia and paronychia, accompanied by increased pigmentation, may follow *Candida albicans* involvement. Brown (1975) has elaborated on this subject.

DRUG-INDUCED CHANGES IN THE NAILS

Dermatologists are familiar with scaly and specific pitting patterns of the nails which have followed the administration of certain drugs, particularly tetracyclines and benoxaprofen. The changes can be misinterpreted as those of fungal infection.

SKIN DISEASE PRODUCING CHANGES IN THE NAILS

The best-known examples would be psoriasis and eczema. Both conditions produce pitting and sometimes discoloration of the nails and again the differentiation from fungal infection may be difficult or even impossible. Lichen planus can cause particularly persistent ridging and atrophy of the nails, and those thus affected are more prone to acute infection.

CONDITIONS MIMICKING INFECTION AROUND THE NAIL

Subungual melanoma is to be remembered. The pain of the rare glomus tumour usually invites the diagnosis of an infection. Subungual exostoses distort the nail and may become secondarily infected, as may subungual fibromata. A mucous cyst produces swelling over the nail germinal matrix and a discrete trough of the nail. Ringworm, usually affecting one hand only, is another condition resulting in deformation of the nails.

PULP SPACE INFECTIONS

Apical pulp space infection

This obvious problem presents little difficulty in management. A collection of pus, nearly always of staphylococcal origin, forms in the apical pulp, most frequently under the extreme distal portion of the nail, the consequence of a foreign body entering the area. Adequate drainage is readily achieved by removing the overlying wedge of nail and any dead keratin overlying the pulp. Early resolution can be anticipated.

Distal, middle and proximal pulp space infections

Early infections

These are often not recognized early enough and there are reasons why that should be so. Again largely of staphylococcal origin, the sequence of events starts usually with the entry of a small foreign body into the pulp, most commonly the distal pulp, less commonly the middle or proximal pulp, for these are the 'working surfaces' of the digits. The majority of patients remember the event. Initially they think little of it. It may be sore but there is nothing much to see. Within 48 hours the affected pulp becomes increasingly painful and within another 48 hours is throbbing and may interfere with sleep. At that stage help is sought. The normal pulp is fluctuant. The physical signs of pulp space infection are those of extreme local tenderness and loss of fluctuance. Such signs should lead to incision over the painful point, using appropriate anaesthesia combined with a finger or arm tourniquet. In the most frequently involved distal pulp the incision should be oblique, to minimize inadvertent division of terminal branches of the digital nerves, a potent cause of troublesome neuromata. Only a small quantity of pus produces the symptoms, so rich is the local nerve supply. A dry dressing and finger splint are indicated.

Late infections

The sight of pus in a pulp should alert the examiner to a more extensive collection, possibly of a 'collar-stud' configuration (*Figure 5.6*) and in these circumstances an X-ray must be taken to determine whether or not there is evidence of bony involvement. Bolton, Fowler and Jepson (1949) have described the natural history of this involvement. Even if none is demonstrated the seriousness of this type of presentation requires more than a simple incision if treatment is to be effective and resolution rapid. The unique properties of pulp skin mean that only dead skin, and particularly dead keratin, may be removed. Bony involvement may necessitate curettage. Such infections should not be left to the uninitiated. Significant morbidity may follow. A more formal exploration under tourniquet is to be recommended and the prescription of adjuvant antistaphylococcal antibiotics will be appropriate until culture and sensitivities are obtained.

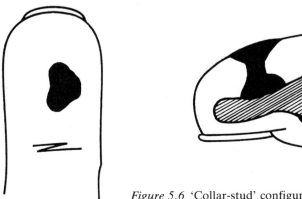

Figure 5.6 'Collar-stud' configuration. For details see text

BOILS OR CARBUNCLES

Almost always due to infection with *Staphylococcus aureus* these occur almost exclusively on dorsal, hair bearing skin and are thus commoner in males. Diabetes must be borne in mind and contaminated sites resulting from drug abuse must also be remembered. (The plight of the addict's hand has been the subject of several reports: McKay, Pascarelli and Eaton (1973), Whitaker and Graham (1973) and Lister (1977).) Incision and drainage should be straighforward, together with appropriate splintage. Antibiotics need only be exhibited when there is significant local reaction or constitutional disturbance.

CELLULITIS

The haemolytic streptococcus is still able to produce serious disability in the hand. The classical signs of spreading redness and ascending lymphangitis characterize the clinical picture. Pus is not formed, but the accumulation of oedema and exudates within confined spaces in the hand can cause great problems. Smith (1977) has reported digital gangrene in association with such an infection. The current tendency is to take these cases too casually. Benzylpenicillin remains the drug of choice but it should be administered in large doses by the intravenous route, while the hand is splinted in the 'position of safe splintage' and elevated. Hospitalization is therefore necessary, but usually only for 48 hours, after which penicillin may be administered orally, and by then gentle mobilization is likely to be appropriate. Other bacteria have been implicated including *Haemophilus influenzae* (Scott, German and Boswick, 1981). Failure of the usual rapid response to penicillin therapy should therefore alert suspicions.

TENDON SHEATH INFECTION

The haemolytic streptococcus is the commonest culprit, though others have been implicated. Hamlin and Sarris (1939) described seven cases due to gonococcal involvement. The propensity for streptococcal infection when occurring in this site to be followed by dense and disastrous adhesion formation make prompt diagnosis and effective treatment mandatory if such sequelae are to be avoided. Infection can follow the entry of a foreign body into the digit but this is by no means always the case. Physical signs consist of swelling of the affected digit, sometimes redness but more particularly marked local tenderness when the tendon sheath is palpated, together with extreme pain when any attempt is made to move any of the digital joints. Urgent exploration of the tendon apparatus, preferably by two incisions to allow thorough irrigation and possibly instillation of antibiotics, is to be recommended. Needless to say this must be undertaken using regional or general anaesthesia and an exsanguinating tourniquet. Parenteral penicillin should be prescribed. Splintage should be for a short period only since stiffness is the overriding problem. The early institution of supervized movement as well as forms of dynamic splintage seek to minimize this problem.

WEB SPACE INFECTION

Commonly following the entry of staphylococci into callosities or blisters on the volar aspect of the metacarpophalangeal (MCP) joint, the resultant pus and soft tissue reaction produces its main visible effect on the dorsum of the hand where the skin is thin and distensible. The affected digits become separated and the resultant picture is that of the so-called 'frog hand'. Local tenderness is, of course, maximal over the volar aspect of the web. Surgical drainage is mandatory. The tendon sheaths and neurovascular bundles that form the natural boundaries to the space are vulnerable at such procedures, particularly since the normal anatomy is likely to be both distorted and discolored as a result of the infection. Regional or general anaesthesia must therefore be used and the procedure carried out under a tourniquet. The web space may be approached by either a volar or a dorsal incision. This author prefers to use both, preserving a bridge of vital web skin between the two. Some form of local drainage may be left in the wound. Packing of long lengths of fine ribbon gauze into such cavities is not desirable, as not only does it tend to perpetuate the cavity but the pain resulting from removal of such tightly packed gauze within the hand is indescribable. I had such an infection treated in that way 25 years ago and can still remember the dread of having the gauze pulled out daily!

THENAR AND PALMAR SPACE INFECTIONS

Seemingly less common nowadays these infections are hence more likely to be incorrectly diagnosed or inadequately treated. The shaft of the middle finger metacarpal is the origin of the adductor pollicis muscle and this structure therefore divides the deep part, or space, of the palm into a radial (thenar) space and an ulnar (palmar) space. The serious nature of any infection becoming established within either of these spaces is self-evident due to their contents, flexor tendons and neurovascular bundles. Once diagnosed, immediate drainage under proper conditions must be undertaken. As this is likely to be due to staphylococci, appropriate antibiotic therapy should also be instituted.

SEPTIC ARTHRITIS

Though uncommon, the serious effects upon articular cartilage which result from its exposure to bacteria, particularly staphylococci, mean that effective treatment is a matter of considerable urgency if such effects are to be prevented. In practice the diagnosis is not infrequently arrived at late. The reason for this is that a relatively common mechanism by which such an infection comes about is that in which the dorsal skin overlying the metacarpophalangeal or proximal interphalangeal joint, stretched tight with the hand in a clenched fist position, is broken when a punch is thrown at the mouth. The organism may be varied and their true and serious nature missed. Punch actinomycosis has been described by both Burrows (1945) and Winner (1960). Rarer still is a more recent report by Schmidt and Heckman (1983) in which the offending organisms was *Eikenella corrodens*. Animal bites can also produce the complication of septic arthritis and *Pasteurella multocida* arthritis was mentioned by Mitchell, Travers and Barraclough (1982). The skin edges are both contused and contaminated and the true extent of the injury, whereby the dorsal aspect of one of those joints has also been broached and hence inoculated with bacteria, is not at first appreciated. Moreover the patient may either be drunk or obstreperous when seen in the accident department, and the wound overlooked, or present some time after the event, since the wound was small and not obviously serious. If such wounds are seen early and treated with respect, contaminated and devitalized skin excised, the wound irrigated, broad-spectrum antibiotics started, and the wound subsequently closed by delayed suture, such complications can be avoided. More often the presentation is one of overt infection of the joint – a wound exuding pus, and a stiff, swollen and extremely painful joint. Treatment must be along the same lines, but persistent stiffness and secondary osteoarthritis are more likely to be the result. Septic arthritis due to pseudomonas in heroin addicts was reported by Gifford *et al.* (1975).

GRANULOMATOUS LESIONS

Pyogenic granuloma

Though this may represent a frustrated local attempt to get rid of a foreign body, many patients will not recall its entry and indeed this is by no means always the cause. The clinical presentation is that of an exuberant localized sphere of granulation tissue, surrounding which there is little if any local reaction. Normally moist, it may become secondarily infected and thus covered with a thin layer of seropus. Treatment consists of curettage. Chemical or electrical cautery to its 'base' should stop troublesome oozing.

Orf

The macroscopic appearance differs significantly from that of a pyogenic granuloma. The lesion is flatter, looking rather like a shallow vesicle, itself filled with 'quiet' granulation tissue. A surrounding 'halo' of redness is usual. Once suspected, the history of contact with sheep should clinch the diagnosis since the virus responsible resides in their incisor teeth. The lesion is self-limiting and no specific treatment is required.

MALIGNANT MELANOMA

Amelanotic varieties, particularly if complicated by superficial sepsis, may masquerade as pyogenic granuloma. Though rare, it should be standard practice to send all granulomata for histological analysis. A recent communication from Kerl, Trau and Ackerman (1984) describes differentiating features between melanotic naevi and malignant melanomata occurring in the nail-beds and elsewhere.

TUBERCULOSIS

Involvement of the wrist and hand in this disease has been the subject of a number of publications (Robins, 1967; Smith and Leffert, 1975; Leung, 1978; Benkeddache and Gottesman, 1982a; Urovitz, 1982b; Bush and Schneider, 1984). The commonest way by which this condition presents in the hand is in the form of chronic flexor synovitis, otherwise called compound palmar ganglion. The swelling thus produced restricts digital movement and its proximal extension will lead to carpal tunnel compression (Lee, 1985). Synovectomy combined with antituberculous chemotherapy is required.

Tuberculous dactylitis

Tuberculous dactylitis is much commoner in children than in adults. The intraosseous presence of tuberculous granulation tissue leads to thinning and expansion of matacarpals or proximal phalanges, producing a characteristic radiological appearance. This consists of marked thinning of the cortex, a mottled or spongy appearance of the medullary canal, which is itself greatly expanded, and sometimes perforation of the cortex. The epiphyses are not involved. This has been described as 'spina ventosa'. Despite the alarming appearance treatment with antituberculous drugs and adjuvant splintage is usually followed by resolution and remodelling. Surgery should be restricted to dealing with abscesses, and with soft tissue or intra-articular extensions of the granulomatous process.

INFECTIONS WITH UNUSUAL ORGANISMS

Erysipeloid

Caused by the organism *Erysipelothrix rhusiopathiae*, the infection is commonest amongst butchers. A small cut on a digit is followed by the development of fairly well-circumscribed cellulitis, of a rather browner hue than that seen with streptococcal infection. Less virulent than the haemolytic streptococcus, ascending lymphangitis and lymphadenopathy is less common. Treatment with penicillin should be curative, but a course of at least ten days' duration is suggested to minimize the likelihood of incomplete eradication and thus recurrence.

Erysipelas

Group A streptococci cause this acute cutaneous infection, sometimes called St Anthony's fire. Commonly presenting with a characteristic butterfly distribution on the face, the infection may occur in the hand. The skin becomes hot and deep pink, the spreading margins are raised, and vesicles or bullae may accompany the cellulitic changes. Penicillin is indicated.

Meleney's synergistic gangrene

This infection, due to a combination of a microaerophilic non-haemolytic streptococcus and an aerobic haemolytic streptococcus, produces an appearance in some ways similar to erysipeloid. The distinguishing feature is that of a progressively enlarging dark or even black margin of necrosis requiring surgical removal. To a systemic penicillin should be added regular local treatment with hydrogen peroxide. Skin grafting may subsequently be necessary.

BITES

Actinomycosis

The hazards of human bites have been discussed under septic arthritis (pages 10 and 11). The problems have been recognized for a long time (Mason and Koch, 1930). To this must be added the rare but serious infection with *Actinomycosis israelii*. Growing saprophytically in the oropharynx, established infection is characterized microscopically by the development of sulphur granules. Penicillin is the antibiotic of first choice. A foreign body may also be responsible (Fayman, Schein and Braun, 1985).

Pasteurella multocida

Infection in the hand may follow the inoculation into the tissues with this organism, most often following a cat bite (Byrne, Boyd and Daley, 1958). Local osteomyelitis may prove troublesome and joint involvement has been mentioned earlier. Erythromycin is the first line drug. *Pasteurella septica* may also infect bites (Lee and Buhr, 1960).

Cat scratch fever

A small local pustule marks the entry point of the virus which causes this condition, a variety of the lymphogranuloma venereum family. Lymphadenopathy is almost invariably present.

Anthrax

The bacillus may enter the hand through a small cut or abrasion. The source is usually sheep or cattle. Initially a small pink lesion, it subsequently enlarges, fills with fluid and may rupture. New lesions occur around a pink macular periphery and the centre then forms a characteristic black eschar. This may be extensive. Pain is not a major feature. Surgical excision of the eschars may sometimes be required for large lesions, though small areas are self-limiting. Systemic penicillin remains the drug of first choice.

HERPES

Herpes simplex can occur in the hand. Herpetic whitlow of childhood is mentioned above (page 102). Infection around the nails may be recurrent. Dentists and dental hygienists may be so bothered (Watkinson, 1982), and endoscopists may be similarly at risk (Shoham, 1979). Small wounds can also be inoculated with the virus. Most often the condition is purely annoying and self-limiting.

ACUTE INFLAMMATORY CONDITIONS

Several of these may present as infections.

Acute calcific tendinitis

Well known to affect the supraspinatus tendon this condition occurs rarely in the hand. The two commonest sites would appear to be the insertion of the finger carpi ulnaris tendon and the insertion of the flexor digitorum profundus tendon. Extreme local pain is the presenting symptom. An X-ray provides the diagnosis (Selby, 1984). (Calcification may occur in the pulps of the fingers in scleroderma; almost always this is associated with other features of the condition and with changes of pulp atrophy.) Splintage and powerful analgesics should control the symptoms which normally subside after four or five days. Occasionally surgical removal of the calcific material becomes necessary.

Gout

Acute gout can present in the hand and may prove difficult to differentiate from septic arthritis, particularly if there is no history and it is non-tophaceous. Soft tissue involvement has been described by both Primm and Allen (1983) and Moore and Weiland (1985).

OTHER INFLAMMATORY ARTHRITIDES

The hand is an uncommon site for acute monoarticular arthritis. Much commoner are the polyarthritic features of rheumatoid arthritis.

Blackthorn synovitis

This is a particularly troublesome condition. The thorn enters the flexor apparatus and excites a most vigorous response in the synovium. The exact mechanism is unknown. Although not particularly painful, swelling and restriction of movement lead the patient to seek attention. Synovectomy should be undertaken but the results can be singularly disappointing. A most vigorous programme of exercises must be instituted as soon as possible and it is probably wise to prescribe an anti-inflammatory drug for at least a month postoperatively.

Venereal infection

The emergence of genital herpes has been mentioned already. The primary chancre of syphilis presents extremely rarely in the hand. An unusual mechanism of infection was reported by Sieff (1946). Sporadic reports of gonococcal hand infection have appeared and one is discussed above in the context of tendon sheath infection (page 105).

Leprosy

It seems right that this awful condition, probably affecting as many as 15 million people worldwide, should be included here. Of course, western hand surgeons see little of this, but the late effects of the condition, which may be lessened by good primary treatment, merit both their attention and interest. Following the success of poliomyelitis vaccination the lepromatous patients represent the largest numerical group for whom tendon transfers may be helpful. Discussion would be inappropriate here.

Secondary infection

This heading serves to act as a final reminder that sepsis in the hand may be consequent upon some underlying pathology. One or two examples have already been given, and to these should be added the presence of foreign bodies. Dorsal hand skin may necrose following over-enthusiastic irradiation. Arsenical keratosis is an example of a specific local chemical effect in the hand, and the condition is almost certainly pre-malignant. Squamous cell carcinomata may ulcerate the skin and mimic granulomatous lesions. This is also described as Bowen's disease. Previously burnt, grafted or ischaemic skin is more vulnerable to injury and less well able to 'cope' with infection.

Postoperative wound infection

The disastrous consequences that follow serious wound infection must be guarded against. Though such infections are thankfully relatively uncommon in the hand this must not result in a relaxed approach to hand surgery, particularly when implants are to be inserted, or where there is to be extensile exposure, as in the surgery of the flexor tendon apparatus. Meticulous skin preparation, draping and surgery are to be encouraged. The prevention of haematomata, the careful application of postoperative dressings and the use of splintage must remain the responsibility of the operating surgeon if morbidity is to be kept at a minimal level. Opinions differ on the place for prophylactic antibiotics in 'elective' hand surgery. Most surgeons would appear to reserve their use for those cases in which foreign materials are implanted, or where prolonged extensile exposure is anticipated.

CONCLUSION

This chapter started with the widely accepted notion that the result of a hand infection will be proportional to the quality of the primary treatment. Common things commonly occur. The 'common' hand infections are common enough and their treatment should be uncomplicated if it is not delayed. It is up to hand surgeons themselves to educate the profession as a whole to ensure that such delays do not happen and that any problems, or 'uncommon' infections, are referred promptly for their attention. Moreover, they should seek to be involved in the primary management of these conditions; too often they are involved at the secondary referral stage only, by which time established complications of infection may be either difficult or sometimes impossible to treat successfully. The price of failure is likely to be significant and protracted disability.

References

BAILEY, D. (1963) *The Infected Hand*. London: H. K. Lewis

BARAN, R. and BUREAU, H. (1981) Surgical treatment of recalcitrant chronic paronychias of the hand. *Journal of Dermatology and Surgical Oncology*, **7**, 106–107

BENKEDDACHE, Y. and GOTTESMAN, H. (1982) Skeletal tuberculosis of the wrist and hand: a study of 27 cases. *Journal of Hand Surgery*, **7**, 593–600

BINGHAM, D. L. G. (1960) Acute infections of the hand. *Surgical Clinics of North America*, **40**, 1285

BOLTON, H., FOWLER, P. J. and JEPSON, R. P. (1949) Natural history and treatment of pulp space infection and osteomyelitis of the terminal phalanx. *Journal of Bone and Joint Surgery*, **31B**, 499

BROWN, H. (1975) Fungus infections of the hand. In *Hand Surgery*, edited by J. E. Flynn, pp. 526–530. Baltimore: Williams and Wilkins

BURROWS, J. H. (1945) Actinomycosis from punch injuries. *British Journal of Surgery*, **32**, 506–507

BUSH, D. C. and SCHNEIDER, L. H. (1984) Tuberculosis of the hand and wrist. *Journal of Hand Surgery*, **9**, 391–398

BYRNE, J. J., BOYD, T. F. and DALEY, A. K. (1958) Pasteurella infection from cats. *Surgery, Gynecology and Obstetrics*, **103**, 57

CARTER, P. R. (1983) *Common Hand Injuries and Infections*. Philadelphia: W. B. Saunders

ENTIN, M. A. (1964) Infections of the hand. *Surgical Clinics of North America*, **44**, 981

FAYMAN, M., SCHEIN, M. and BRAUN, S. (1985) A foreign body related actinomycosis of a finger. *Journal of Hand Surgery*, **10**, 411–412

GIFFORD, D. B., PATZAKIS, M., IVLER, D. and SWEZEY, R. L. (1975) Septic arthritis due to pseudomonas in heroin addicts. *Journal of Bone and Joint Surgery*, **57A**, 631–635

HAMLIN, E. and SARRIS, S. P. (1939) Acute gonococcal tenosynovitis: report of seven cases. *New England Journal of Medicine*, **221**, 228

JARRIS, R. F. and KIRKWOOD, C. R. (1984) Herpetic whitlow in family practice. *Journal of Family Practice*, **19**, 797–801

KANAVEL, A. B. (1905) Study of acute phlegmons of the hand. *Surgery, Gynecology and Obstetrics*, **82**, 749

KANAVEL, A. B. (1933) *Infections of the Hand*. Philadelphia: Lea and Febiger

KERL, H., TRAU, H. and ACKERMAN, A. B. (1984) Differentiation of melanotic naevi from malignant melanomas in palms, soles, and nail beds solely by signs in the cornified layer of the epidermis. *American Journal of Dermatopathology*, **6**, 159–160

KOCH, S. L. (1946) Inflamed and injured tissues need rest. *Surgery, Gynaecology and Obstetrics*, **82**, 749

LAMB, D. W. and KUCZYNSKI, K. (1981) *The Practice of Hand Surgery*. Oxford: Blackwells

LASKIN, O. L. (1985) Acyclovir and suppression of frequently occurring herpetic whitlow. *Annals of Internal Medicine*, **102**, 494–495

LEE, K. E. (1985) Tuberculosis presenting as carpal tunnel syndrome. *Journal of Hand Surgery*, **10**, 242–245

LEE, M. L. and BUHR, A. J. (1960) Dog bites and local infection with *Pasteurella septica*. *British Medical Journal*, **1**, 169

LEUNG, P. C. (1978) Tuberculosis of the hand. *The Hand*, **10**, 285–291

LINSCHEID, R. L. and DOBYNS, J. H. (1975) Common and uncommon infections of the hand. *Orthopaedic Clinics of North America*, **6**, 1063–1104

LISTER, G. (1977) Inflammation. In *The Hand: Diagnosis and Indications*. Edinburgh: Churchill Livingstone

LOWDEN, T. G. (1964) Prevention and treatment of hand infections. *Postgraduate Medical Journal*, **40**, 247–252

McCONNELL, C. M. and NEALE, H. W. (1979) Two-year review of hand infections at a municipal hospital. *American Journal of Surgery*, **45**, 643–646

McKAY, D., PASCARELLI, E. F. and EATON, R. G. (1973) Infections and sloughs in the hands in drug addicts. *The Journal of Bone and Joint Surgery*, **54A**, 629–633

MASON, M. L. and KOCH, S. L. (1930) Human bite infections of the hand. *Surgery, Gynecology and Obstetrics*, **51**, 591–625

MITCHELL, H., TRAVERS, R. and BARRACLOUGH, D. (1982) Septic arthritis caused by *Pasteurella multocida*. *Medical Journal of Australia*, **1**, 137

MOORE, J. R. and WEILAND, A. J. (1985) Gouty tenosynovitis in the hand. *Journal of Hand Surgery*, **10**, 291–295

PILCHER, R. S., DAWSON, R. L. G., MILSTEIN, B. B. and RIDDLE, A. G. (1949) Infection of the fingers and hand. *Lancet*, **1**, 777–783

PRIMM, D. D. and ALLEN, J. R. (1983) Gouty involvement of a flexor tendon in the hand. *Journal of Hand Surgery*, **8**, 863–865

RHODE, C. M. (1961) Treatment of hand infections. *American Journal of Surgery*, **27**, 85

ROBINS, R. H. C. (1952) Infections of the hand. A review based on 1000 consecutive cases. *Journal of Bone and Joint Surgery*, **34B**, 567

ROBINS, R. H. C. (1967) Tuberculosis of the wrist and hand. *British Journal of Surgery*, **54**, 211–218

SCHMIDT, D. R. and HECKMAN, J. D. (1983) *Eikenella corrodens* in human bite infections of the hand. *Journal of Trauma*, **23**, 478–482

SCOTT, F. A., GERMAN, C. and BOSWICK, J. A. (1981) *Haemophilus influenzae* cellulitis of the hand. *Journal of Hand Surgery*, **6**, 506–509

SELBY, C. L. (1984) Acute calcific tendonitis of the hand: an infrequently recognised and frequently misdiagnosed form of periarthritis. *Arthritis and Rheumatism*, **27**, 337–340

SCOTT, J. C. and JONES, B. V. (1952) Results of treatment of infections of the hand. *Journal of Bone and Joint Surgery*, **34B**, 581–587

SHOHAM, M. A. (1979) Herpetic infection of the finger: a risk to the endoscopist. *Gastrointestinal Endoscopy*, **25**, 26–27

SIEFF, B. (1946) Primary syphilis of the hand resulting from trauma sustained on striking an infected subject: a report of four cases. *South African Medical Journal*, **20**, 114

SMITH, R. B. (1977) Streptococcal infection with digital gangrene. *The Hand*, **9**, 279–282

SMITH, R. J. and LEFFERT, R. D. (1975) Tuberculosis of the hand. In *Hand Surgery*, edited by J. E. Flynn, pp. 516–526. Baltimore: Williams and Wilkins

SNEDDON, J. (1969) Dressings in hand sepsis. *British Medical Journal*, **1**, 372–373

SNEDDON, J. (1970) *The Care of Hand Infections*. London: Edward Arnold

UROVITZ, E. P. (1982) Tuberculous dactylitis: a rare entity. *Canadian Journal of Surgery*, **25**, 689–690

WATKINSON, A. C. (1982) Primary herpes simplex in a dentist. *British Journal of Dentistry*, **153**, 190–191

WATSON, N. A. (1985a) Antibiotics in hand infections. *British Medical Journal*, **590**, 492

WATSON, N. A. (1985b) *Practical Management of Musculoskeletal Emergencies*. Oxford: Blackwells

WATSON, N. A. (1986) *Pocket Picture Clinical Guide to Hand Injuries and Infections*. London: Gower

WHITAKER, L. A. and GRAHAM, W. P. (1973) Management of hand infections in the narcotic addict. *Plastic and Reconstructive Surgery*, **52**, 384–389

WINNER, H. I. (1960) Punch actinomycosis. *Lancet*, **2**, 907

6
Skin cover in the hand
David M. Evans

INTRODUCTION

Injury to the skin of the hand threatens function in a number of ways. Tight scars and inelastic skin restrict movement, loss of skin in important tactile areas inhibits function in those areas, and inadequate skin cover compromises the repair process in underlying structures. Delay in healing opens the way for infection and allows the development of granulation tissue which matures into dense scar tissue when healing finally takes place.

The correct approach to the problem of skin loss in the hand demands an understanding of the nature, mechanism, and likely progress of the injury to the skin, and this may not always be self-evident.

Skin loss may be real or apparent; when a laceration is associated with a crushing mechanism the swelling produced may make it impossible or inadvisable to close the skin directly. This apparent skin loss is in fact a temporary requirement for additional skin surface area.

Skin loss may be immediate or delayed. Many untidy lacerations have areas of skin of doubtful viability so that the decision to provide skin replacement has to be deferred until the outcome is clear. Such areas of skin with tenuous blood supply should be handled with care and not subjected to any tension or pressure. If a critical area of skin is involved and the injury involves damage to the vascular supply of the skin a vascular repair may be indicated.

Skin loss may involve full-thickness or partial-thickness injury. This applies mainly to burns and to injuries involving friction.

Finally, decisions concerning treatment must take into account the particular function of the area of the skin damaged. Some areas may be regarded as critical from this point of view, including the tactile digital pulps, the skin of the first web space, palmar skin at joint creases, and thin skin overlying extensor tendons and joints.

CLOSURE OF SKIN DEFECTS

In most situations primary closure of wounds gives the best prospect for early healing. In untidy injuries involving extensive tissue damage or contamination it

114

may be wise to pursue the well-tried policy of delayed primary closure. This requires that all measures are taken short of wound closure, including excision of dead tissue and removal of all foreign material, stabilization of fractures and repair of divided structures where conditions are suitable. The wound is dressed, splinted and elevated for 2–5 days, after which it is inspected and closed by the appropriate method. Provided closure is achieved within this time granulation tissue does not form and healing proceeds in exactly the same way as after primary closure. This policy can also be applied to injuries in which skin viability is in doubt, in which case a second look after 3–5 days allows further wound excision if necessary and delayed primary skin closure. There is probably no place for a deliberate policy of secondary closure of full-thickness skin defects in the hand, although this may be necessary where a previous attempt at primary closure has failed.

The surgeon has at his disposal a wide spectrum of techniques of wound closure. In general the simplest and most reliable method appropriate to a particular defect is used and the indications for more complex or time-consuming methods should be very clear.

Leaving wounds open

There are occasions when a deliberate policy of allowing a wound to close spontaneously can give a satisfactory result. Small areas of skin loss on the fingertips of infants can be treated in this way (Das and Brown, 1978), but if this policy is applied to larger defects or to older patients the distortion of surrounding tissues, particularly those supporting the nail, will result in an unacceptable deformity. Occasionally skin crease wounds or incisions in the palm can be left open, and provided they are precisely within the skin crease healing to a fine scar will occur.

Direct closure

This is only appropriate when there is no significant skin loss. When the wound cannot be closed primarily due to swelling, elevation may allow delayed primary closure once the swelling has settled. It is always unwise to close wounds under tension. In some areas of the hand it may appear that there is redundant skin which can be mobilized to close the wound. For example, with the fingers fully extended the skin on the dorsum of the hand is lax. If this is placed under tension, however, there is no spare skin to allow flexion of the metacarpophalangeal (MP) joints and except in the very old there is rarely any spare skin in this area.

Free skin grafts

In the majority of situations where additional skin is required to close a wound on the hand, a free skin graft will be the method of choice. Skin grafts can take on any surface with sufficient vascularity to sprout capillary loops and vascularize the graft, and therefore all but the smallest areas of exposed bone, tendon or cartilage require skin cover with its own vascularity. Split skin grafts are the safest and simplest to use in post-traumatic skin defects and can be applied to defects of any size. Small grafts may be taken from the ulnar border of the hand (Patton, 1969) and have the advantage of similarity to the skin that has been lost in thickness and texture, particularly when dealing with skin loss on the volar aspect of the hand. Great care should be taken in cutting a skin graft from this site; provided it is only partial thickness no scarring will result. It is wise to use a proper skin graft knife rather than a free blade. Because of the thick keratin layer it is possible to cut a graft so thin that it has no dermis in it, in which case the graft will have a tendency to contract and there will be more scarring. An alternative source of skin for palmar cover is the non-weightbearing instep area of the foot (Nakamura, Nambak and Tsuchida, 1984). Donor site morbidity is said to be slight, but some scarring may be encountered.

Larger skin grafts can be taken from further up the arm or from the thigh or buttock. The arm has the advantage of convenience but it is not acceptable to inflict an unsightly skin-graft donor site on the forearm of a patient who might be distressed by it in order to avoid the minor inconvenience of preparing an alternative donor site. In elderly patients there may be something to be said for taking skin from the inner or outer aspects of the upper arm to avoid immobilization and bandaging of the leg, particularly in patients who may have increased susceptibility to deep venous thrombosis. For large areas of skin graft the thigh is the ideal donor site. In many situations meshing the skin graft allows it to adapt to the contours of the recipient site and permits escape of fluid which might otherwise collect beneath the graft. Usually a mesh-graft would be left unexpanded but if a large area is being covered elsewhere on the body there may be a shortage of skin, and expanded mesh grafts give a satisfactory result under these circumstances. This would generally only apply to the grafting of burns. In pigmented skin the mesh holes may produce hypertrophic scarring to a far greater extent than would occur otherwise. Small skin grafts are best kept in place with a tie-over pack but this may not be appropriate for larger or inconveniently shaped areas, in which case a well-applied dressing and splint can immobilize the graft satisfactorily. When resurfacing a large complex surface like the whole dorsum of the hand and fingers the three-dimensional aspect has to be considered. Hurwitz and White (1978) have found glovemaking patterns useful to place the connecting scars between grafts in the optimal position.

Degloving injuries pose a special problem in that the skin viability is uncertain. If there is dermal bleeding at the free edge of an open degloving injury it is reasonable to lay the skin back without suturing it (London and Clarke, 1959; Elliott, Hoehn and Stayman, 1979). Intravenous fluorescein gives a good indication of skin perfusion when the damaged area is viewed by ultraviolet light (McGrouther and Sully, 1980). Areas considered unlikely to survive can be used as a source of primary skin graft (*Figure 6.1*), either full-thickness if the area involved is small and the bed clean and healthy, or by shaving large areas of split skin from the flap. It helps to stretch the skin over large gauze swabs while cutting the graft (Goris and Nicolai, 1982). It is unwise to use degloved skin as a free graft it it is crushed or damaged (Sanguinetti, 1977). Flap cover may be required if important structures are exposed (*see below*, and Stranc, 1973). Finally, in the management of degloving injuries the possibility of compartment compression within an intact fascial envelope must be borne in mind.

Full-thickness skin grafts have a place in skin cover on the hand and are more widely used in elective skin replacement than in the post-traumatic situation. The advantage of a full-thickness skin graft is conferred by the preservation of dermis across the grafted area. This allows the skin to retain its normal texture and elasticity and also results in far less scar tissue and less tendency to contract. Wolfe

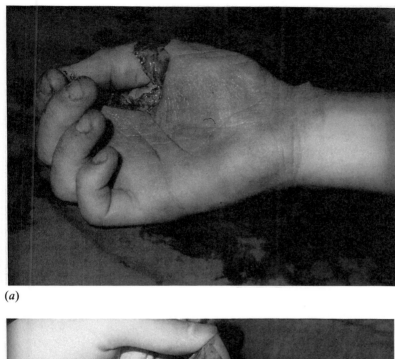

(a)

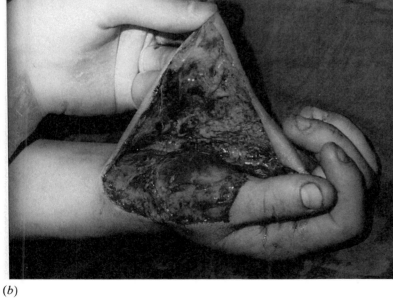

(b)

Figure 6.1 (a) Degloving injury of the palm; (b) with undermining to the ulnar border of the hand

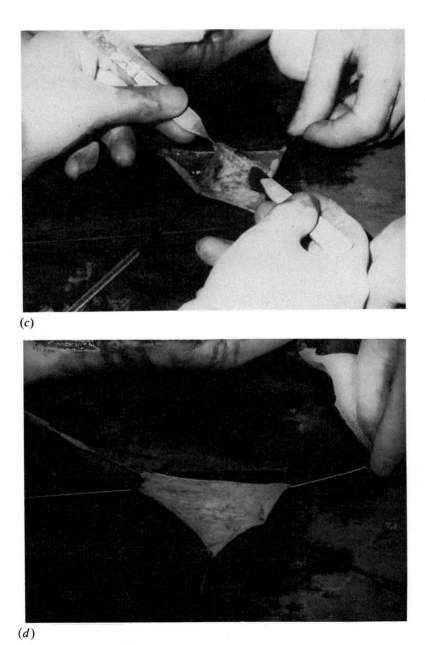

(c)

(d)

Figure 6.1 (c) and (d) It was clear that the skin of the thenar eminence was not perfused, and this was therefore excised and defatted by sharp dissection, taking care to leave no fat attached to the dermis. Note that the graft is stretched out on a flat board to stabilize it

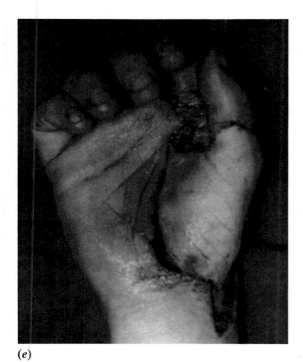

(e)

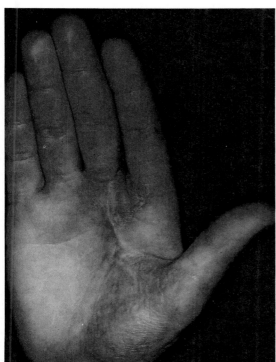

(f)

Figure 6.1 (*e*) When replacing such a graft it should not be sutured to the free edge of the undermined skin but to the underlying bed, so that fluid from under the flap drains over, not under, the graft. Remaining areas are grafted, and undermined skin must not be sutured under tension. (*f*) A successful palmar Wolfe graft retains the best qualities of palmar skin

grafts therefore have their place, particularly on the palm of the hand and in the web spaces. When full-thickness grafts are used to resurface palmar defects in small children excellent sensory recovery can be expected with tactile gnosis of a quality approaching that of normal palmar skin. Skin loss on the fingertips with preservation of underlying pulp tissue is also a good situation for full-thickness skin grafts, and in this situation the ideal skin would have the same characteristics as the skin that is missing. Small full-thickness grafts can be taken from the ulnar side of the hand (Schenck and Cheema, 1984) and it may occasionally be justified in a critical tactile area to use a graft from the pulp of a toe. Most full-thickness grafts however are taken from the groin crease where it is important to avoid hair-bearing skin. An area up to 5 cm wide can be taken and still allow direct closure in the groin. Under particular circumstances post-auricular skin is also useful. There are few areas on the upper limb where full-thickness skin is freely available.

The take of Wolfe grafts is more vulnerable than that of split skin grafts where adverse factors exist. It is vitally important to achieve full haemostasis and to provide adequate immobilization of the graft to its bed. At the first dressing Wolfe grafts always appear blistered and discoloured and it is not uncommon for a small portion of the graft to fail to take. If this happens in a critical area it is advisable to excise the non-viable part of the graft as soon as the outcome can be confidently predicted, and replace it with another graft of appropriate thickness.

When raising Wolfe grafts it is customary to remove the fat layer from the graft as cleanly as possible. This removes much of the subdermal vascular plexus, and Tsukada (1980) has pointed out that the deliberate preservation of the plexus, inevitably with a film of fat also, improves the texture and elasticity of the graft, without compromising the pick-up of circulation. Grafts revascularize by a dual process of ingrowth of capillaries and direct anastomosis between open vessels of graft and bed. The latter may be enhanced by the preservation of the subdermal plexus.

With all free skin grafts the placing of marginal scars is an important factor to take into consideration. Any longitudinal scar in the palmar aspect of the hand or fingers will give rise to a contracture. This can be avoided by adjusting the defect to take the margin of the skin graft on to the side or dorsal aspect of the finger, and it is even justifiable on occasions to sacrifice a small amount of skin in order to achieve this. When grafting children's hands it is wise to move towards the thicker type of skin graft or Wolfe graft whenever possible as this will allow for better growth than a split skin graft.

Skin flaps

A skin flap is required when the underlying bed is not suitable for a free graft, or when the contraction that inevitably takes place in a graft could lead to limitation of movement. On occasions a flap may be chosen when it is known that subsequent surgery will be required for underlying structures. The choice of flap technique depends on the size and site of the defect.

Local flaps

Small defects can usually be repaired by movement of local skin as a transposition or rotation flap. This has the advantage of using skin of like quality and of confining the scarring to the injured area. In designing and raising local flaps it is important to consider the effect of the procedure on the area from which the skin is taken. Usually this has to be closed by a split skin graft, but occasionally direct closure is possible. Local flaps may be useful on the dorsum of the hand, in the web spaces and particularly for small defects on the dorsum of the proximal interphalangeal (PIP) joint.

Local flaps are easily raised on the dorsum of the hand because of the layer of loose areolar tissue beneath the skin. There is actually less skin available for movement as a flap than there would appear to be since some laxity of the skin is necessary to be taken up when the hand is clenched into a fist. Rotation flaps are designed on a scale several times larger than the area to be covered, the basis of the design being that a large flap will only need a small expansion proportionate to its size to fill the defect whereas a small flap might have to expand by 50 per cent or more of its size for the same area. Rotation flap donor areas can usually be closed directly. Large local flaps need a skin graft on the donor area, but careful design of small ones may allow direct closure with the tension placed at 90° to the line of tension created by moving the flap into the primary defect. There are various designs for such flaps, but the principle of the rhomboid flap, well described by Lister and Gibson (1972), is frequently applicable.

Small transposition flaps are useful on the dorsal aspects of the fingers, especially for small defects exposing the extensor mechanism or joint (Gibraiel, 1977; Green and Dominguez, 1979; Smith, 1982a; Thompson, 1977). The flag flap (Iselin, 1973; Lister, 1981) is more mobile because the pedicle is narrowed down to a few millimetres (*Figure 6.2*). Iselin maintains that the arterial supply is through the dermal vascular network, derived from the volar digital arteries, and not through larger arteries from the dorsal metacarpal system. He emphasizes the need to preserve longitudinal dorsal veins in the pedicle to ensure survival of the flap. Because of its mobility the flap can reach adjacent dorsal, lateral and volar areas easily, on the same or neighbouring digit, but has to be raised with care to avoid damage to its vascular supply, and no tension can be applied.

The Moberg advancement flap (Moberg, 1964; Posner and Smith, 1971) is useful in the management of thumb pulp loss when proximal volar skin is undamaged

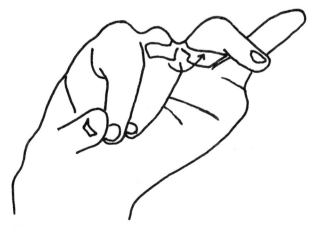

Figure 6.2 An example of the Iselin 'flag flap', taken from the dorsum of the middle finger to fill a volar defect on the ring finger. The narrow pedicle makes this a freely mobile flap

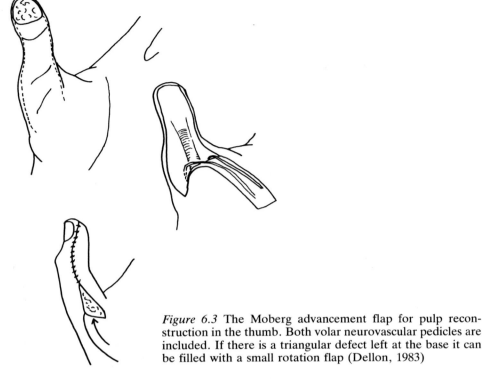

Figure 6.3 The Moberg advancement flap for pulp reconstruction in the thumb. Both volar neurovascular pedicles are
included. If there is a triangular defect left at the base it can
be filled with a small rotation flap (Dellon, 1983)

(*Figure 6.3*). It is an axial flap containing both digital vessels and nerves.
Advancement of the flap may leave two triangular gaps which can be filled by two
local transposition flaps (Dellon, 1983). Because innervated skin is advanced
excellent sensation is preserved on the thumb tip. Macht and Watson (1980)
showed that this can be safely employed in the fingers also, provided that the flap is
dissected by teasing the neurovascular bundles away from the finger without
dividing dorsal branches, otherwise fingertip necrosis is possible. For this reason
many have avoided using this flap for fingertip reconstruction. Ognuro (1983)
described a local flap from the dorsum of the thumb to repair small tip losses.

An alternative innervated local flap for thumb cover is the transposition flap
from the radial side of the index finger, incorporating branches of the radial nerve
and artery (Rae and Pho, 1983; Stern, Kreilein and Kleinert, 1983). A lengthened
version of this flap has been used for thumb reconstruction (Rybka and Pratt, 1979)
and it also provides an excellent first web reconstruction (*Figure 6.4*). When
releasing the first web-space all tight structures have to be released at the same time
as the additional skin is provided. The adductor origin is separated from the third
metacarpal shaft through a thenar crease extension of the web-releasing incision,
and the first dorsal interosseous attachment to first metacarpal may also need
division. The skin flap is raised from the dorsal aspect of the second metacarpal
area, exposing the first dorsal interosseous, but dissection of the flap stops as soon
as the line of the first web space is reached. The tip of the flap comes from the
dorsum of the index finger up to proximal interphalangeal joint level. As the first
web space opens up the flap moves radially with the thumb, and flops over to

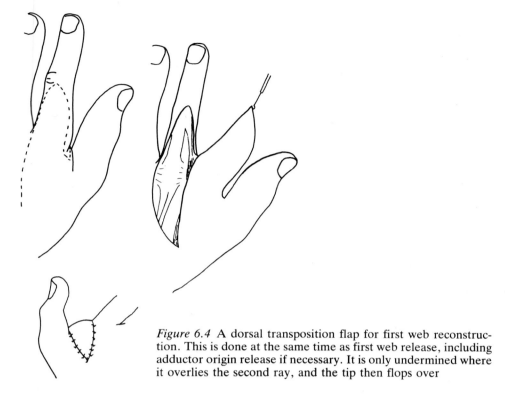

Figure 6.4 A dorsal transposition flap for first web reconstruction. This is done at the same time as first web release, including adductor origin release if necessary. It is only undermined where it overlies the second ray, and the tip then flops over

loosely fill the open web. The secondary defect is grafted. It is wise to hold the web space apart with an intermetacarpal K-wire for two weeks.

Shortage of skin in the web-spaces of the fingers usually results from burns, and the skin is often tight in all directions. A number of local flaps have been used in this area (Lister and Gibson, 1972; Shaw *et al.*, 1973). If there is generalized skin shortage a free graft is needed in the secondary defect.

Island flaps

When the pedicle of a skin flap can be reduced to little more than the principal blood vessels supplying it, the mobility and adaptability of the flap is greatly increased. Where a tactile area is being resurfaced sensory nerve supply has to be included in the pedicle. Island flaps may be used in any situation requiring full-thickness skin cover, where the local anatomical arrangements allow the isolation of an area of skin on a vascular pedicle without detriment to the remaining tissues which are deprived of vascular input from the artery that has been used.

Fingertip injuries

Small V-Y island flaps are well established as a means of closure of certain types of fingertip loss. The volar V-Y flap (Atasoy *et al.*, 1970) is suitable for terminal pulp losses in which the length of remaining volar skin is greater than the length dorsally

– that is, the line of amputation faces in a dorsal direction. This method of reconstruction is only appropriate when sufficient length of nail matrix and underlying phalangeal support will remain to allow adequate nail growth. Dissecting these small island flaps is a difficult procedure because it is necessary to divide all fibrous tissue connections between the flap and surrounding skin while preserving small terminal branches of the digital vessels and nerves. It is important to make the flap long enough to include a number of these branches on either side and dissection has to proceed until the flap will advance easily over the fingertip to meet the nail bed without tension. As well as the lateral dissection the flap is undermined at the skeletal plane to provide adequate mobility. If the flap is tethered it will pull back to its original position during healing and distort the shape of the nailbed, leaving a hook nail. If the distal edge of the flap is concave the two distal corners can be sutured to each other, causing the flap to assume a cup shape (Furlow, 1984). Lateral island flaps can be used as described by Kutler (1947), and have to be mobilized in a similar fashion. They are inevitably smaller and leave a finger-tip criss-crossed by scar tissue. Weston and Wallace (1976) have reported satisfactory results in a series of V-Y island flaps of the volar, oblique and double lateral design.

An alternative approach which provides innervated skin cover on a more mobile pedicle is the triangular island flap from one side of the fingertip based on one neurovascular pedicle, and dissected completely free apart from the pedicle (Pho, 1979; Venkataswami and Subramanian, 1980). This can be applied to more awkwardly shaped defects than the V-Y island flap will cover. If the flap is designed with zigzag edges which interdigitate as the flap advances distally the position of the skin is well maintained postoperatively and a straight volar scar is avoided (*Figure 6.5*). Joshi (1974a) described an island flap taken from the dorsolateral aspect of the finger or thumb, based on the digital neurovascular bundle through its dorsal branches. The bundle has to be dissected to the base of the finger, and the flap donor site covered with a skin graft.

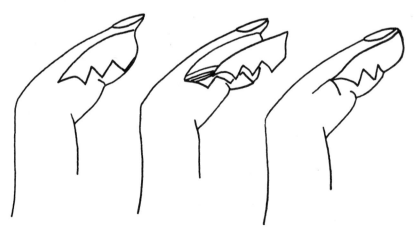

Figure 6.5 A modified design for an island flap to reconstruct distal digital pulp; the step cuts interdigitate and help to hold the new position, and avoid a straight volar scar

Neurovascular island flaps taken to other areas of the hand

Before raising a neurovascular island flap for transfer to another area it is essential to check that the remaining digital artery has not been damaged by previous trauma. The commonest use for this flap (Littler, 1956) is for thumb pulp replacement or to provide a sensate island of skin on a thumb that has been reconstructed from flap skin without innervation. The free innervated toe pulp transfer has supplanted this technique to some extent. The flap can also be used for other areas in the hand, for example the weight-bearing ulnar margin of the hand can be reinnervated using an island flap from the middle finger in a patient with complete anaesthesia in the ulnar territory. For the thumb the usual donor finger is the ring finger, most popularly from the ulnar side, although there are advantages in taking a flap from the radial side of the finger. As one moves towards the ulnar side of the hand the ulnar pulp becomes more important than the radial pulp because this is the skin which is in contact with a horizontal surface while using the hand in the usual writing position. It is unusual for the radial pulp of the ring finger to be used for thumb to fingertip pinch. It is also possible that by taking the flap from the median nerve distribution its mobility when moving to the radial side of the hand would be a little greater than a flap tethered by its digital nerve to other branches of the ulnar nerve. When dissecting the flap it is most important to take the dissection down to the origin of the digital artery from the superficial palmar arch and to dissect the digital nerve free from the branch to the neighbouring finger down to the same level. In this way kinking and tension at the point where the pedicle turns can be avoided. When the flap is tunnelled through to the thumb the tunnel must be wide enough to accommodate the flap and the pedicle without difficulty. It is advisable to leave a trailing suture on the flap so that the island of skin can be brought back to the palm with ease if this proves to be necessary because of inadequate dissection. If this precaution is not taken it is difficult to retrieve the flap without danger to the pedicle. This is a precaution that one should take with any island flap that is tunnelled to another position. When a narrow flap has been used it may be possible to close the defect on the donor finger directly, otherwise a skin graft is required, preferably full thickness.

Henderson and Reid (1980) reported a long-term review of 20 neurovascular island flaps, and found adequate sensation for tactile gnosis in 19. Only five had achieved any reorientation of sensation, a point in favour of a reconstructive technique involving nerve suture to a digital nerve in the recipient area. This either involves division of the nerve to the island flap and resuture to the digital nerve of the thumb, or the use of a neurovascular free flap from a toe (*see below*).

Distally based radial forearm island flap

This flap, otherwise known as the Chinese flap, has enjoyed popularity both as an island flap within the hand and as a free flap for more distant reconstruction (Fatah and Davies, 1984; Foucher *et al.*, 1984a; Muhlbauer, Herndl and Stock, 1982). The principle on which it is based is readily appreciated when the radial artery is divided in the forearm and the force of flow from the two ends observed. The generous double arch system within the hand ensures good flow from the distal cut end in all but 4 per cent of people. A less traumatic demonstration can be used clinically in the form of Allen's test, which should always be carried out before dividing the radial artery in the preparation of a radial forearm flap. In this test the radial and ulnar arteries are occluded by digital compression and blood squeezed out of the hand by fist clenching. Release of each artery in turn is followed by rapid vascular refill when the vessel is patent. If there is delay from either vessel then a radial forearm flap is not an appropriate technique. Provided that this precaution is observed there need be no concern about the arterial supply of a distally based island flap with the pedicle dissected along the path of the radial artery right through into the first web space, and even into the palm. If the arterial circulation is examined in the way outlined there is no need for arteriography. Venous drainage, however, is less secure, due to the presence of valves in the venae comitantes on which the flap depends. The fact that such a system ever works is a matter of some surprise and in practice the distal island flap is reasonably reliable provided there has not been trauma to the venae comitantes. It is therefore not enough to establish continuity of the radial artery from the wrist through the first web space into the palm, since an injury in the web space could disrupt the veins without occluding the artery. Two theories have been put forward to explain the mechanism of retrograde flow in the venae comitantes. Firstly there are known to be cross-connections between the two veins that are usually present and these may bypass sections containing valves (Lin, Lai and Chiu, 1984). A more intriguing theory has been suggested by Timmons (1984) who has observed that anaesthetized or denervated veins in the forearm lose valvular competence and thus allow retrograde flow.

The radial forearm island flap can be used to resurface dorsal or palmar defects of considerable size. In elderly patients, or if a very large flap is raised, it may be advisable to carry out an additional venous anastomosis using a vein at the proximal end of the superficial venous system (Godfrey *et al.*, 1984). The flap has also been used for thumb reconstruction, in which case a vascularized cortical bone graft from the radius can be included with the skin (Foucher *et al.*, 1984b).

In planning the flap it is important to take into account the length of vascular pedicle required to bridge the distance from the point where it pivots to the point of entry into the flap in its final position. After measuring the precise distance the length of pedicle should be increased by 50 per cent to allow for elastic recoil after dissection since any attempt to pull the pedicle out to its original length is likely to result in vascular spasm. A similar allowance for shrinkage should be made in calculating the size of the flap which cannot be pulled out to its original dimensions when it is sutured in its new position. This principle applies to all flap surgery, particularly island and free flaps.

In raising the flap great care should be exercised to preserve the connections between the vascular pedicle and the flap. This is achieved by raising the flap as a fasciocutaneous unit, starting on the lateral extremities of the flap and dissecting from each side towards the radial artery at the subfascial plane. When approaching from the ulnar side the key structure to identify is flexor carpi radialis, and as soon as this tendon is reached it is carefully dissected free from its overlying fascia and retracted in an ulnar direction. The radial artery and its accompanying veins can be clearly seen and elevated from the underlying bed, maintaining all fascial and vascular connections between the vessels and the flap. When approaching from the radial side, brachioradialis is similarly identified and retracted radially to bring the dissection into the plane deep to the radial artery. On this side there is the added complication of the superficial branch of the radial nerve. Although it passes through part of the flap between the deep fascia and the skin, it is quite possible to preserve the nerve and its distal branches while raising the flap.

When the whole flap and its underlying pedicle have been elevated, they remain attached proximally and distally by the radial artery and veins, and the proximal vessels may be divided. Distal dissection of the vascular pedicle is a difficult manoeuvre involving retraction of the overlying tendons of abductor pollicis longus and extensor pollicis brevis and the radial nerve, to free the radial artery and venae comitantes as they pass distally into the anatomical snuffbox, beneath extensor pollicis longus as they enter the first web space from its dorsal aspect. Small vascular branches have to be divided carefully and great care must be used to avoid damage to the venae comitantes. The dissection continues until the flap can move into its new position without any kinking or tension on the pedicle. If the flap is to be tunnelled to its new site the tunnel must be wide enough to thread the flap through without difficulty. The radial forearm flap has been criticized on account of its donor site, and careless dissection of the fascia over the tendons of flexor carpi radialis and brachioradialis can result in failure of the graft to take over these tendons, which may become exposed and slough. This is less common in younger patients and can be avoided by careful preservation of the paratenon. If necessary, part of the muscle belly of flexor pollicis longus can be gently advanced to cover part of the exposed tendons. The donor site is closed with a thick split skin graft, held in place with a tie-over pack.

There is some disagreement as to the advisability of using this flap in view of the fact that it does reduce the arterial input to the hand. Cavalier use of the flap in the absence of the usual pattern of arterial arches in the palm could result in gangrene of part of the radial side of the hand, but a much more likely and less easily identified complication may be relative ischaemia of the hand giving rise to claudication, possibly some years later, and the possible development of cold intolerance, although this is generally regarded as a complication more of neurological than vascular insult. When the flap is used as a free flap (*see below*) it is possible to insert a reversed vein graft in the gap in the radial artery. Undoubtedly in some patients this will thrombose due to the small pressure difference that can exist at the two ends of the graft in a patient with a good anastomotic system in the hand.

When a distally based island flap is used it is not possible to reconstitute the radial artery directly, but a vein graft could be taken from the proximal cut end of the radial artery to the cut end of the artery emerging from the flap when its new position brings the distal end proximal.

In spite of these reservations, the radial island flap does provide a large area of skin immediately, reliably and fairly simply (*Figure 6.6a* and *b*).

The donor site is grafted, and leaves an unsightly scar which might be objectionable in, for example, a young woman. To avoid the skin defect it is possible to turn back thin skin flaps and dissect out the deep fascia together with the radial pedicle, producing a vascularized fascial flap, the surface of which has to be grafted (Soutar and Tanner, 1984).

Island flaps with a vein only

The idea of providing venous drainage, but no arterial input, to an island flap challenges accepted principles of flap surgery, but evidence is accumulating that this may be a sound technique under some circumstances (Baek *et al.*, 1985). Possibly the Iselin flag flap (Iselin, 1973), which has good venous drainage but doubtful arterial supply, was an early demonstration of this principle.

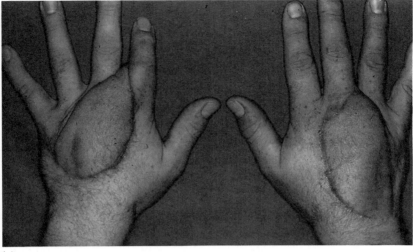

(*a*)

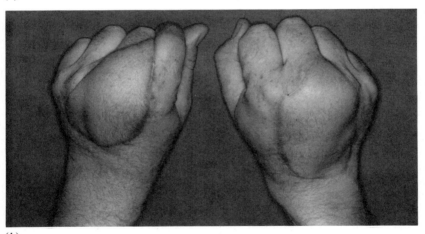

(*b*)

Figures 6.6 (*a*) and (*b*) Use of bilateral radial forearm island flaps for immediate (*right*) and one week delayed (*left*) resurfacing of dorsal degloving injuries caused by a bus fanbelt. Immediate tendon grafting was also carried out on the right, and delayed reconstructive bone and tendon surgery beneath the flap on the left

Distant pedicle flaps within the hand

In fingertip injuries where there is greater loss of pulp tissue than skeletal length, and sufficient nail support is preserved, a cross-finger flap·or thenar flap may be indicated. The cross-finger flap provides sufficient skin of good quality for reconstruction of the whole fingertip pulp, although wherever possible the use of local innervated full thickness skin is preferable. Flaps which involve immobilization of the fingers, particularly in a flexed position, are best avoided in the elderly, in view of the risk of permanent stiffness, and this particularly applies to the thenar flap where the finger has to be flexed acutely into the palm. Miller (1974) found no problems with joint stiffness in patients with injury only to the single fingertip repaired with a thenar flap. This flap is useful in children and has the advantage that no skin graft is required, and the donor site is inconspicuous.

Cross-finger flap

This is a well-established procedure, so only important points of technique will be mentioned. The flap is usually taken from the middle segment of the finger, avoiding if possible the pad of skin over the proximal interphalangeal joint, although under some circumstances it is acceptable to use this skin also. It is preferable to take the flap from the longer of the two fingers available when other factors allow choice. The flap is raised at a level just superficial to the paratenon of the extensor mechanism and it is important to preserve this and to avoid it drying out. It is helpful to divide Cleland's ligament in the base of the flap to allow the skin to transfer without tension on to the neighbouring finger. As with all flaps the dimensions must be generous to allow for skin elasticity. As well as the more usual laterally based flap for fingertip pulp, it is possible to raise the flap obliquely or proximally or distally based in particular situations. In addition to fingertip defects the cross-finger flap can be used to cover more proximal skin defects on the flexor surface and when used as a subcutaneous (Atasoy, 1982) or reverse dermis flap (Pakiam, 1978) the flap can cover extensor surface defects also. In this case the flap is raised after removing the epidermal and superficial dermal layers of the skin. The flap is then hinged on its pedicle to bring the exposed deep dermal surface into contact with the bed to be covered. This leaves the exposed subcutaneous surface of the flap to be skin grafted in continuity with the defect on the donor finger. For defects on the index finger tip a cross-finger flap from the dorsum of the thumb may be used (Atasoy, 1981).

The donor site of the cross-finger flap is closed with a free skin graft, preferably full-thickness skin from the groin. When suturing the flap into its new position tension should be avoided on its margins. It is helpful to place a strong suture between the two fingers themselves at either end of the flap pedicle. The latter is divided at a second procedure 10–14 days after the first. If there is ample skin the fourth side of the flap can be sutured in place, but it is unwise to dissect it at this stage in order to close the wound directly, and if there is any difficulty it is safer to use a small skin graft to achieve healing on the pedicle. It is easy to produce a necrotic skin edge at this time.

The thenar flap

This is taken not from the broad surface of the thenar eminence but from the area of the palmar crease running oblique to the transverse axis of the thumb at the metacarpal phalangeal joint level. This flap is most commonly used to repair transverse loss of the tip of the index or middle fingers and is particularly useful for providing support for the distal nail because the flap can be designed with enough length to stand slightly proud of the level of the nail, thus allowing for subsequent shrinkage during healing. The donor defect can generally be closed directly, although Melone, Beasley and Carstens (1982) recommend the use of a small Wolfe graft, and it is helpful to make one side of the flap longer than the other at its base. When the defect is sutured in the line of the crease the flap will turn to face the defect if this is the desired effect, and the gap left after division of the pedicle, 10–14 days later, remains narrow. In order to allow the flap to adopt its new position without tension the proximal interphalangeal joint of the finger has to be flexed to 90°, and the thumb needs to rest in an opposed position. One or two stronger sutures should be used to hold the position of the fingertip relative to the palm. This avoids tension on the flap. When there is a distal deficit in the nail-bed the free edge of the flap which comes up to the level of the nail matrix is best left raw so that epithelialization can take place from the edge of the supporting matrix which has a specialized function of adhering to the growing nail plate. If there is an area of exposed bone at the distal nail-bed it is sometimes possible to tease a small amount of fat from the undersurface of the flap and bring it to lie on the raw phalangeal surface.

With both thenar and cross-finger flaps it is essential to hold the fingers in the appropriate position with a splint, at least for the first week.

Local muscle flaps for soft tissue cover have been little used within the hand itself. Abductor digiti minimi has been used to cover the carpal tunnel area (Milward, Stott and Kleinert, 1977). Other muscles have been used in the proximal forearm (Hodgkinson and Shepard, 1983) including brachioradialis, flexor digitorum superficialis and flexor carpi ulnaris. Fasciocutaneous flaps are also available in the forearm, particularly the antecubital flap (Lamberty and Cormack, 1983).

Distant pedicle flaps

To some extent distant pedicle flaps have been superseded by single stage free flaps, although there are situations in which distant flaps are still useful for resurfacing large areas of skin loss. The disadvantages of distant flaps are the immobility and dependency that are required during the period of attachment, and the length of time taken to complete the reconstruction, much of it in hospital. It is difficult to give rigid indications for the use of the pedicle flaps in favour of free flaps and the decision to use such a flap is usually made when conditions favouring the use of a free flap are lacking. If there are problems in finding suitable vessels, or vascular problems are anticipated, for example in patients with arterial disease or even in heavy smokers, the balance may be tipped in favour of a pedicle flap. Similarly if later microvascular reconstruction is planned, for example a free toe transfer, one might prefer to avoid dissection of blood vessels when achieving primary skin cover if those vessels are going to be required later. Multiple small defects can sometimes only be satisfactorily covered by the use of multiple distant flaps. Morris (1981) described the use of small reverse dermis distant flaps for small defects requiring soft tissue cover. The donor skin is de-epithelialized and the raw surface sutured to it, giving maximum contact. After 1–2 weeks the area of the flap is detached from its bed, having picked up good blood supply from its dermal contact. The exposed raw surface is grafted. The advantage is the shorter attachment time.

McGregor (1979) gives a clear overview of the development of distant flaps for use in the hand.

The groin flap

One advantage of the groin flap in particular is that the distal part of the flap that is attached to the hand can be raised thinner than any free flap, especially in young people, and the use of a groin flap in this way may avoid the need for subsequent surgery to thin a bulky flap (*Figure 6.7a* and *b*).

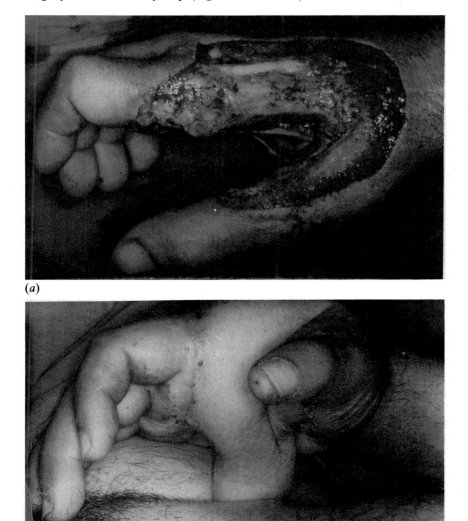

(*a*)

(*b*)

Figure 6.7 (*a*) The use of a pedicle groin flap to reconstruct the first web space, denuded by skin necrosis following a high pressure injection injury. (*b*) Shows the flap in place, illustrating the amount of thinning that is possible, and the freedom of movement allowed by the long pedicle

Although Shaw and Payne (1946) described a similar flap, the groin flap was popularized by McGregor and Jackson (1972), and at that time represented a significant advance in the management of hand trauma with skin loss (May and Bartlett, 1981). It had great advantages over currently used random pattern flaps in that the territory of skin available was considerably in excess of the standard 1 : 1 length–width ratio, with the dual advantages of a larger area of skin and greater length and mobility of the pedicle. The axial vascular arrangement, consisting of the superficial circumflex iliac artery and vein, is responsible for the reliability of this flap, but also reduces the speed with which new vascular connections are made around its margins, making it necessary to 'delay' the flap by dividing its axial vessels some time before separating it completely. Since this is now a relatively uncommon operation it may be unfamiliar to surgeons who have trained in the free flap era and therefore the surgical technique will be described in detail.

The central axis of the flap lies along a line parallel to, and 2 cm below, the inguinal ligament. In order to allow direct closure of the groin defect the maximum width of the flap is 10 cm in an adult, but greater width is available if the donor defect is to be skin grafted. In length the flap can be extended to the mid-lateral line at least, and in many cases it can extend a short distance on to the back, although the area beyond the mid-lateral line will only have random-patterned blood supply, with decreased reliability. The flap is raised from its lateral end, and here the full thickness of subcutaneous fat need not be included with the skin. As soon as the dissection reaches the level of the lateral margin of sartorius it is necessary to move to the deep fascial plane. Before reaching the medial border of sartorius the deep fascia should be incised so that the perforating superficial circumflex iliac artery is included with the flap. This will only be assured if the anterior sartorius fascia remains with the skin. Sartorius muscle is retracted laterally and the deep fascia is again incised at the medial limit of the sartorius compartment to take the dissection into the femoral triangle. The muscular branch entering sartorius has to be divided (Schlenker, 1980). The superficial circumflex iliac artery need not be visualized, but will automatically remain with the skin. It is not usually necessary to extend the dissection any further medially when raising a pedicled groin flap. The proximal pedicle can then be tubed, taking care to avoid circumferential tension. If the incisions marking the sides of the flap reach a different point medially a spiral is introduced to the seam, and this helps to prevent tension (Schlenker, 1980). If the lower incision is longer the raw surface of the distal end of the flap faces downwards, and vice versa.

The donor defect is closed by flexing the hip and the knee, and the distal part of the flap is sutured to the defect in the hand. It is usually necessary to commence attachment at the least accessible part of the flap, that is the point where the seam opens out into the raw undersurface. The distal free edge of the flap is then sutured last. It is most important that the flap is sutured without any tension and that no haematoma accumulates beneath it. Postoperative management requires close supervision of the position of the arm, which can be restrained with carefully placed elastoplast straps, keeping a cotton wool pad in the axilla, which otherwise becomes very sore. Within a few days the position is more easily maintained by the patient and freer mobility can be allowed. As soon as the tension of the donor scar allows it, the hip can be extended and the patient can start to walk with the hand still attached to the flap. Because the flap has a dominant axial blood supply it is advisable to divide the main feeding vessels by a 'delay' procedure under local anaesthetic a few days before separating the flap from its pedicle. It is reasonable to carry out this delay 2½ weeks after flap attachment, provided good primary healing has occurred, and to divide the flap between three and four weeks. It is not safe to apply even the slightest tension to the remaining free edge of the flap after separation, and it is often better to leave this wound open for several days and carry out a delayed primary closure after the new vascular arrangements of the flap have become established. Inevitably flaps become oedematous during the weeks following healing and the use of pressure garments and physiotherapy may be required to prevent this becoming established. It is safe to carry out secondary surgery beneath the flap within a few weeks of complete healing, but the longer the flap is left the easier it is to work with, and the more safely can it be thinned. Thinning a flap should be carried out with caution and in stages, to avoid separating too much of its attachment at one time.

For very extensive defects of both surfaces of the hand a large bilobed flap may be used to resurface both on one pedicle (Smith, 1982b). The design of this flap uses the diverging superficial external iliac and superficial epigastric vessels which support a groin flap and inferiorly based lower abdominal flap raised with a common pedicle in the groin. It is likely that the donor site will be large enough to require some split skin graft to close it. Alternative approaches to this problem have included simultaneous bilateral groin flaps (Heath *et al.*, 1983), a groin flap and tensor fascia lata myocutaneous flap from the same side (Watson and McGregor, 1981), and two flaps from the adjacent surfaces of the opposite upper arm and chest, both hinged forward to lie on either side of the injured hand (Smith and Furnas, 1976). Reinisch, Winters and Puckett (1984) have included with a groin flap a block of iliac crest as a vascularized bone graft to restore skeletal continuity. For more proximal upper limb defects the abdominohypogastric flap can be used (Schlenker, Atasoy and Lyon, 1980). This lies above the inguinal ligament and parallel to the groin flap, and is supplied by branches of the deep and superficial inferior epigastric arteries.

Other distal pedicle flaps are available and may, under special circumstances, still be applicable. They include cross-arm flaps, which are usually raised on the opposite upper arm, the position and size being designed to fit exactly into the defect, allowing for shrinkage. Dolich, Olshansky and Babar (1978) have shown that the radial nerve can be included and sutured to a sensory nerve in the recipient area. Another application of the cross-arm flap is its use as a 'flap graft' (Colson *et al.*, 1967). A bipedicle strap-like flap is raised and the central part due to cover the defect is thinned so as to remove all subcutaneous fat but leave all dermis. Mercer (1985) has shown that even large flaps of this type can usually survive even on a poor underlying surface, and they probably take partly as a full thickness skin graft, and partly through slow perfusion from the pedicles. The great advantage is that no thinning procedures are needed later.

The deltopectoral flap is another axial pattern flap and has the advantage over the groin of being placed higher in the body, therefore avoiding dependency of the hand during attachment. The pectoralis major myocutaneous island flap has been used as a distant flap for the upper limb (Luce and Gottlieb, 1982) but has little application. For very large defects extending the full length of the forearm, random pattern abdominal flaps are occasionally useful because large areas of skin can be raised without a preliminary delay procedure, provided that the base of the flap is very wide.

Microvascular free flaps

Free flap transfer, first reported by Taylor and Daniel (1973), is now a standard procedure in most plastic surgery units. Free flaps are used in many circumstances where full thickness skin cover is required, and have the advantage of being completed usually in a single stage, avoiding unwanted immobilization of the hand, and introducing new blood supply into the injured area rather than parasitizing existing blood supply (Daniel and Weiland, 1982). The choice between a free flap and a conventional pedicle flap may not be easy (Cannon, 1981), but as experience and confidence increase, the advantages given above tend to outweigh the disadvantages more and more, these being length of operative time, technical difficulty, need for equipment, and the risk that failure means total, not partial, failure.

The development of free tissue transfer in hand surgery has been traced by Chase (1984). Several donor sites are available and they each have features which make them applicable to different circumstances.

Successful and reliable use of free flap transfers requires considerable experience and familiarity with the surgical techniques involved and the complications which can occur. Anaesthetic techniques are no less important (Apps *et al.*, 1985), and the success of the procedure may depend on the maintenance of body temperature, blood volume, cardiac output and peripheral blood flow. Any significant technical problem can threaten the viability of the entire flap, whereas a technical problem in conventional flaps and grafts will more often lead only to partial failure. Smoking by the patient has an adverse effect on the behaviour of blood vessels after anastomosis, and heavy smoking in the period immediately prior to surgery may tip the balance in favour of a traditional method of skin transfer rather than a free flap. The indications for free flaps in the hand may be less frequent than in reconstructive surgery in other areas of the body, particularly the lower limb and the head and neck, and it is therefore desirable that free tissue transfers to the hand should be carried out by surgical teams performing microvascular reconstruction regularly in other areas of the body.

The situations requiring free tissue transfer in the hand include small skin defects, large skin defects, loss of sensory skin, and the need for skin cover combined with other reconstructive procedures, particularly of tendon and bone.

Small skin defects

If an area of skin loss is too large to close directly and requires full-thickness skin cover to avoid contracture or exposure of important structures, the lateral arm free flap provides the necessary tissue with probably the least morbidity of the donor site (Katsaros *et al.*, 1984). The flap is based on the posterior radial collateral artery (PRCA) which is situated beneath the lateral intermuscular septum in the lower part of the upper arm, and sends branches to the skin between the leaves of the septum. The septum lies on a line from the lateral epicondyle to the insertion of deltoid, and the skin area to be used should be placed so that the septum bisects it.

The flap is raised as a fasciocutaneous flap by dissecting beneath the deep fascia of triceps and brachialis (*Figure 6.8*). It is best to carry out the initial dissection from behind as this exposes the vascular pedicle at an early stage and allows the surgeon to dive deeply at the lateral intermuscular septum and include the vessels

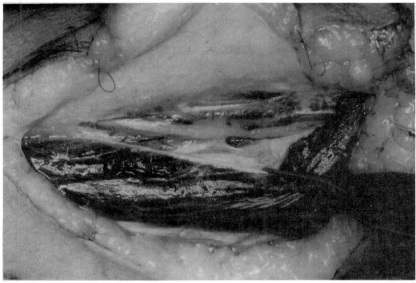

(*a*)

Figure 6.8 Dissection of a lateral arm free flap. (*a*) Dissection of a flap on the left arm; the posterior (lower) half of the flap has been raised subfascially, revealing triceps, the lateral intermuscular septum (held), the radial nerve above it, and just above that the vascular pedicle entering the flap towards the left. Note the temporary sutures tethering the skin of the flap to the deep fascia to prevent shearing

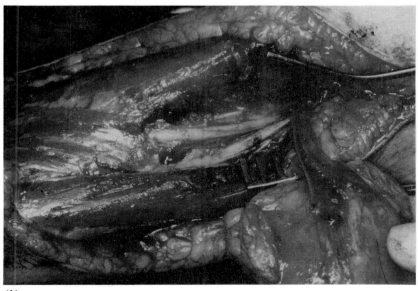

(*b*)

Figure 6.8 (*b*) The dissection completed, with the flap held downwards and the pedicle sweeping into it, diverging from the radial nerve

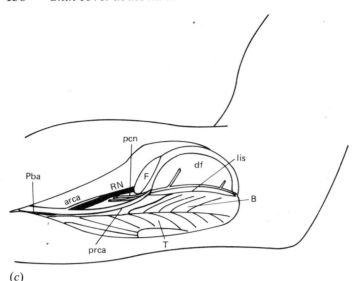

(c)

Figure 6.8 (c) Shows diagrammatically the flap's anatomy, drawn for the right arm. The elbow is to the right, the shoulder would be to the left. pba = profunda brachii artery, arca = anterior radial collateral artery, prca = posterior radial collateral artery, RN = radial nerve, F = flap, df = deep fascia, lis = lateral intermuscular septum, B = brachioradialis, T = triceps

with the flap. The posterior radial collateral artery is the continuation of the profunda brachii artery, which enters the lateral compartment of the arm together with the radial nerve. The posterior radial collateral artery, its vein and the lateral antebrachial cutaneous nerve diverge posteriorly from the radial nerve as they approach the level of the deep fascia. Once the pedicle has been identified, the anterior half of the flap can be raised subfascially from brachialis, and the lateral intermuscular septum divided deeply. As the vessels are followed proximally through an extended incision they become larger and deeper and a pedicle several centimetres long with good vessels can be isolated.

As with all free flap transfers, the ideal arterial anastomosis is an end-to-side arrangement (Ikuta *et al.*, 1975; Godina, 1979) which provides the most reliable haemodynamic system, because any tendency to spasm in the recipient vessel opens the side-hole in the artery wider. There is usually little difficulty in finding a recipient vessel in the upper limb. The venous anastomosis may be end-to-side or end-to-end. Vascular anastomoses must be without tension, and great care is needed to ensure a comfortable lie of the vessels with no twisting or compression. If recipient vessels are not close enough for tension-free anastomosis, reversed vein grafts should be interposed. The skin must be sutured without tension and it is not uncommon to find that part of the circumferential wound of a free flap must be left open to avoid tension, and the defect closed with a temporary skin graft.

The other free flap donor site that may be considered for smaller skin defects is the scapular flap (Barwick, Goodkind and Serafin, 1982; Gilbert and Teot, 1982; Hamilton and Morrison, 1982; Mayou, Whitby and Jones, 1982; Urbaniak *et al.*, 1982; Santos, 1984), or parascapular flap (Fissette, Lahaye and Colot, 1983; Nassif *et al.*, 1982), and the reader is referred to these articles for details of technique. The flap has thicker skin and slightly more subcutaneous tissue than the lateral arm flap, and the patient has to be turned on to the side for the dissection, but the donor site is acceptable and can be closed directly if the flap is less than 12 cm wide. It is usually oriented transversely across the scapula, but can be more vertically placed, running down the lateral border of the scapula. The flap is based on the circumflex scapular vessels as they pass out of the axilla medial to triceps. A long pedicle can be traced to the thoracodorsal vessels, though Gahhos, Tross and Salomon (1985) recommend an additional axillary incision for safe dissection of the pedicle.

Large skin defects

The latissimus dorsi myocutaneous flap provides as large a surface area of skin as one could possibly require in the hand, but it is bulky, particularly when folded, and may therefore require later thinning. One way of circumventing this problem is to use the muscle as a free transfer without skin (Bailey and Godfrey, 1982). The surface area available is less, but usually enough, and the muscle is covered with a split skin graft. The skin surface is that of a graft rather than a flap. Denervated muscle does atrophy fairly rapidly, then stabilizes (Hagerty, Bostwick and Nahai, 1984), but there may still be too much bulk, in which case thinning is a problem because the grafted surface cannot be safely reflected as a thin flap and the muscle may have to be shaved down and regrafted. As an alternative to the latissimus dorsi flap, the territory of the scapular flap can be extended, with grafting of the donor site then being a requirement.

The free groin flap may be considered (Harii *et al.*, 1975; Ohmori and Harii, 1975; Daniel and Faibisoff, 1979; Shah, Garrett and Buncke, 1979), but the pedicle is short and the vessels small. Familiarity with the later generation of large-vessel, long-pedicle free flaps makes the groin flap unattractive, although the donor scar is more acceptable than most, being easily closed directly in most cases.

Taylor, Corlett and Boyd (1984) advocate the inferiorly based rectus abdominis myocutaneous flap. This tends to be bulky, and sacrifice of rectus abdominis may be a disadvantage.

Sensate skin replacement

Skin replacement in important tactile areas should be innervated if possible, and free flaps are valuable in this respect. The lateral upper arm flap can be reinnervated by anastomosis of the lateral cutaneous nerve of the arm, which has to come with the flap anyway, to a suitable cutaneous nerve in the recipient area. Similarly the dorsalis pedis flap (McCraw and Furlow, 1975; Ohmori and Harii, 1976; Robinson, 1976) can be innervated by anastomosis of the superficial peroneal nerve, although many fibres of this nerve pass right through the flap. The dorsalis pedis flap relies on small branches to the overlying skin arising from the artery itself, and of the first dorsal metatarsal artery (1st DMA) which is its continuation distally towards the first web space. Man and Acland (1980) have shown that such branches are most reliably present in the distal third of the flap, from the first dorsal metatarsal artery, and comparatively few are present in the central part of the flap. Occasionally the first dorsal metatarsal artery is absent, in which case the skin may receive inadequate blood supply from the dorsalis pedis artery.

When raising this flap great care must be taken to include the dorsalis pedis artery and first dorsal metatarsal artery with the skin, by dissecting deeply between extensor hallucis longus and extensor digitorum longus of the second toe. The artery and its veins are lifted away from the periosteum of the cuboid and first metatarsal, and the vessels that pass through into the plantar aspect of the foot are divided deep in the intermetacarpal space. Venous drainage of the flap is through the superficial system, usually the long saphenous vein.

Paratenon must be carefully preserved over the extensor tendons, and the graft used to resurface the defect should be carefully packed into the deep crevices. Poor take of the graft over tendons or periosteum has given this flap a bad name, since the unstable scarring that results can be very troublesome, particularly in older patients. With care, and good patient selection, this problem can be avoided.

For first web space reconstruction a free flap from the first web space of the foot can be prepared as a more distal dorsalis pedis flap (Doi and Hattori, 1980), and a similar flap has been described to resurface tactile areas of the thumb and fingers (May *et al.*, 1977; Morrison *et al.*, 1978; Strauch and Tsur, 1978). Alternatively, neurovascular free pulp flaps from the toes may be considered (Buncke and Rose, 1979; Stern, Kreilein and Kleinert, 1983). Foucher *et al.* (1980) have described a number of ingenious custom-made composite transfers from the toes to the hand, including a neurovascular island flap with some nail-bed and distal phalanx for partial thumb reconstruction (*Figure 6.9*). The quality of sensory recovery that can be expected is excellent. The nerve repair can be carried out under ideal conditions with no tension, and in some cases the final two-point discrimination in the reconstructed area may be better than that of the toe skin in its original location.

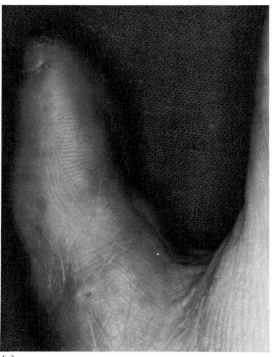

Figure 6.9 (*a*) A short, insensitive, poorly padded thumb following a crush injury under a 5 tonne crane

(a)

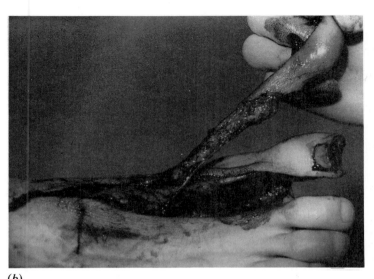

(b)

Figure 6.9 (b) Shows a composite flap raised from the big toe including lateral innervated skin, part of the distal nail matrix and the underlying tip of the distal phalanx

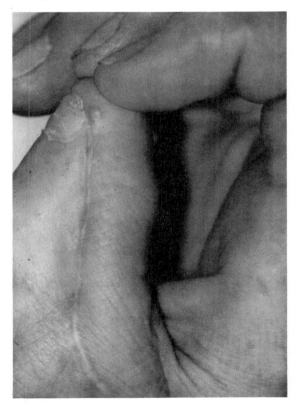

Figure 6.9 (c) After transfer to the hand and neurovascular anastomosis there was good sensory recovery and the patient uses his longer sensate thumb much more effectively

(c)

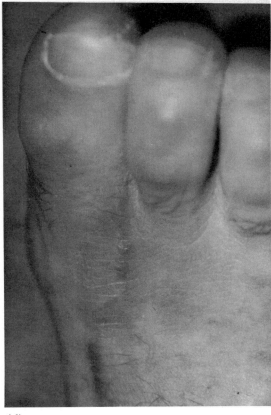

Figure 6.9 (*d*) The scarring on the foot is minimal and the disability nil

(*d*)

A large area of sensate skin can be provided by the tensor fasciae latae flap (Mathes and Buchanan, 1979; O'Hare, Leonard and Brennan, 1983) using the lateral femoral cutaneous nerve, but this is more suitable for use in the lower limb as the flap is bulky, and a large area of sensitive skin is seldom required in the hand. The other possible donor site is the opposite free forearm flap (Muhlbauer, Herndl and Stock, 1982), but many patients would prefer not to have extensive scarring on the opposite limb. Occasionally an opportunity is presented to use a free flap from an amputated part to preserve stump length when replantation is not appropriate. May and Gordon (1980) described such a case when a palmar free flap based on the ulnar vessels allowed preservation of a below-elbow stump.

Composite free tissue transfer

Free skin flaps may be raised to include multiple vascularized tendon grafts in their gliding mechanisms (*Figure 6.10*, which shows a dorsalis pedis flap with long toe extensor tendons), vascularized bone, and toe proximal interphalangeal joint with skin, although here the skeletal reconstruction is the essential part of the procedure.

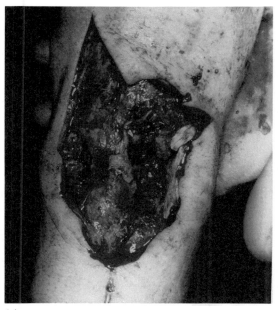

(a)

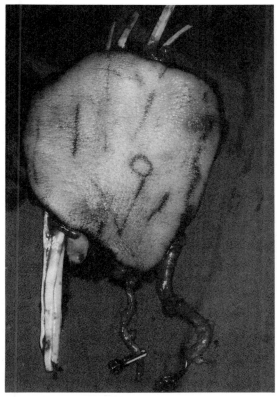

(b)

Figure 6.10 (a) The situation following open reduction and internal fixation of a distal radial fracture that had been complicated by loss of skin and extensor tendons due to necrosis following the primary reduction and ˙immobilization. (b) Shows a composite dorsalis pedis free flap including four long extensor tendons with their gliding mechanisms. The dorsalis pedis artery and larger long saphenous vein can be seen

142

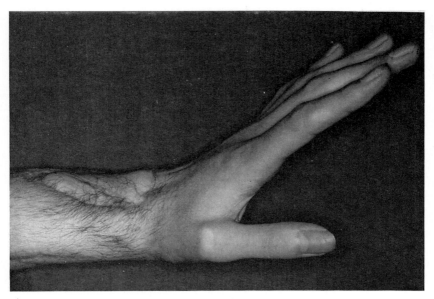

(*c*)

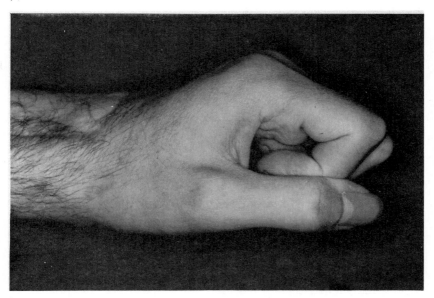

(*d*)

Figure 6.10 (*c*) The early result in flexion and (*d*) full extension shows good active tendon function, achieved in a single-stage procedure

Monitoring

Although a trained eye can usually discern problems in the circulation of a flap through the colour changes, it is useful to have some objective monitoring system. Temperature comparison with nearby skin is simple and reliable (Leonard, Brennen and Colville, 1982). The photoplethysmograph (Harrison, Girling and Mott, 1981) and laser doppler (Jones, 1985) are more informative but require elaborate equipment. When only muscle has been transferred, stimulation with a low power nerve stimulator causes a twitch which dies out if the circulation stops, and this can be reliably observed by nursing staff (Batchelor, Kay and Evans, 1982).

CONCLUSION

The most appropriate choice of technique for replacement of a significant area of missing skin can only be made against a wide background of familiarity with all techniques available. Those faced with important decision-making either in the acute situation or in elective cases have an obligation to achieve this familiarity, or to ensure that the patient falls into appropriate hands in time for the right choice to be made, and this is usually earlier rather than later.

Acknowledgements

I thank my secretary, Mrs Rita Hanson, for typing tirelessly, and Mrs Jean Tyler for the photographic prints.

References

APPS, C., COX, R. G., MAYOU, B. J. and SENGUPTA, P. (1985) The role of anaesthetic management in enhancing peripheral blood flow in patients undergoing free flap transfer. *Annals of the Royal College of Surgeons of England*, **67**, 177–179

ATASOY, E. (1980) The cross thumb to index finger pedicle. *Journal of Hand Surgery*, **5**, 572–574

ATASOY, E. (1982) Reversed cross finger subcutaneous flap. *Journal of Hand Surgery*, **7**, 481–483

ATASOY, E., IOAKIMIDIS, E., KASDAN, M. L., KUTZ, J. E. and KLEINERT, H. E. (1970) Reconstruction of the amputated fingertip with a triangular volar flap. *Journal of Bone and Joint Surgery*, **52A**, 921–926

BAEK, S-M., WEMBERG, H., SONG, Y., PARK, E. G. and BILLER, H. F. (1985) Experimental studies in the survival of venous island flaps without arterial inflow. *Plastic and Reconstructive Surgery*, **75**, 88–95

BAILEY, B. N. and GODFREY, A. M. (1982) Latissimus dorsi muscle free flaps. *British Journal of Plastic Surgery*, **35**, 47–52

BARWICK, W. J., GOODKIND, D. J. and SERAFIN, D. (1982) The free scapular flap. *Plastic and Reconstructive Surgery*, **69**, 779–785

BATCHELOR, A., KAY, S. and EVANS, D. (1982) A simple and effective method of monitoring free muscle transfers: a preliminary report. *British Journal of Plastic Surgery*, **35**, 343–344

BUNCKE, H. J. and ROSE, E. H. (1979) Free toe-to-fingertip neurovascular flaps. *Plastic and Reconstructive Surgery*, **63**, 607–612

CANNON, B. (1981) Flaps old and new. *Journal of Hand Surgery*, **6**, 1–2

CHASE, R. A. (1984) The development of free tissue transfer in hand surgery. *Journal of Hand Surgery*, **9A**, 463–477

COHEN, B. E. and CRONIN, E. D. (1983) An innervated cross-finger flap for fingertip reconstruction. *Plastic and Reconstructive Surgery*, **72**, 688–697

COLSON, P., HOUOT, R., GANGOLPHE, M. *et al.* (1967) Use of thinned flaps (flap-grafts) in reparative hand surgery. *Annales Chirurgie Plastique*, **12**, 298–310

DANIEL, R. K. and FAIBISOFF, B. (1979) Free flap transfers for upper extremity reconstruction. *Annals of the Academy of Medicine of Singapore*, **8**, 440–444

DANIEL, R. K. and WEILAND, A. J. (1982) Free tissue transfers for upper extremity reconstruction. *Journal of Hand Surgery*, **7**, 66–76

DANIEL, R. K., TERZIS, J. and MIDGLEY, R. D. (1976) Restoration of sensation to an anesthetic hand by a neurovascular flap from the foot. *Plastic and Reconstructive Surgery*, **57**, 275–280

DAS, S. K. and BROWN, H. G. (1978) Management of lost fingertips in children. *The Hand*, **10**, 16–27

DELLON, A. L. (1983) The extended palmar advancement flap. *Journal of Hand Surgery*, **8**, 190–194

DOI, K. and HATTORI, S. (1980) Free neurovascular flap from the first web space of the foot for reconstruction of the mutilated hand. *The Hand*, **12**, 130–136

DOLICH, B. H., OLSHANSKY, K. J. and BABAR, A. H. (1978) Use of a cross-forearm neurocutaneous flap to provide sensation and coverage in hand reconstruction. *Plastic and Reconstructive Surgery*, **62**, 550–558

ELLIOTT, R. A., HOEHN, J. G. and STAYMAN, W. (1979) Management of the viable soft tissue cover in degloving injuries. *The Hand*, **11**, 69–71

EMMETT, A. J. J. (1974) Finger resurfacing by the multiple subcutaneous pedicle or louvre flaps. *British Journal of Plastic Surgery*, **27**, 370–374

FATAH, M. F. and DAVIES, D. M. (1984) The radial forearm island flap in upper limb reconstruction. *Journal of Hand Surgery*, **9B**, 234–244

FISSETTE, J., LAHAYE, T. and COLOT, G. (1983) The use of the free parascapular flap in mid palmar soft tissue defects. *Annals of Plastic Surgery*, **10**, 235–238

FLATT, A. E. (1957) The thenar flap. *Journal of Bone and Joint Surgery*, **39B**, 80–85

FOUCHER, G. and BRAUN, J.-B. (1979) A new island flap transfer from the dorsum of the index to the thumb. *Plastic and Reconstructive Surgery*, **63**, 344–349

FOUCHER, G., MERLE, M., MANEAUD, M. and MICHON, J. (1980) Microsurgical free partial toe transfer in hand reconstruction: a report of 12 cases. *Plastic and Reconstructive Surgery*, **65**, 616–626

FOUCHER, G., VAN GENECHTEN, F., MERLE, M. and MICHON, J. (1984a) A compound radial artery forearm flap in hand surgery: an original modification of the Chinese forearm flap. *British Journal of Plastic Surgery*, **37**, 139–148

FOUCHER, G., VAN GENECHTEN, F., MERLE, M. and MICHON, J. (1984b) Single stage thumb reconstruction by a composite forearm island flap. *Journal of Hand Surgery*, **9B**, 245–248

FURLOW, L. T. (1984) V-Y 'cup' flap for volar oblique amputation of fingers. *Journal of Hand Surgery*, **9A**, 750–753

GAHHOS, F. N., TROSS, R. B. and SALOMON, J. C. (1985) Scapular free-flap dissection made easier. *Plastic and Reconstructive Surgery*, **75**, 115–118

GATEWOOD, A. (1926) A plastic repair of finger defects without hospitalization. *Journal of the American Medical Association*, **87**, 1479

GIBRAIEL, E. A. (1977) A local finger flap to treat post-traumatic flexion contractures of the fingers. *British Journal of Plastic Surgery*, **30**, 134–137

GILBERT, A. and TEOT, L. (1982) The free scapular flap. *Plastic and Reconstructive Surgery*, **69**, 601–602

GODFREY, A. M., POOLE, M. D., ROWSELL, A. R. and ROHRICH, R. J. (1984) Local transposition of a distally based island forearm flap to close a complicated excisional wrist defect in a nonagenarian: some anatomical and clinical considerations. *British Journal of Plastic Surgery*, **37**, 493–495

GODINA, M. (1979) Preferential use of end-to-side arterial anastomoses in free flap transfers. *Plastic and Reconstructive Surgery*, **64**, 673–682

GORIS, R. J. A. and NICOLAI, J. P. A. (1982) A simple method of taking skin grafts from the avulsed flap in degloving injuries. *British Journal of Plastic Surgery*, **35**, 58–59

GREEN, D. P. and DOMINGUEZ, O. J. (1979) A transposition skin flap for release of volar contractures of a finger at the MP joint. *Plastic and Reconstructive Surgery*, **64**, 516–520

HAGERTY, R., BOSTWICK, J. and NAHAI, F. (1984) Denervated muscle flaps: mass and thickness changes following denervation. *Annals of Plastic Surgery*, **12**, 171–176

HAMILTON, G. G. L. and MORRISON, W. A. (1982) The scapular free flap. *British Journal of Plastic Surgery*, **35**, 2–7

HARII, K., OHMORI, K., SHUHEI, T. *et al.* (1975) Free groin skin flaps. *British Journal of Plastic Surgery*, **28**, 225–237

HARRISON, D. H., GIRLING, M. and MOTT, G. (1981) Experience in monitoring the circulation in free flap transfers. *Plastic and Reconstructive Surgery*, **68**, 543–553

HEATH, P. M., JACKSON, I. T., COONEY, W. P. and MORGAN, R. G. (1983) Simultaneous bilateral staged groin flaps for coverage of mutilating injuries of the hand. *Annals of Plastic Surgery*, **11**, 462–468

HENDERSON, H. P. and REID, D. A. C. (1980) Long term follow up of neurovascular island flaps. *The Hand*, **12,** 113–122

HODGKINSON, D. J. and SHEPARD, G. H. (1983) Muscle musculocutaneous and fasciocutaneous flaps in forearm reconstruction. *Annals of Plastic Surgery*, **10,** 400–407

HURWITZ, P. J. (1980) The many-tailed flap for multiple finger injuries. *British Journal of Plastic Surgery*, **33,** 230–232

HURWITZ, D. J. and WHITE, W. L. (1978) Application of glove design in resurfacing the dorsum of the hand. *Plastic and Reconstructive Surgery*, **62,** 385–389

IKUTA, Y., WATARI, S., KAWAMURA, K. *et al.* (1975) Free flap transfers by end-to-side arterial anastomosis. *British Journal of Plastic Surgery*, **28,** 1–7

ISELIN, F. (1973) The flag flap. *Plastic and Reconstructive Surgery*, **52,** 374–377

JONES, B. M. (1985) Predicting the fate of free tissue transfers. *Annals of the Royal College of Surgeons of England*, **67,** 62–70

JOSHI, B. B. (1974a) A local dorsolateral island flap for restoration of sensation after avulsion injury of the fingertip pulp. *Plastic and Reconstructive Surgery*, **54,** 175–182

JOSHI, B. B. (1974b) Sensory flaps for the degloved mutilated hand. *The Hand*, **6,** 247–254

JOSHI, B. B. (1976) A sensory cross finger flap for use on the index finger. *Plastic and Reconstructive Surgery*, **58,** 210–213

KATSAROS, J., SCHUSTERMAN, M., BEPPU, M., BANIS, J. C. and ACLAND, R. D. (1984) The lateral upper arm flap: anatomy and clinical applications. *Annals of Plastic Surgery*, **12,** 489–500

KLEINMAN, W. B. and DUSTMAN, J. A. (1981) Preservation of function following complete degloving injuries of the hand: use of simultaneous groin flap, random abdominal flap and partial thickness skin graft. *Journal of Hand Surgery*, **6,** 82–89

KUTLER, W. A. (1947) A new method for fingertip amputation. *Journal of the American Medical Association*, **133,** 29–30

LAMBERTY, B. G. H. and CORMACK, G. C. (1983) The antecubital fasciocutaneous flap. *British Journal of Plastic Surgery*, **38,** 428–433

LEONARD, A. G., BRENNAN, M. D. and COLVILLE, T. (1982) The use of continuous temperature monitoring in the post-operative management of microvascular cases. *British Journal of Plastic Surgery*, **35,** 337–342

LIN, S-D., LAI, C-S. and CHIU, E. C. (1984) Venous drainage in the reverse forearm flap. *Plastic and Reconstructive Surgery*, **74,** 508–512

LISTER, G. D. (1981) The theory of the transposition flap and its practical application in the hand. *Clinics in Plastic Surgery*, **8,** 115–127

LISTER, G. D. and GIBSON, T. (1972) Closure of rhomboid skin defects: the flaps of Limberg and Dufourmentel. *British Journal of Plastic Surgery*, **25,** 300–314

LISTER, G. D., McGREGOR, I. A. and JACKSON, I. T. (1973) The groin flap in hand injuries. *Injury*, **4,** 229–239

LITTLER, J. W. (1956) Neurovascular pedicle transfer of tissue in reconstructive surgery of the hand. *Journal of Bone and Joint Surgery*, **38A,** 917

LONDON, P. S. and CLARKE, R. (1959) Severe accidental flaying. *Journal of Bone and Joint Surgery*, **41B,** 658–670

LUCE, E. A. and GOTTLIEB, S. F. (1982) The pectoralis major island flap for coverage in the upper extremity. *Journal of Hand Surgery*, **7,** 156–159

MACHT, S. D. and WATSON, H. K. (1980) The Moberg volar advancement flap for digital reconstruction. *Journal of Hand Surgery*, **5,** 372–376

MAN, D. and ACKLAND, R. D. (1980) The microarterial anatomy of the dorsalis pedis flap and its clinical applications. *Plastic and Reconstructive Surgery*, **65,** 419–423

MATEV, I. B. (1980) Tactile gnosis in free skin grafts in the hand. *British Journal of Plastic Surgery*, **33,** 434–439

MATHES, S. J. and BUCHANAN, R. T. (1979) Tensor fascia lata: neurosensory musculocutaneous free flap. *British Journal of Plastic Surgery*, **32,** 184–187

MAY, J. W. and GORDON, L. (1980) Palm of hand free flap for forearm length preservation in nonreplantable forearm amputation: a case report. *Journal of Hand Surgery*, **5,** 377–380

MAY, J. W. and BARTLETT, G. P. (1981) Staged groin flap in reconstruction of the pediatric hand. *Journal of Hand Surgery*, **6,** 163–171

MAY, J. W., CHAIT, L. A., COHEN, B. E. and O'BRIEN, B. Mc. (1977) Free neurovascular flap from the first web of the foot in hand reconstruction. *Journal of Hand Surgery*, **2,** 387–393

MAY, J. W., GALLICO, G. G., JUPITER, J. and SAVAGE, R. C. (1984) Free latissimus dorsi muscle flap with skin graft for treatment of traumatic chronic bony wounds. *Plastic and Reconstructive Surgery*, **73,** 641–649

MAYOU, B. J., WHITBY, D. and JONES, B. M. (1982) The scapular flap – an anatomical and clinical study. *British Journal of Plastic Surgery*, **35,** 8–13

McCRAW, J. B. and FURLOW, L. T. (1975) The dorsalis pedis arterialised free flap. *Plastic and Reconstructive Surgery*, **55**, 177–185

McGREGOR, I. A. (1979) Flap reconstruction in hand surgery: the evolution of presently used methods. *Journal of Hand Surgery*, **4**, 1–10

McGREGOR, I. A. and JACKSON, I. T. (1972) The groin flap. *British Journal of Plastic Surgery*, **25**, 3–16

McGROUTHER, D. A. and SULLY, L. (1980) Degloving injuries of the limbs: long-term review and management based on whole-body fluorescence. *British Journal of Plastic Surgery*, **33**, 9–24

MELONE, C. P., BEASLEY, R. W. and CARSTENS, J. H. (1982) The thenar flap – an analysis of its use in 150 cases. *Journal of Hand Surgery*, **7**, 291–297

MERCER, D. (1985) The dermal flap-graft. Paper read at joint meeting of The British Society for Surgery of the Hand and the Eastern Mediterranean Hand Society, Cairo, March 1985

MILLER, A. J. (1974) Single fingertip injuries treated by thenar flap. *The Hand*, **6**, 311–314

MILWARD, T. M., SCOTT, W. G. and KLEINERT, H. E. (1977) The abductor digiti minimi flap. *The Hand*, **9**, 82–85

MIURA, T. (1973) Thumb reconstruction using radial-innervated cross-finger pedicle graft. *Journal of Bone and Joint Surgery*, **55A**, 563–569

MOBERG, E. (1964) Aspects of sensation in reconstructive surgery of the upper extremity. *Journal of Bone and Joint Surgery*, **46A**, 817–825

MORRIS, A. M. (1981) Rapid skin cover in hand injuries using the reverse dermis flap. *British Journal of Plastic Surgery*, **34**, 194–196

MORRISON, W. A., O'BRIEN, B. Mc, MACLEOD, A. M. and GILBERT, A. (1978) Neurovascular free flaps from the foot for innervation of the hand. *Journal of Hand Surgery*, **3**, 235–242

MUHLBAUER, W., HERNDL, E. and STOCK, W. (1982) The forearm flap. *Plastic and Reconstructive Surgery*, **70**, 336–342

NAKAMURA, K., NAMBA, K. and TSUCHIDA, H. (1984) A retrospective study of thick split thickness plantar skin grafts to resurface the palm. *Annals of Plastic Surgery*, **12**, 508–513

NASSIF, T. M., VIDAL, L., BOVET, J. L. and BAUDET, J. (1982) The parascapular flap: a new cutaneous microsurgical free flap. *Plastic and Reconstructive Surgery*, **69**, 581–600

OGNURO, O. (1983) Dorsal transposition flap for reconstruction of lateral or medial oblique amputations of the thumb with exposure of bone. *Journal of Hand Surgery*, **8**, 894–898

O'HARE, P. M., LEONARD, A. G. and BRENNAN, M. D. (1983) Experience with the tensor fasciae latae free flap. *British Journal of Plastic Surgery*, **36**, 98–104

OHMORI, K. and HARII, K. (1975) Free groin flaps: their vascular basis. *British Journal of Plastic Surgery*, **28**, 238–246

OHMORI, K. and HARII, K. (1976) Free dorsalis pedis sensory flap to the hand with microneurovascular anastomoses. *Plastic and Reconstructive Surgery*, **58**, 210–213

PAKIAM, A. I. (1978) The reversed dermis flap. *British Journal of Plastic Surgery*, **31**, 131–135

PATTON, H. S. (1969) Split skin grafts from hypothenar area for fingertip avulsions. *Plastic and Reconstructive Surgery*, **43**, 426–429

PHO, R. W. H. (1979) Local composite neurovascular island flap for skin cover in pulp loss of the thumb. *Journal of Hand Surgery*, **4**, 11–15

POSNER, M. A. and SMITH, R. J. (1971) The advancement pedicle flap for thumb injuries. *Journal of Bone and Joint Surgery*, **53A**, 1618–1621

RAE, P. S. and PHO, R. W. H. (1983) The radial transposition flap. A useful composite flap. *The Hand*, **15**, 96–102

REINISCH, J. F., WINTERS, R. and PUCKETT, C. L. (1984) The use of the osteocutaneous flap in gunshot wounds of the hand. *Journal of Hand Surgery*, **9A**, 12–17

ROBINSON, D. W. (1976) Microsurgical transfer of the dorsalis pedis neurovascular island flap. *British Journal of Plastic Surgery*, **29**, 209–213

ROSE, E. H. (1983) Local arterialized island flap coverage of difficult hand defects preserving donor digit sensibility. *Plastic and Reconstructive Surgery*, **72**, 848–857

RYBKA, F. J. and PRATT, F. E. (1979) Thumb recostruction with a sensory flap from the dorsum of the index finger. *Plastic and Reconstructive Surgery*, **64**, 141–144

SANDZEN, S. C. (1982) Dorsal pedical flap for resurfacing a moderate thumb-index web contracture release. *Journal of Hand Surgery*, **7**, 21–24

SANGUINETTI, M. V. (1977) Reconstructive surgery of roller injuries of the hand. *Journal of Hand Surgery*, **2**, 134–140

SANTOS, L. F. (1984) The vascular anatomy and dissection of the free scapular flap. *Plastic and Reconstructive Surgery*, **73**, 599–603

SCHENCK, R. R. and CHEEMA, T. A. (1984) Hypothenar skin grafts for finger-tip reconstruction. *Journal of Hand Surgery*, **9A**, 750–753

SCHLENKER, J. D. (1980) Important considerations in the design and construction of groin flaps. *Annals of Plastic Surgery*, **5**, 353–357

SCHLENKER, J. D., ATASOY, E. and LYON, J. W. (1980) The abdominohypogastric flap – an axial pattern flap for forearm coverage. *The Hand*, **12**, 248–252

SHAH, K. G., GARRETT, J. C. and BUNCKE, H. J. (1979) Free groin flap transfer to the upper extremity. *The Hand*, **11**, 315–320

SHAW, D. T. and PAYNE, R. L. (1946) One stage tubed abdominal flaps. Simple pedicle tubes. *Surgery, Gynaecology and Obstetrics*, **83**, 205–209

SHAW, D. T., LI, C. S., RICHEY, D. G. and NEHIGIAN, S. H. (1973) Interdigital butterfly flap in the hand (the double-opposing Z-plasty). *Journal of Bone and Joint Surgery*, **55A**, 1677–1679

SMITH, P. J. (1982a) A sliding flap to cover dorsal skin defects over the proximal interphalangeal joint. *The Hand*, **14**, 271–278

SMITH, P. J. (1982b) The Y-shaped hypogastric-groin flap. *The Hand*, **14**, 263–270

SMITH, R. C. and FURNAS, D. W. (1976) The hand sandwich. *Plastic and Reconstructive Surgery*, **57**, 351–354

SOUTAR, D. S. and TANNER, N. S. B. (1984) The radial forearm flap in the management of soft tissue injuries of the hand. *British Journal of Plastic Surgery*, **37**, 18–26

STERN, P. J., KREILEIN, J. G. and KLEINERT, H. E. (1983) Neurovascular cutaneous flaps for the management of radiation-induced fingertip dermal necrosis. *Journal of Hand Surgery*, **8**, 88–93

STRANC, M. F. (1973) Severe degloving injury of the upper limb. *The Hand*, **5**, 76–78

STRAUCH, B. and TSUR, H. (1978) Restoration of sensation to the hand by a free neurovascular flap from the first web space of the foot. *Plastic and Reconstructive Surgery*, **62**, 361–367

TAKAMI, H., TAKAHASHI, S. and ANDO, M. (1983) Use of the dorsalis pedis free flap for reconstruction of the hand. *The Hand*, **15**, 173–178

TAYLOR, G. I., CORLETT, R. J. and BOYD, J. B. (1984) The versatile deep inferior epigastric (inferior rectus abdominis) flap. *British Journal of Plastic Surgery*, **37**, 330–350

TAYLOR, G. I. and DANIEL, R. K. (1973) The free flap: composite tissue transfer by microvascular anastomosis. *Australia and New Zealand Journal of Surgery*, **43**, 1–3

THOMPSON, R. V. S. (1977) Closure of skin defects near the proximal interphalangeal joint – with special reference to the patterns of finger circulation. *Plastic and Reconstructive Surgery*, **59**, 77–81

TIMMONS, M. J. (1984) William Harvey revisited: reverse flow through the valves of forearm veins. *Lancet*, 394–395

TSUKADA, S. (1980) Transfer of free skin grafts with a preserved subcutaneous vascular network. *Annals of Plastic Surgery*, **4**, 500–506

URBANIAK, J. R., KOMAN, L. A., GOLDNER, R. D., ARMSTRONG, N. B. and NUNLEY, J. A. (1982) The vascularized cutaneous scapular flap. *Plastic and Reconstructive Surgery*, **69**, 772–778

VENKATASWAMI, R. and SUBRAMANIAN, N. (1980) Oblique triangular flap: a new method of repair for oblique amputations of the fingertip and thumb. *Plastic and Reconstructive Surgery*, **66**, 296–300

WATSON, A. C. H. and McGREGOR, J. C. (1981) The simultaneous use of a groin flap and a tensor fascia lata myocutaneous flap to provide tissue cover for a completely degloved hand. *British Journal of Plastic Surgery*, **34**, 349–352

WESTON, P. A. M. and WALLACE, W. A. (1976) The use of locally based triangular skin flaps for the repair of fingertip injuries. *The Hand*, **8**, 54–58

WOOD, M. B. and IRONS, G. B. (1983) Upper extremity free skin flap transfers: results and utility compared with conventional distant pedicle flaps. *Annals of Plastic Surgery*, **11**, 523–526

WRAY, R. C., WISE, D. M., YOUNG, V. L. and WEEKS, P. M. (1982) The groin flap in severe hand injuries. *Annals of Plastic Surgery*, **9**, 459–462

7
Tendon injuries
J. E. Kutz and D. L. Bennett

INTRODUCTION: STRUCTURE, METABOLISM AND MECHANICAL PROPERTIES

A tendon is a specialized form of connective tissue that links muscle to bone. Primarily its function is to transmit muscular tension into motion and useful work. Secondarily, a tendon eliminates the bulk of muscle from the joint(s) over which it acts, concentrates muscular pull on a small bony insertion, and in some cases allows a muscle to act over several joints with the aid of fibrous pulleys (Elliott, 1965).

Grossly, a tendon is a white cord composed primarily of bundles of collagen (Grant and Prockop, 1972). It is circumferentially surrounded by a thin sheet of fibrous tissue called epitenon. A tendon begins at the muscle–tendon junction where myofibrils interdigitate with fibrils of the tendon (Elliott, 1965). Next it passes through loose areolar connective tissue called paratenon. As it continues distally it courses through potential concavities (wrist and finger joints) where it can change direction. Here the tendon is surrounded by a fibrosseous tunnel and is lined by a synovial membrane. Finally it inserts into bone by passing through four histological zones – tendon, fibrocartilage, mineralized fibrocartilage, and bone (Cooper and Misol, 1970).

The organic components of tendon include collagen, proteoglycans, and elastin. Collagen, the major constituent of tendon, comprises between 75 and 85% of its dry weight (Lowry, Gilligan and Katersky, 1942). The collagen is arranged in bundles running parallel to the longitudinal axis of the tendon until the tendon enters the pulley system. Field (1971) demonstrated at this level that the tendon fibers enter into counter-rotating spirals which help minimize distortion and ischemia in an area where the tendon is subject to high compressive forces. Proteoglycans comprise between 9.2 and 3.5% of the dry weight of tendon (Gillard *et al.*, 1977). Their concentration is greatest in areas of high pressure, that is, the pulley system. Histological examination of the tendon at this level reveals chondrocyte-like cells lying in a matrix which stain metachromatically (suggesting the presence of proteoglycans) (Greenlee, Beckham and Pike, 1975; Lundborg, 1976). Small, poorly developed elastic fibers comprise about 2% of the dry weight of tendon (Lowry, Gilligan and Katersky, 1942). There is no evidence of reticulin in mature tendon (Elliott, 1965).

Tenocytes, the predominant cells, are sparsely distributed among the collagen fibers. They arise from immature mesenchymal cells and during growth produce the bulk of the secreted organic material (Greenlee, Beckham and Pike, 1975). In mature tendon the tenocyte is relatively inactive, with minimal capacity for mitosis or protein synthesis (Weiner and Peacock, 1971). The metabolic rate of tendon is quite low (0.1 µl oxygen/unit weight/h) (Peacock, 1959), and is lower still if the tendon is immobilized (Birdsell, Tustanoff and Lindsay, 1966).

Tensile strength of tendons in adult cadavers carried from 8700 to 18 000 lbs/in^2 (60–124 Pa) (Cronkite, 1936). In an experimental model when the entire muscle–tendon system is loaded, rupture occurs at the musculotendinous junction. When just the tendon–bone system is loaded, rupture occurs at the bony attachment (Welsh, MacNab and Riley, 1971). Clinically, this is borne out as it is rare to see a tendon rupture within its substance as the result of an avulsion injury.

Summary

(1) Tendons are composed primarily of collagen with small amounts of proteoglycan and elastic fibers.
(2) Tenocytes (mature fibroblasts) are the dominate cell and have minimal metabolic activity and limited synthetic capacity.
(3) Tensile strength in adult tendon is quite high.

NUTRITION

As the result of a classical textbook published by Koellicker in 1850, tendons were considered to be avascular. In the early part of the 20th century, Mayer (1916) demonstrated in a series of cadaver injection studies that tendons have a definite blood supply. His basic findings still hold true and have been substantiated by numerous investigators (Edwards, 1946; Brockis, 1953; Peacock, 1959; Smith, 1965; Schatzker and Branemark, 1969; Young and Weeks, 1970; Caplan, Hunter and Merklin, 1975; Lundborg, Myrhage and Rydevik, 1977).

Flexor tendon nutrition can be divided into four zones: the musculotendinous junction, the zone between the musculotendinous junction and the sheath, the zone where the tendon passes through the fibrous flexor sheath, and the zone where the tendon inserts into bone (*Figure 7.1*). Each zone has its own nutritional characteristics and will be discussed in more detail below.

At the musculotendinous junction vessels running within the substance of muscle continue into tendon (Edwards, 1946). In addition to this longitudinal system, there are extrinsic vessels which divide near the junction with one branch going into muscle and the other into tendon (Schatzker and Branemark, 1969). Peacock (1959), using radioisotopes, noted that vessels coming in at the musculotendinous junction supplied only the proximal one-third of tendon.

Moving distally, the tendon passes through a loose, fatty connective tissue, rich in elastic fibers called paratenon (Mayer, 1916; Edwards, 1946; Brockis, 1953; Smith, 1965; *Figure 7.2*). At frequent intervals blood vessels passing through the paratenon enter the tendon and penetrate it or run longitudinally along its surface. Within the tendon the vessels run as a basic unit – a single arteriole and one or two venules (Caplan, Hunter and Merklin, 1975).

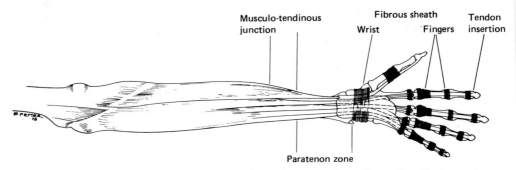

Figure 7.1 Nutritional zones of flexor tendons: the musculotendinous junction, paratenon zone, fibrous sheath, and bony insertion of a flexor tendon. Each have their own nutritional characteristics

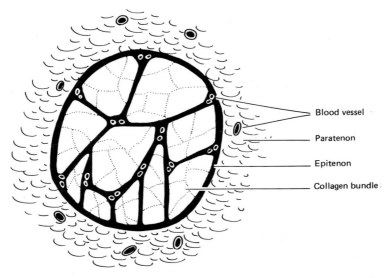

Figure 7.2 Cross-section of tendon in paratenon zone: paratenon is loose areolar connective tissue carrying blood vessels which nourish a tendon

As the flexor tendons pass over the wrist and finger joints their course changes direction and they enter a potential concavity. Anterior displacement of the tendons (bowstringing) during flexion is prevented by the transverse carpal ligament (at the wrist) and a fibrous sheath (over the fingers). Surrounding the tendons at this level is a synovial membrane containing fluid which is a proteinaceous dialysate of blood plasma. Synovial fluid lubricates and nourishes the tendon. In this zone, tendon nutrition comes from *two* sources – synovial fluid and blood vessels (*Figure 7.3*).

Within the sheath, *extrinsic* tendon blood supply comes in through the vincula (Brockis, 1953; Zancolli, 1968; Leffert, Weiss and Athanasoulis, 1974; Lundborg, Myrhage and Rydevik, 1977), filmy condensations of synovium containing blood

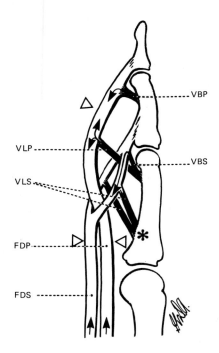

VBP

VLP

VBS

VLS

FDP

FDS

Figure 7.3 Main vascular supply of tendons in the flexor digital sheaths. Vascular inflow is indicated by arrows, and the poorly vascularized segments are indicated by triangles. The inconstant vinculum longus of the superficialis is shown by an asterisk. (From Kleinert, Stillwell and Netscher, 1985)

vessels which arise from one or both of the digital arteries. The vincula brevia (two in number) are constant. The proximal vinculum brevis supplies the superficial flexor, arises from the neck of the proximal phalanx and inserts into the dorsal surface of the tendon just proximal to its insertion into the middle phalanx. The distal vinculum brevis supplies the deep flexor and arises from the volar surface of the neck of the middle phalanx and inserts into the dorsal surface of the tendon just proximal to its insertion into the base of the distal phalanx.

The vinculum longus, which supplies the profundus tendon, is more slender and variable in location. Most commonly it is an extension of the proximal vinculum brevis and inserts into the dorsal surface of the overlying profundus tendon at the level of the proximal interphalangeal joint (Carter and Mersheimer, 1966).

In addition to the vincular system, Lundborg has demonstrated an *intrinsic* microvascular system arising from synovial vessels and from longitudinal vessels originating in the palm (Lundborg, Myrhage and Rydevik, 1977).

Thus, within the fibrous flexor sheath, there are two systems of blood supply – the extrinsic vincular and intrinsic systems. Despite this seemingly abundant blood supply, vessels are sparse and the volar 1 mm (a third to a quarter the thickness of the tendon) is avascular (Chaplin, 1973; Lundborg, Myrhage and Rydevik, 1977; *Figure 7.4*). In addition, because of the segmental nature of the blood supply, there are watershed zones which are virtually avascular (Young and Weeks, 1970; Lundborg, Myrhage and Rydevik, 1977). An experimental study with baboon tendons revealed a scant vascular system in the intact tendon with relatively avascular areas. Following injury, however, vascular dilatation occurs along the tendon and the vincula and significantly contributes to the intrinsic healing capability of the tendon (DeKlerk and Jonck, 1982). Clinically, when dealing with a

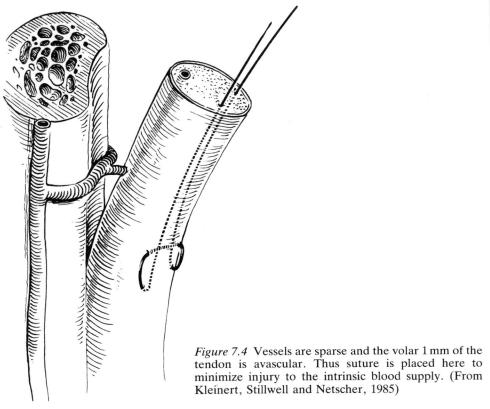

Figure 7.4 Vessels are sparse and the volar 1 mm of the tendon is avascular. Thus suture is placed here to minimize injury to the intrinsic blood supply. (From Kleinert, Stillwell and Netscher, 1985)

flexor tendon laceration within the sheath, one should strive to preserve the vincula and to place suture material in the volar (avascular) portion of the tendon to avoid strangulating more dorsally located vessels.

The fourth zone of the tendon nutrition is at the insertion of tendon into bone. Here periosteal vessels penetrate the tendon.

Synovial fluid is also important in tendon nutrition, particularly in the volar avascular zone and in the relatively avascular watershed areas of the tendon. Though the exact role of synovial fluid in the nutrition of human tendons is not established, investigators have shown experimentally that devascularized tendons remain viable if they stay in contact with synovial fluid (Eiken, Lundborg and Rank, 1975; Matthews, 1976; Lundborg, Myrhage and Rydevik, 1977; McDowell and Snyder, 1977; Lundborg and Rank, 1978; Manske, Whiteside and Lesker, 1978; Manske, Birdwell and Lesker, 1978; Manske *et al.*, 1978; Lundborg and Rank, 1978; Lundborg, Holm and Myrhage, 1980; Lundborg *et al.*, 1980; Manske and Lesker, 1982, 1983). Metabolites from the synovial fluid diffuse into the tendon. In the dog and rabbit diffusion may be the principal source of tendon nutrition within the digital sheath, while in chickens and primates perfusion and diffusion are both important (Manske and Lesker, 1983). During tendon surgery, many authors believe the sheath should be preserved (Lundborg, Myrhage and Rydevik, 1977).

Using a variety of animal models and *in vitro* experiments, several investigators have found that tendons have an intrinsic potential to heal (Lowry, Gilligan and Katersky, 1942; Lindsay and Thomson, 1959; Lundborg, 1976; McDowell and Snyder, 1977) and Thomson found when studying chickens that the epitenon was the most proliferative structure in the repair process and the sheath contributed very little (Lindsay and Thomson, 1959). A second line of evidence supporting intrinsic tendon healing comes from two groups of investigators who preserved the integrity of the sheath by retracting the profundus tendon proximal to the sheath, partially dividing it, and then the tendon was allowed to go into the sheath (Matthews and Richards, 1974, 1975; McDowell and Snyder, 1977). The animals were serially sacrificed and it was found that tendons healed in the absence of adhesions or vascular ingrowth from the surrounding sheath. Thus, Matthews and Richards (1975) proposed that tendon repaired with suture and held immobilized allowing extrinsic healing produced the greatest adhesion formation as per Potenza's (1962) study. They felt that in his study suturing the tendon and the injury to the sheath necessary to join the tendons together so compromised tendon nutrition that the cells, even if they survived, were unable to participate in the repair. Lundborg (1976) divided and repaired rabbit flexor tendon and then placed the repaired tendon in the knee joint. Not only did the tendon survive (presumably through synovial nutrition) but the juncture healed and resisted rupture. It was concluded that the tenoblasts secreted collagen which bridged the repair. In subsequent investigation Lundborg found that surrounding the repaired tendon by a dialyzing membrane to prevent cell seeding from the synovium impeded fibroplasm of the superficial layer only slightly, and the tendon still possessed the ability to heal this layer and bridge the suture gap.

In 1984 Manske and his associates demonstrated histological and biochemical evidence of viability and repair of whole tendon segments of four different animals (Gelberman *et al.*, 1984; Manske and Lesker, 1984a, 1984b; Manske *et al.*, 1984). They provided biochemical evidence for an increase in the number of tendon cells, increased collagen production and the incorporation of labelled prolene into the tendon. They also observed phagocytosis and differentiation of fibroblasts from the epitenon of culture rabbit tendons while the endotenon was the primary source of collagen synthesis. Becker demonstrated that the cells from culture chicken tendons contained fibroblast that could proliferate, migrate into a defect in the tendon and synthesize collagen. All of these studies indicate the importance of intrinsic healing from the tendon. Though controversial, the value of maintaining a synovial environment to support the diffusional pathways of tendon nutrition is implied.

There exists a third school of investigators who have found tendon repair to be a combination of extrinsic (peritendinous tissue) and intrinsic (tenoblastic) healing. In 1932 Mason and Shearon published a monumental work on tendon repair. Using dogs, they noted that at five days postrepair the sheath had produced a fibroblastic bridge between the tendon similar to fracture callus. At 2–3 weeks postrepair the extrinsic 'callus' remodelled to allow for tendon gliding while tenocytes began to proliferate allowing for intrinsic healing. Flynn and Graham (1962, 1965), studying dogs, had similar findings.

Peripheral adhesions are present in many clinical repairs. They may represent extrinsic fibroblastic activity necessary for tendon healing, an inflammatory response not involved in the healing process or even an extension from the intrinsic healing process to the periphery (Manske *et al.*, 1984). In most clinical situations healing probably involves both mechanisms to varying degrees.

TENSILE STRENGTH DURING TENDON HEALING

Regardless of the technique and suture material used in tenorrhaphy, tensile strength over a period of time follows a characteristic pattern (Mason and Allen, 1941; Urbaniak, Cahill and Mortenson, 1975). Over the first 3–5 days there is a rapid diminution in tensile strength because the tendon ends soften. For the next 5–7 days there is a slow increase in strength, although the tendon ends are still soft and subject to rupture if a longitudinal stress is applied. Thereafter, tensile strength increases more rapidly, particularly if there is protected mobilization.

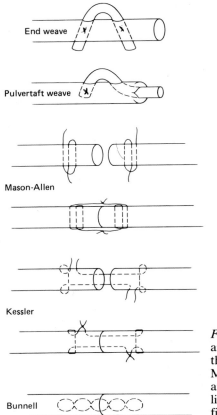

End weave

Pulvertaft weave

Mason-Allen

Kessler

Bunnell

Figure 7.5 Types of tenorrhaphies: the Pulvertaft and end weave are strong but cannot be used where the tendon passes through a narrow sheath. The Mason–Allen, Kessler and Bunnell tenorrhaphies are not as strong but allow gliding through regions of limited space such as the carpal tunnel and fibrous finger flexor sheaths

Urbaniak found stainless steel to be the strongest suture material available and the tensile strength of all suture material was diminished by knotting and manipulation. End-weave and fish-mouth produced the strongest tenorrhaphies and were recommended for areas where there is paratenon. The Mason–Allen, Bunnell, and Kessler repairs (where initial strength is dependent upon the strength of the suture material itself) are moderately strong and were recommended for areas of limited space (*Figure 7.5*).

PRINCIPLES OF PRIMARY REPAIR

Repair of divided flexor tendons in zone 2 was for years regarded as contraindicated. The term 'no man's land' was applied because of the dismal results at that time surrounding primary repair. The experienced hand surgeons preferred to perform delayed tendon grafting (Bunnell, 1922; Boyes, 1950; Rank and Wakefield, 1950; Pulvertaft, 1956, 1958; Bunnell, 1964; Boyes, 1971; Boyes and Slack, 1971; Verdan, 1972).

The advantages of tendon grafting were that a fresh surgeon would be electively performing the procedure with a fresh team. There was no anastomosis within the flexor digital sheath, only the smooth surface of a tendon graft. The clinical parts of the procedure were performed in accessible areas – namely the distal pulp and the palm. Pulvertaft and Boyes reported a success rate of 70–80% with secondary grafting (Boyes, 1950; Rank and Wakefield, 1951; Pulvertaft, 1956). This includes patients who were able to flex to within 2.5 cm of the distal palmar crease and who had less than 40° combined interphalangeal joint restriction of extension. To achieve this they stressed the importance of a supple hand, gentle surgery, and a cooperative patient. However, these excellent results were not always achieved by other surgeons. Problems such as joint stiffness, lack of active range of motion, inability to fully extend the finger due to short grafts, cold intolerance, and sensory impairment all detracted from the results of tendon grafting. This pessimism yielded to faint optimism as Verdan (1960), Kleinert, Kutz *et al.* (1967) championed a return to primary repair.

The advent of new suture techniques and materials enabling strong, non-reactive anastomoses, the improved general availability of technically competent hand surgeons, the increased use of magnification by those performing the repair with the associated use of finer instruments, and especially the use of early motion following repair, contributed to the increasingly successful use of primary tendon repair.

Zone 2 – 'no man's land'

Zone 2 is that portion of the fibrosseous digital canal which is occupied by both flexor tendons. It extends from the proximal edge of the A4 pulley. Within this area the profundus and superficialis tendons interweave in a complex and close relationship. Minimal swelling of their epitenon is sufficient to impair free motion of both tendons. The tendons are like a piston entering the cylindrical fibrosseous canal, but with an even finer clearance. The margin for error in tendon repair is thus very small in this region. Only meticulous technique, minimal operative trauma, and precise anastomosis will result in the restoration of the tendon's gliding function. It was common practice in the past to excise portions of the flexor sheath in the belief that it was an impediment to the ingrowth of tissue from the surrounding elements that was necessary for healing (Potenza, 1962). The use of early mobilization partially negated this argument as only flimsy adhesions form between the sheath and tendon injury site. Current evidence indicates that the synovial fluid and sheath are important in tendon nutrition and should be preserved to improve healing (Lundborg, 1976; Manske, Whiteside and Lesker, 1978; Lundborg and Rank, 1980; Lundborg, Holm and Myrhage, 1980; Lundborg *et al.*, 1980; Lister, 1983). Eiken has recommended the incision and closure of tendon sheath during primary repair (Eiken *et al.*, 1980). Its closure following tenorrhaphy may significantly contribute to the retention of fluid, thus aiding in gliding as well as nutrition. With this in mind, exploration and opening of the sheath should be approached in such a fashion as to allow reconstruction following repair.

Zone 2, like zone 1, may be subdivided into two areas: a proximal area with rigid unyielding A1 and A2 pulleys making access to divided tendons difficult; and a distal area with a soft, pliable roof in the region of A3, A5 pulleys and cruciate fibers. The distal area provides easy access to divided tendons and the digital sheath may be opened as a laterally based L or funnel-shaped trapdoor.

Proximally the A1 pulley can be divided and left unrepaired if necessary. It is nearly impossible to repair a longitudinal incision in the A2 and A4 pulleys because of their close approximation to the underlying tendon. This should be avoided. The areas between the A2 and A4 pulleys and distal to the A4 pulley are selected for exposure to the injured tendon.

Between the A1 and A4 pulleys the tendons are in complex relationship to one another. Entering the proximal end of the digital sheath, the flat and wide superficialis is volar to the wider profundus. At the distal end of the A2 pulley the superficialis has split into two halves, which spiral around and deep to the profundus to join up in a chiasm at the level of the proximal interphalangeal joint and the volar plate. Half of the fibers from each superficialis slip decussate and join the remaining fibers of the other slip. Both slips continue distally to be inserted on to bony ridges along the sides of the volar aspect of the middle phalanx. The distal limit of the insertion is at the level of the A4 pulley. A double long vinculum with its attendant blood supply enters the superficialis chiasm at its proximal end, with a short vinculum originating in the area of the volar pouch of the proximal interphalangeal joint entering at the distal edge of the chiasm. From this a long vinculum to the profundus takes origin.

Thus, within zone 2, a simple laceration can produce much damage. Not only may the tendons and sheath be divided, but also the vinculae providing blood supply to the tendons. The volar plates or pouches may be opened. Division of the vinculae has three effects on tendon repair:

(1) tendon nutrition and healing is impaired;
(2) bleeding into the digital sheath can lead on to granulation tissue and subsequent fibrosis, producing firm unyielding adhesions; and
(3) loss of the restraining effect of the intact vinculae allows retraction of the tendon ends.

Another less frequently observed effect can be noted by those who perform delayed primary repairs. If the tendon is lacerated at a site far removed from a vinculum, its end becomes rounded off and remains lying free within the digital sheath. However, in cases where the tendon is lacerated close to its vinculum, granulation tissue can creep into the tendon end from the site of vincular damage and cause the tendon stump to adhere to the digital sheath. This prejudices the result of a delayed primary or secondary repair.

The complexity of zone 2 provides the surgeon attempting primary repair with many problems. The proximal area makes access difficult; the superficialis is flat and is technically difficult to suture, and there is little room to spare for gliding of a swollen repair site. In addition, a satisfactory pulley must be retained. The distal area is more susceptible to injury, being covered by less subcutaneous tissue and having a more flimsy roof in the digital sheath. Here damage to the vinculae and volar plate may complicate the issue. Such problems require the highest standards of surgical technique to obtain good results and should only be undertaken by those who are well trained in hand surgery (Mason, 1940; Rank and Wakefield, 1950, 1951; Kelley, 1959; Kleinert *et al.*, 1967; McFarlane, Lamon and Jarvis, 1968; Kessler and Missim, 1969; Kessler, 1973; Kleinert *et al.*, 1973; Green and Niebauer, 1974; Jenson and Weibly, 1974; Kutz and Cohen, 1975; Lister *et al.*, 1977; Ejeskar, 1980a, 1980b; Earley and Milward, 1982).

TECHNIQUE

In achieving good results with primary repair, certain principles must be adhered to. The wound should be a clean cut laceration with no crushing element and should be less than six hours old. Many will attempt repair even in less ideal circumstances. In the series of 156 severed flexor tendons reviewed by Lister *et al.* (1977), contamination was not a contraindication to primary repair provided the wounds were thoroughly irrigated with Ringer's lactate and 0.5% neomycin sulphate solution within six hours after injury.

Exposure should be kept to the minimum required for suture of the tendon ends. The wound usually needs only to be extended in a distal direction to retrieve the distal end, and extension should follow well-established principles of exposure in the hand. We prefer the Bruner technique to a midlateral approach. If the fingers were straight at the time of injury the site of tendon division will be directly deep to the wound. If the fingers were grasping the object which severed them, the site of the distal tendon end may be as much as the full excursion of the tendon, distal to the wound (up to 4.5 cm). Proximal extension of the wound may be necessary to retrieve the proximal end if the injury was sustained with the fingers in extension or if violent muscular contraction was occurring at the time of division, and the tendon has retracted proximal to a nearby pulley.

The tendon ends should be delivered in an atraumatic fashion and handled similarly. The outside surface should not be grasped or touched, and fine instruments should be used to grip the core of the divided tendon. The distal end may be delivered by flexion of the interphalangeal joints beyond the wound, and the proximal end by flexing the wrist and milking the palm or even using an Esmarch bandage. More often than not some form of tendon retriever has to be used proximally. A no. 25 gauge hypodermic needle is then used to retain the delivered tendon ends in the absence of tension.

A strong suture of 4-0 non-absorbable, non-reactive, braided material should be used. The heavier braided synthetics have the advantage of being easier to hold and knots are suitable. Extreme caution should be exercised in order to avoid damaging the suture material as it is upon its integrity that the suture junction will rely. In the series from Louisville a modified Bunnell suture was employed, although since that time two of the authors have changed to using a Kessler modification of the Mason–Allen technique in the belief that a better grip is obtained. Urbaniak's studies have shown that, although the Bunnell and Kessler sutures have the same strength initially, this is not so later when the Kessler suture retains up to three times the strength of the Bunnell suture during the healing phase (Urbaniak, Cahill and Mortenson, 1975). It also prevents loss of the suture material to the surrounding sheath and buries the knot in the central core of the tendon. A criss-cross type of suture may jeopardize the vascularity of the tendon ends. The Kessler suture, if used, should be inserted toward the volar surface of the tendon as the main vessels lie more dorsally. Whichever technique is used it is important to obtain a good grip on both tendon ends so that the inevitable subsequent softening of the two ends does not reduce the grasp of the holding suture. At least 3 cm of each end should be grasped by the suture. The suture should be inserted loosely so that there is no bunching up of the grasped ends. In tendons with bunched-up anastomoses, the resulting increased diameter may seriously impair the gliding ability of the tendon junction.

Lister (1983) has outlined good guidelines for determining where to open the sheath following exposure (*Figure 7.6*). If the tendon is located beneath the A2 or A4 pulley the finger is flexed to see how much of the tendon can be exposed proximal to the dense annular pulley. If 1 cm can be exposed the entire repair can

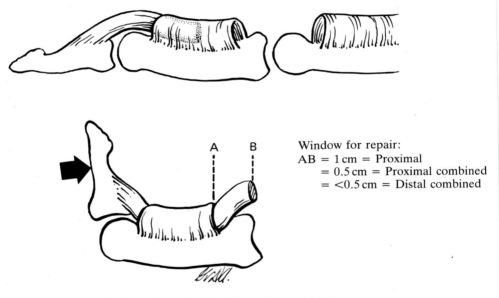

Window for repair:
AB = 1 cm = Proximal
   = 0.5 cm = Proximal combined
   = <0.5 cm = Distal combined

Figure 7.6 Flexor tendon sheath incision (From Lister, 1983)

be accomplished in a rectangular window proximal to the annular pulley. If only 0.5–1 cm can be exposed a window must be opened distal to the annular pulley and the first half of the core stitch passed through the distal tendon in this window with the remainder of the repair accomplished in the proximal window. If less than 0.5 cm can be produced through the proximal window the first pass of the core suture must be passed through the proximal portion of this tendon with the remainder of the repair accomplished through a distal window.

Following placement of the core stitch, a careful running 'epitenon' suture of 6-0 nylon or Tircon will ensure a smooth external surface within the anastomotic site. This prevents the dangers of frayed everted edges catching and perhaps splitting the tendon longitudinally. Each bite of the running suture should grasp only about

1 mm of the tendon surface and may be converted to a Lembert suture to ensure absence of everted edges. The tendon should be rotated to allow the deep surface to be similarly sutured. Following this, a running suture of 6-0 or 7-0 absorbable suture is used to repair the sheath.

This technique is easily applied to the profundus, but the flattened superficialis is more difficult to deal with. It should be repaired if divided and where it lies deep to the profundus a figure-of-eight suture with the knot adjacent to bone is more effective than the previously described technique. An epitenon suture to smooth out the volar surface is still of value.

Prior to approximating the tendon after the core stitch, the tourniquet is released to study the intrinsic blood supply. The availability of intrinsic bleeding can be beneficial in postoperative care. If adequate supply is present in both the distal and proximal ends of the tendon, primary healing will usually take place in 3–4 weeks. If the blood supply is present in either the distal or proximal tendon ends, healing will require a period of 4–6 weeks. When the laceration lies in the watershed area, healing requires 8–10 weeks. Postoperative management will be controlled by these factors.

Preservation of the pulley system during the initial exposure, particularly the A2 and A4 pulleys, prevents the development of bowstringing which reduces grip strength and tendon excursion. Careful closure of the sheath will reduce the chances of the anastomosis catching on it, and improve nutrition.

After completion of the tenorrhaphy and sheath repair it is particularly important to put the repaired tendon through a full range of passive movement, holding the wrist flexed while doing so. This shows the tendon's ability to glide freely within the tendon sheath and reassures the surgeon that there is no anatomical obstruction to smooth tendon function subsequently.

Before closure of the wound meticulous hemostasis is achieved. A bipolar coagulator is useful here. The wound is irrigated, all clots removed, and the skin closed with 6-0 nylon suture.

The fingers are left free of any constricting dressing from the distal palmar crease to the fingertips in order to allow early active extension against the resistance of a dynamic elastic splint. This form of controlled mobilization is commenced immediately when the patient has recovered from the effects of axillary block anesthesia or general anesthesia. The rubber bands are attached to the fingernails by a double loop of 2-0 suture. The position of the wrist and fingers within the splint is best achieved by holding the arm above the elbow and allowing the wrist to flex with the forearm pronated. In this position the hand falls naturally into the correct position for the dorsal plaster splint. This should extend from the fingertips to the proximal forearm, being well molded around either side of the wrist. The wrist should be in 20° less than full flexion, and the fingers should be capable of full interphalangeal extension, with a 40° block to full metacarpophalangeal extension. The splint is retained in position by both a Kling and an elastic bandage. The dynamic elastic bands are passed through safety pins in the palm and attached at the mid-forearm (*Figure 7.7*). The elastic bands should be tight enough to passively flex the interphalangeal joints but lax enough to allow full interphalangeal extension. Thus, during the first few days postoperatively, they may require daily adjustment; 20 min spent with the patient during each of the early postoperative days may well save 20 weeks later. It is at this time that the results are obtained, and it is usually possible to predict with accuracy which patients will do well within 72 hours following surgery.

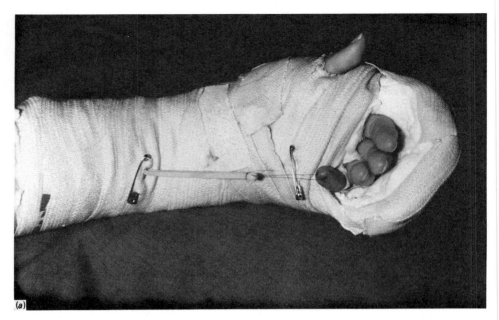

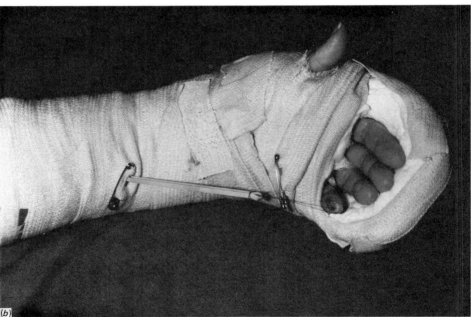

Figure 7.7(a) and (*b*) Following flexor tendon repair the patient is placed in a dorsal plaster splint from the fingertips to the proximal forearm, allowing full interphalangeal extension with a 40° block to full metacarpophalangeal extension. The splint is held in place by both a Kling and an elastic bandage. The rubber band traction attached at the palm and mid-forearm should allow the patient to passively flex the interphalangeal joints, but be lax enough to allow full interphalangeal extension

During the first three weeks the patient is encouraged to actively extend the fingers until they touch the plaster splint. They then relax and allow the dynamic bands to return their fingers to a resting position of interphalangeal flexion. It is at this stage that flexion contractures of the proximal interphalangeal joints should be avoided by checking that these joints are being fully extended during the active extension exercises. If this is not occurring then a metacarpophalangeal extension block should be inserted to ensure that all the extension force is transmitted to the proximal interphalangeal joints. If a lack of full extension is noted at the distal interphalangeal joint the dynamic elastic may be shifted proximal to this joint with a splint to prevent contracture.

Splintage is discarded at 3–6 weeks depending upon the intrinsic blood supply at the repair site. The anastomosis is still protected for two more weeks. The wrist is free but dynamic elastics remain attached to the wrist. Active extension and passive flexion are continued. At five weeks, active unresisted flexion is commenced. Flexion against resistance may be commenced at six weeks, but passive extension should be avoided until eight weeks postoperatively. At this stage a joint jack at night and a Capener during the day can be used to correct any tendency towards a flexion contracture.

ELECTROMYOGRAPHIC (EMG) STUDIES OF DYNAMIC SPLINTAGE

This technique of early controlled mobilization was introduced to enable the repaired tendon to acquire only the flimsy type of adhesions during its healing phase. Thus, movement would be unrestricted and any adhesions forming would be so flimsy that their rupture would occur upon full use of the digit concerned. During active extension there is no tension on the anastomotic site in the flexor tendon. If EMG probes are inserted into the profundus bellies and the belly of the extensor digitorum communis, and the muscular activity occurring during the use of the splint is studied, tracings show absence of activity in the profundus during active finger extension. Contraction of one group of muscles against resistance promotes simultaneous relaxation of their antagonists. These studies were performed by Lister *et al.* (1977).

Principles of the technique

The essential criteria of this technique are:

 (1) Avoid tension during repair and mobilization.
 (2) Performed only if there is a clean, incised wound.
 (3) Atraumatic surgical technique.
 (4) Fine instrumentation and magnification.
 (5) Appropriate suture material.
 (6) Meticulous restoration of tendon continuity and gliding function.
 (7) Meticulous hemostasis.
 (8) Maintain pulleys and close the sheath.
 (9) Immediate controlled mobilization.
(10) A technically proficient surgeon.

If they are followed, good or excellent results should be obtained in 80% of patients. Both tendons should be repaired when both are divided.

Primary repair is not a new technique. Bunnell reported his results in 1947. His suture at a distance was an attempt to overcome some of the problem. Subsequent reports gave details of poor range of motion (Kelly, 1959). The technique was abandoned in favor of tendon grafting until Verdan (1960, 1972) developed a technique of primary repair using a proximal blocking transfixation pin which allowed for a tension-free anastomosis immobilized for three weeks. These results were as good as those obtained by Boyes and Pulvertaft using grafting techniques. However, primary repair returned the patient to work in a much shorter period of time than tendon grafting. Kleinert (Kleinert, Kutz and Cohen, 1975; Kleinert *et al.*, 1967, 1973) introduced early controlled active mobilization following primary repair. We feel this has been instrumental in the successful management of these injuries. We now believe that primary repair even in less than ideal circumstances accompanied by subsequent tenolysis gives results equal to or better than tendon grafts and shortens the period of time that the patient is incapacitated. In this respect, it is interesting to note that Fetrow (1967) reported an incidence of tenolysis of 16% of grafted patients.

We feel that postoperative mobilization is necessary to achieve good results in primary tendon repair in zone 2. Mobilization may also be achieved by the technique popularized by Duran (Duran and Houser, 1975). They mobilize first the proximal then the distal interphalangeal joint through passive extension. Complete extension is prevented by a splint. The independent extension not only prevents adhesions from the surrounding tissue but also moves the injured tendons away from each other. This is done ten times in two to three sessions per day early following the repair under the supervision of an occupational therapist. Active extension is permitted at five weeks and active flexion the following week. Duran's results are unexcelled. Strickland and Glogovac, 1980, in repairing 50 consecutive digits in 37 patients, used the method described by Duran in 25 digits, and compared the results with 25 digits treated by 3½ weeks of immobilization followed by a program of gradually increasing motion. In the immobilization group, there were four ruptures (16%), no excellent results, 12% good results, 28% fair and 44% poor. In the early mobilization group there were 86% excellent, 20% good, 26% fair and 24% poor results. All procedures were performed by one surgeon.

The beneficial effects of stress and motion on tendon function have been demonstrated in a number of experimental and clinical studies (Hernandez *et al.*, 1967; Kessler and Missim, 1969; Furlow, 1972; Kleinert *et al.*, 1973; Duran and Houser, 1975; Matthews and Richards, 1976; Gelberman *et al.*, 1980; Strickland and Glogovac, 1980). Recently Gelberman *et al.* (1982) have demonstrated experimentally that early mobilized tendons in dogs have improved strength as demonstrated by greater ultimate failure load, increased angular rotation and linear excursion when compared to delayed mobilization or immobilized animals. They also demonstrated that early controlled passive motion improves the quality of the biological repair response by stimulating intrinsic healing and restoring the gliding surfaces when compared to the immobilized group (Gelberman *et al.*, 1983).

In some cases of contaminated lacerations due to biological materials, for example in the use of a butcher's knife where there is a large inoculum of gram-negative aerobic and anaerobic bacilli, we may rest the digits for the first week and commence mobilization when it is apparent that the wound has settled without infection. We have on occasion mobilized these hands immediately but usually have regretted it. These patients will benefit from the use of one of the cephalosporins, which are administered when the patient is seen in the emergency room, and continued postoperatively. Admission to the hospital, bedrest, and elevation with the use of intravenous antibiotics is on occasion a wise precaution.

Our approach to tendon injuries in 'no man's land' could be summarized as follows.

In fresh wounds, whether simple or complex, primary repair should be attempted unless there is substantial tissue loss requiring a graft for tendon reconstruction, skin flap coverage, and nerve and arterial grafts. In wounds up to 4 weeks old end-to-end tendon repair can be attempted. If at exploration this proves impossible, a tendon graft can be used. In older injuries a graft is the procedure of choice. If the injury is old and complex with a grossly disturbed fibrosseous tunnel, then two-stage tendon grafting is indicated.

DELAYED PRIMARY OR SECONDARY REPAIRS

Mark Iselin (1958) pointed out that nothing would be lost by thoroughly preparing a patient for tenorrhaphy at a time when a fresh and experienced team was available to work under more ideal circumstances. He introduced the concept of the 'delayed emergency' (Carter and Mersheimer, 1966; Madesen, 1970; Salui, 1971). A primary repair is one that is prepared within 24 h of injury. A delayed primary repair is one that is performed up to the time that the wound edges can no longer be bluntly separated (about two weeks). In an early secondary repair the wound has healed and must be incised. This period extends until about five weeks following the repair. The results of delayed primary and early secondary repair should be equivalent to primary repair. This concept of delayed primary or secondary repair is not applied to superficial wounds, hemorrhages, dislocations or displaced fractures. When viability is questioned, exploration needs to be immediate. One finding of particular interest was the fact that crushed wound edges were fit for closure in 56 out of 71 cases after an appropriate delay. Certainly immediate closure might create tension and cause more skin loss in some such cases. Infection did not present a problem. Iselin leaves the wound open after thorough cleaning and repairs the tendons up to three weeks after injury. Other authors, including Schneider and Hunter (1975), prefer to close the wound after cleansing and repair the tendons up to three weeks after injury. They reported 25 patients with 31 flexor injuries involving both tendons in 'no man's land'. In their review, 68% achieved a total active range of motion exceeding 200°; 26% were regarded as failures and 20% later required tenolysis. There were no wound complications. Tsuge, Ikuta and Matsuishi (1977) found no effect on results of delay up to 90 days following trauma. Ejeskar (1980a) found no detriment of delay up to 30 days. After that, the delay had a negative effect on the outcome of the repair. Other authors have found primary repair superior to secondary repair.

It is our experience that the greatest value of this technique is where a suitable team is unavailable for primary repair. It means that in less well-staffed and equipped peripheral hospitals, wounds may simply be cleansed, irrigated, closed, and then the patients referred to a centre that specializes in hand surgery. In this way, many more patients than before will be able to benefit from the advantages of primary repair (Arkin and Siffert, 1953; Iselin, 1958; Carter and Wersheimer, 1966; Madesen, 1970; Salvi, 1971).

Zone 1

Zone 1 extends from the distal insertion of the profundus to the site of the superficialis insertion. Verdan divides it into a proximal area beneath the A4 pulley in which lies the profundus alone and a distal area over the volar aspect of the distal interphalangeal joint with a roof of thin synovial tissue. Injuries at this level may be sharply incised wounds or due to hyperextension avulsion injuries.

Tendon interruption in zone 1 diminishes grip strength and abolishes active distal interphalangeal flexion. Pinch is weakened. With strong attempted pinch the distal interphalangeal joint will give way and the fingertip becomes hyperextended. Occasionally a retracted profundus stump may produce mechanical blockage of the superficialis, restricting full flexion of the finger. The retraction of the profundus may cause the production of a lumbrical plus finger (Littler, 1960; White, 1960; Parkes, 1971). Loss of profundus function may cause painful hyperextension of the distal interphalangeal joint with grip. In the little finger the superficialis is often absent and injury to the profundus produces a finger incapable of active flexion.

Clean wounds more than 1–1.5 cm from the profundus insertion are suitable for primary repair and provide the best results. They are accomplished as already described. Surgery here is difficult technically due to the A4 pulley. If a sharp laceration has been sustained in flexion, the distal end may be well clear of the A4 pulley, but the proximal end may have retracted proximal to it. Thus, delivery of the proximal stump may be exceedingly difficult, requiring opening of the sheath proximally as a trapdoor based laterally with sacrifice of the A3 pulley. Only in extremely difficult cases may the A4 pulley, normally 10 mm in length, be shortened to 5 mm without adverse effect on function. However, because of the obvious technical difficulties that tendon division at this level present, some surgeons would advance the profundus if the division is within 1.5 cm of the insertion to the distal phalanx, at the midpoint of the distal phalanx. This technique will eliminate the suture line from the fibrosseous canal. Any advancement exceeding this will most likely produce inability to fully extend the interphalangeal joints. Some of the distal profundus stump may require resection to prevent a bulky obstruction to the A4 pulley causing inability to fully flex the distal interphalangeal joint.

The surgical technique of advancement is not difficult. The wound is enlarged, the proximal stump delivered and retained in the wound by the use of a Keith needle. A 4-0 Prolene or steel suture on a double needle is inserted into the tendon in a lazy loop fashion, obtaining at least 2 cm of tendon in the grasp of the suture. A distal osteoperiosteal flap is raised from the volar surface of the distal phalanx. The proximal stump is placed deep to this and retained in place by passing the ends of the suture around either side of the distal phalanx and out through the nail distal to the lunula. Here it is tied over a button. The osteoperiosteal flap is sutured over the site of the tendon insertion and to the tendon, using 5-0 braided, non-absorbable suture.

Occasionally patients will present late following a zone 1 injury whether it be due to a laceration or an avulsion. In such cases the profundus has often retracted far proximally along the finger. The tendon ends may be frayed and adherent with the opportunity for delayed secondary repair or tendon advancement having both been lost. If the bed within the fibrosseous tunnel is reasonable, tendon grafting could be performed. Tendon grafting in the presence of an intact superficialis is an extremely difficult procedure. Although some good results have been reported, often the effort is not justified. Many authors have advised against the procedure.

Certain patients require active motion at the distal interphalangeal joint. This includes those involved in crafts involving the molding of soft substances as in pottery, or the fingering of keys as in playing musical instruments or typing. In well-motivated, young patients with such demands, it may be justifiable to graft through the intact superficialis. Fibrosis and collapse of the fibrosseous tunnel may necessitate two-stage tendon grafting using a silicone rod. This can be successful in most patients. Occasionally, a patient will present with poor distal interphalangeal joint motion (less than 30°). It is essential to achieve virtually full range of passive motion prior to tendon grafting. This may require a superficialis tenolysis with the insertion of a rod followed by vigorous passive and active exercises until a supple finger is achieved. If the superficialis is involved in extensive scar tissue, and poor proximal interphalangeal joint movement persists despite intensive physiotherapy and surgery, then it may have to be resected prior to the insertion of a rod. However, in these cases the superficialis has almost certainly been damaged itself. The surgeon must never sacrifice an intact undamaged superficialis.

For patients who will put less stress on the active use of their distal interphalangeal joints, some sort of stabilizing procedure may be adequate even though there will be some loss of grip strength and dexterity. These procedures should be regarded as salvage measures where the profundus cannot be repaired and when the superficialis is strong and provides 90° of the proximal interphalangeal flexion. The methods available are tenodesis or capsulodesis, which retain the ability for passive distal interphalangeal flexion by the adjacent digits, or fusion of the joint in slight flexion.

Closed avulsion of the profundus from its insertion

The profundus insertion is complex and extensive. Often such avulsions occur in sports where an opponent's jersey is grasped at high speed. The profundus has superficial and deep bands. The deep fibers are inserted centrally and the superficial fibers fan out to be inserted laterally. The attachment is spread out along the proximal half of the phalanx and the proximal insertion is limited by a transverse ridge which acts as a fulcrum over which the tendon gains increased mechanical advantage. The fibers may simply be avulsed, in other words, stripped off their insertion, or may detach a portion of bone, producing an avulsion fracture.

Robins and Dobyns (1975) point out that when the deep fibers are avulsed with bone, the fragment is usually large; with the superficialis fibers the fragment is small and laterally placed. Multiple fragments indicate avulsion of all the fibers. Bohler (cited in Carroll and Metch, 1970) has noted that 50% of avulsed fracture fragments also have the profundus with the free fragment.

Powerful muscle contraction at the time of injury may pull the detached tendon through the superficialis bifurcation, producing a painful swelling in the finger or palm. Flatness over the middle phalangeal pulp and an inability to flex the distal interphalangeal joint are present. If a large bone fragment is impacted in the decussation of the superficialis, proximal interphalangeal flexion and extension may be impaired. Tendons avulsed without bony fragments are inserted by the technique described under advancement except, of course, the tendon is the correct length. Sometimes the tendon may have ruptured its vincula when it retracted, producing bleeding and subsequent granulation tissue within the fibrosseous tunnel. Resultant fibrosis and tunnel collapse may necessitate tendon grafting in one or two stages.

All of these avulsion fractures tend to be intra-articular and therefore, if comprising over 30% of the articular surface, particularly require careful fixation. Large fragments (over 30% of articular surface) with tendon attached require both careful K-wire fragment fixation as well as the use of a pullout wire through the tendon that is sutured dorsally over a button on the nail. If the tendon is not attached to the fragment, then both tendon and bone need to be fixed as above in turn. A small avulsed fragment may be excised and the tendon reattached to the terminal phalanx directly. Small, free avulsed fragments are best treated this way.

Zone III – the lumbrical origin

This corresponds to Verdan's zone 5, centered on the middle of the palm and extending from the distal edge of the carpal tunnel to the proximal edge of the fibrosseous tunnel. In this region the lumbrical muscles take origin from the profundi and lie alongside the tendons. The palmar fascia and its vertical septa are in close relationship to each tendon group.

This area is a relatively favorable one although not as favorable as the area proximal to the wrist. Primary repair is the rule in this region. Some authors recommend repairing only the profundus if both tendons are lacerated at the same site. If the wound was sustained while the tendons were flexed then there will be injuries at different levels in the two tendons. An arbitrary difference of 1 cm has been stated to decrease the likelihood of the repaired tendons cross-uniting. It has also been suggested that the vertical septa and palmar fascia covering the extent of excursion of the site of tenorrhaphy should be resected. Such arguments may well apply to the hand immobilized after primary repair; they do not apply to hands undergoing immediate controlled mobilization (Verdan, 1960; Verdan and Crawford, 1971).

In long-standing cases tendon grafting may prove necessary should there be loss of tendon substance or severe retraction.

Zone IV – the carpal tunnel

This area contains the profundi and superficialis tendons to the index, middle, ring and little fingers, flexor pollicis longus, and lying superficial to them all – the median nerve. To the ulnar and superficial side lie the ulnar nerve and artery in Guyon's canal.

It is rare for injuries to occur to the carpal tunnel as the structures are for the most part well protected. Often, however, injuries just proximal to the wrist crease sustained with the wrist in flexion may well require the division of the volar carpal ligament to retrieve the distal tendon ends. Primary repair of nerves and tendons is performed in this area. If possible, it is wise to retain a small portion of the volar carpal ligament intact to serve as a pulley, preventing bowstringing of the tendons when the wrist is immobilized in flexion. Some authors advocate complete division of the roof of the carpal tunnel during exposure and subsequent immobilization in only mild flexion. This places the repaired tendons in a more precarious situation as contraction of their muscle bellies is capable of producing tension at the repair site.

Repair of part of the volar carpal ligament after tenorrhaphy, or leaving part intact during exposure, will enable the surgeon to flex the wrist postoperatively without fear of wound dehiscence with the tendons dislocating from the carpal tunnel volarly. In this flexed position muscle belly activity cannot exert tension forces on the anastomosis site. We tend to use dynamic flexor bands and institute early active motion even in the presence of primary nerve repairs.

Zone V – proximal to the carpal tunnel

In this region most of the important structures lie to the ulnar side of the palmaris longus – the area which tends to be exposed when the outstretched hand tries to protect you from a fall. Injuries here tend to be severe, involving multiple tendons and the median nerve. The ulnar nerve can also be involved, leaving a hand with intrinsic paralysis and no sensation. Occasionally, the level of injury may be multiple as in attempted suicide cases. The priorities for repair are the restoration of profundus function to all fingers and superficialis to the index and flexor pollicis longus. Nerve repair may require grafting, and restoration of the profundi may require bridge grafts of sublimis. Beasley recommends that the wrist flexors need not be repaired as their short excursion is soon filled with scar tissue affording some wrist control. He feels that the flexed position following repair makes regaining extension difficult. Our policy is to repair the wrist flexors; they provide for a stable, well-controlled wrist and the flexed position will be used in any event to protect the finger flexors. Dynamic bands and early motion are instituted for the finger flexors.

In the more proximal region of the forearm where the muscle bellies are superficial, damage will lead to adherent scar tissue which moves with muscular contraction. Careful closure of the antebrachial fascia may help prevent this, but usually this is not possible due to swelling of the muscle bellies. Some authors advocate resection of the antebrachial fascia over the area of repair.

Flexor tendon injuries in the thumb

The flexor pollicis longus follows a sinuous course from the forearm to the distal phalanx of the thumb. In the forearm and wrist it is encased in its own tendon sheath. It may rarely be partially united to the index profundus. Proximal to the wrist, it has a 3–4 cm muscle-free segment which Urbaniak has used for lengthening of the tendon (Urbaniak, Cahill and Mortenson, 1975). From the distal wrist crease to the metacarpophalangeal joint, it runs deep to the roof of the carpal tunnel and the thenar muscles and is thus well protected. From the level of the flexion crease of the metacarpophalangeal joint distally, the flexor pollicis longus is very superficial and in close relationship to both digital nerves. In the more proximal area, these digital nerves and the motor branch to the thenar muscles take origin. Exposure in the well-padded thenar area must be cautious. Luckily, lacerations are more frequent distal to the metacarpophalangeal joint or proximal to the carpal tunnel. Exposure should be along accepted lines. Urbaniak, Cahill and Mortenson (1975), in an excellent study of 57 patients with divided flexor pollicis longus tendons, found it wise to treat injuries at different levels in different ways. Distal to the metacarpophalangeal joint, they advocate either direct repair or advancement and lengthening of the flexor pollicis longus proximal to the transverse carpal ligament. At the most distal part, advancement without lengthening may be possible. Within the confines of the thenar region, tendon grafting is advocated. Surgical exposure is difficult although Bruner (1967, 1973) performs direct repair. Nonetheless, the proximal annular ligament and the distal carpal tunnel restrict access. Proximal to the wrist crease, repair is performed primarily.

In a study in animals Urbaniak compared the different methods of repair. There were more viable tenocytes in the advanced and lengthened tendons than in the free grafts. There were fewer adhesions about the advanced and lengthened tendons than about the grafts.

In the thumb, the long vinculum is more often absent than present and this form of nutrition is of less significance. Retraction of the divided tendon due to loss of the restraining action of the vinculum is, however, more common.

When the muscle belly of flexor pollicis longus is damaged directly or denervated, a tendon transfer is of use. The sublimis to the ring finger may be used as a motor.

Active distal joint flexion is desirable for the finer types of pinch. However, it is not essential for good function. Occasionally in the rheumatoid patient an arthrodesis may be used to provide stability. However, this stability is obtained by sacrificing the flexion power of the thumb giving poor key pinch and poor ability to pick up small objects.

Complex injuries

The question to be asked is when an injury complex enough to make primary tendon repair unwise? Any substantial loss of tissue, either tendon or skin, is in most situations a contraindication to primary tendon repair. Loss of tendon substance exceeding 1 cm requires a graft, either in one or two stages. Skin loss requiring flap coverage is also not suitable for primary repair of underlying tendon injuries in 'no man's land' as the skin loss will often also be associated with loss of tendon substance.

Nerve damage requiring direct repair does not adversely influence the results of primary tenorrhaphy. Injuries requiring nerve grafting would be unusual in the presence of a clean-cut tendon laceration. The same is true of arterial damage requiring grafts. Vessel damage followed by arterial repair is associated with poorer than average results (Lister *et al.*, 1977). This may be related to interference with tendon nutrition or to the accompanying trophic changes associated with neurovascular interruption.

Skeletal injury may include fracture of a phalanx or joint dislocation with or without articular fracture. At the phalangeal level transverse stable fractures may be immobilized effectively by the interosseous wiring technique. This will allow primary tendon repair and the use of early controlled mobilization. Periosteal closure on the floor of the fibrosseous tunnel is of primary importance in such injuries. Dislocations, unless due to sharp division of the volar plate and collateral ligaments, are not often associated with tendon injuries suitable for primary repair. Profundus avulsion from its insertion should be repaired immediately. Sharp bony lacerations involving the articular surface must be carefully, internally fixed. Often K-wires will suffice. These are not contraindications to primary tenorrhaphy. The joint should be fixed so as to allow movement – the prime function of both tendons and joints. Severe intra-articular damage may require arthroplasty or arthrodesis – whichever is appropriate.

The most complex of all the injuries we deal with are cases requiring revascularization or replantation. We do not hesitate to perform primary repairs in these cases.

Tenolysis

This is the surgical release of adherent tendons from their surrounding tissues. It is a frequent secondary procedure following tendon suture or grafting. Postoperative edema and stiffness will produce secondary adhesions. Crush injuries with or without fractures will also produce adhesions. Infection and burns may do the same. Adhesions are the commonest cause of failed primary repairs or tendon grafts. Up to 18% of Pulvertaft's (1956) grafts required tenolysis and up to 12% of Lister's *et al.* (1977) series of primary repairs needed subsequent tenolysis.

The timing of tenolysis is controversial. Some regard a minimum delay of three months following tendon repair or six months following a graft. Others advocate a long delay. Weeks and Wray (1976), however, showed that 85% and 90% of the range of active motion at one year was present within 22 weeks of I and II stage grafting, respectively. Thus, 5–6 months post-surgery seems appropriate timing for tenolysis in patients whose passive range exceeds their active range in the involved digits.

Tenolysis is a major undertaking complicated occasionally by tendon or graft rupture. The postoperative care needs to be as well supervised as that of a primary repair or graft. A cooperative patient is essential. The use of local anesthesia aids this by allowing the patient to immediately see the increase in active motion following surgical lysis of the adhesions.

Under tourniquet, the whole length of the involved digit is opened, preferably by a Bruner approach. The sheaths are widely excised, leaving only the pulleys. The tendons are tested for their ability to glide beneath the pulleys. Following tendon repair only a localized adhesion may need to be released, but after grafting the whole length of the graft requires release. The surgical release of these adhesions diminishes the vascularity of the tendon and subsequent rupture is more likely. All tenolyses must be protected from active flexion against resistance for eight weeks. The postoperative regime is as for primary repair or grafts. If performed under axillary block or general anesthesia, proximal pull must be exerted after lysis of the adhesions to confirm that this will produce the full range of preoperative passive flexion.

Various attempts have been made to reduce the recurrence of postoperative adhesions. Our group tends to use active exercises against dynamic flexion bands, commencing early in the postoperative phase.

Boyes used silicone inlays and Bunnell (1964) and others have suggested fascial strips. It is more than likely that some of these act as foreign bodies while others simply obstruct revascularization of the tendon junction. Cortisone is of unproven value, although triamcinolone does have specific effects on wound healing which may be useful. Kleinert *et al.* continue to use triamcinolone as does Ketchum (1971) and others (Carstam, 1953; Wrenn, Goldner and Markee, 1954; James, 1959).

Fetrow (1967) and Whitaker, Strickland and Ellis (1977) have improved the function of the hand in 50% of their cases. This appears to correspond with the experience of others. Following attempted and failed tenolysis, the finger may require a two-stage tendon graft. Arthrodesis is rarely indicated or in extreme cases a useless digit can be amputated.

EXTENSOR TENDONS

Injury to extensor tendons is common and occurs far more frequently than flexor tendon injuries. They are flat, thin, relatively exposed structures with little superficial skin coverage which are in close relation to underlying bones and joints on the dorsum of the hand. Soft tissue and intratendinous connections prevent separation of tendon ends in the hand following laceration. The deficit detectable on physical examination may be minimal, and too often extensor tendon injuries are missed in the emergency department, particularly partial injuries. Pain with resisted motion and decreased strength will invariably be noted in injured tendons. The degree of extension lag varies with the level of injury. The safest and surest method to ascertain injury to the extensor mechanism is by direct inspection in a well-lit operating room.

Despite the caution of many authors, these injuries are still lightly regarded, leading to avoidable complication (Kelly, 1959; Entin, 1960; Littler, 1960; Fetrow, 1967; Littler, 1967; Tubiana, 1968; Blue, Spira and Hardy, 1976; Lovett and McCalla, 1983). Extension is not as critical as flexion and a minor loss is acceptable, but these injuries can have as serious an effect on hand function as flexor injuries. The goal of extensor tendon repair is to restore extension, but grasp is the most important hand function and is never sacrificed for extension. Repair of these injuries by the least experienced member of the surgical team is ill-advised; they require as much knowledge and skill as do flexor injuries to obtain excellent results.

The mechanical balance of the extensor is complex, and precise. Restoration of continuity following injury is necessary for a favorable result. It is much simpler to restore the tendon immediately following injury than to wait until scar and contracture have altered its delicate mechanism (McFarlane and Hampole, 1973). We manage all open extensor tendon injuries in the operating room. These wounds are afforded all the attention and detail as are other hand injuries.

There is no uniformly well-accepted, descriptive classification system for injuries involving the extensor tendon. An acceptable approach is to divide the extensor tendon system into zones based on the general location or the deformity that results.

Distal forearm

Injuries that occur proximal to the retinaculum of the wrist will do well if the suture line does not impinge upon the retinaculum during excursion (*Figure 7.8*). Physical examination is insufficient for evaluating the injury. The wound must be thoroughly explored and all tendons and injuries identified. This is particularly true in stab or glass injuries, as an innocuous wound may conceal extensive involvement. If the laceration occurs distal to the musculotendinous junction the tendon will retract into the muscle. Gentle exploration of the muscle proximally may produce a tendon end suitable for suture (Lovett and McCalla, 1983). If the tendon is not repaired in this case, an extension lag will result, increasing over time

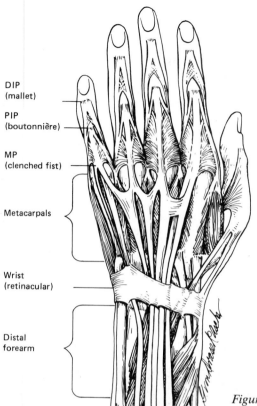

DIP
(mallet)

PIP
(boutonnière)

MP
(clenched fist)

Metacarpals

Wrist
(retinacular)

Distal
forearm

Figure 7.8 Anatomy of the extensor
mechanism is illustrated by regions

as tendon interconnections stretch and become displaced. Figure-of-eight sutures
of 4-0 braided, non-absorbable material are used in the tendon substance. If the
injury occurs proximal to the musculotendinous junction a fibrous tissue raphe in
the muscle belly from which the tendon originates should be identified and the
tendon reapproximated to it using similar sutures (Doyle, 1982). Absorbable
sutures of 3-0 or 4-0 are used in the muscle substance, taking care to avoid
devascularizing the muscle with the suture. A few interrupted 5-0 absorbable
sutures are commonly used to approximate the muscle fascia.

Postoperative splinting is critical and its importance is emphasized to the patient.
Only the involved fingers need to be splinted; but for patient comfort and ease of
splint fabrication the immediately adjacent fingers may be included. The wrist is
splinted at approximately 45° of extension, the metacarpophalangeal joint at
approximately 15° of flexion, and the interphalangeal joints are flexed slightly. An
injured proprius tendon has no interconnection to the other tendons and separate
splinting will not cause any difficulty. If a communis tendon is injured freeing the
uninvolved fingers will allow them to assume a more flexed posture. Interconnections pull the repair distally and provide tendon relaxation. Splinting is continued
for 4–6 weeks. For two additional weeks the patient is placed in a dynamic
extension splint and flexion against resistance is encouraged.

Wrist level

Repair of extensor tendons at the level of the wrist is not without controversy. The extensor retinaculum most influences extensor repair in this area. This is a thick fibrous fascial investment overlying the radial dorsal and ulnar aspects of the wrist joint, containing six synovium-lined retinacular compartments which are traversed by 12 extensor tendons (Palmer *et al.*, 1985). Recent experimental evidence indicates that a significant portion of the extensor tendon nutrition in this area occurs from diffusion, much as occurs in the flexor tendons (Manske, Ogata and Lesker, 1985). The average width of the retinaculum is 4.9 cm with variations from 2.9 cm to 8 cm (Palmer *et al.*, 1985). The most important portion of the retinaculum from a biomechanical point of view is that part directly overlying the wrist joint, approximately 1 cm in width. Preservation of this portion of the retinaculum will prevent unsightly bowstringing (Palmer *et al.*, 1985). Complete sacrifice of the retinaculum will cause bowstringing, some extension loss, and patients will invariably be unsatisfied. It has long been our policy to preserve a portion of the retinaculum in this area.

Completely lacerated tendons here will promptly retract proximal to the wound and are difficult to locate without adequate extension of the wound or a more proximal incision. A tendon retriever is useful for tendons located beneath the retinaculum.

These injuries have all the attendant complications of flexor tendon injuries in zone 2 and should be respected as such. Multiple tendon involvement at this level is particularly troublesome; as Peacock and Van Winkle (1970) noted, they will heal

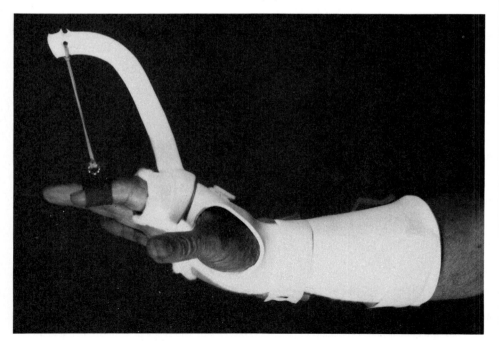

Figure 7.9 Dynamic extension may be necessary in extensor tendon injuries at the retinacular area to prevent restrictive adhesion beneath the retinaculum

by a common coagulum; adherence to surrounding tissue will cause a loss of motion. A portion of the retinaculum may be opened to prevent impingement by the tendon repair, preserving 1 cm to prevent bowstringing. A core suture of 4-0 non-absorbable, braided material, placed as for the flexor tendons, is used. Following the core stitch, 6-0 or 7-0 absorbable suture in a simple running fashion, or a Lembert modification is used to smooth the repair site. Loupe magnification is a must.

Lacerations of the abductor pollicis longus or the wrist extensors close to the bony insertion are repaired with core suture as described if a sufficient stump remains, but if this is not possible the tendon is firmly reattached to bone with a 3-0 or 4-0 non-absorbable, braided suture. Elevating the periosteum and removing a small portion of the cortex will facilitate healing and firm reattachment to bone. Injury to these tendons is easily missed; they are specifically examined when exploring wounds near them.

Postoperative management is cautious. If only the wrist extensors are involved, the wrist is immobilized for 4 weeks with slight deviation to the involved side. Gentle active motion is encouraged for 2–3 weeks, followed by progressive passive exercises if necessary.

With extensor injury of the fingers the involved digits are immobilized. The wrist is splinted in 45° of extension and the metacarpophalangeal joints in 15–20° of flexion. At 3–5 weeks dynamic extension is applied to the injured fingers and active motion is encouraged to lessen the chance of restrictive adhesions (*Figure 7.9*).

Repair is usually possible here until 2½ weeks following the injury; after this shortening of the muscle can prevent an end-to-end repair. There is no loss, however, in checking the excursion of the muscle to see if repair is feasible, even at 6 weeks following injury. If primary repair is not possible, an appropriate tendon transfer is accomplished.

Metacarpal area

Complete division of finger extensors distal to the junctura will result in a significant extension lag while more proximal division is not as predictable (*see Figure 7.8*). The only functional loss with proprius division is independent extension of the involved index or small finger. Complete or partial injury is heralded by pain and weakness, but reliable assessment of the injury must include operative exploration (Lovett and McCalla, 1983). Communis tendons divided proximal to the junctura and all divided proprius tendons will retract while the junctura prevent retraction in more distal communis injuries. Injuries early or late are managed as injuries at the wrist. Extensor tendons become more flat and thin over the metacarpals and are best approximated with 4-0 non-absorbable sutures in a figure-of-eight fashion. Their superficial location frequently leads to annoying skin adhesions after injury; these will resolve with physiotherapy and only rarely require surgical intervention.

Splinting is identical to that described for the more proximal injuries. Mobilization at 3–5 weeks in a dynamic extension splint is important to help regain complete finger flexion, particularly in crush injuries where underlying adhesions are more common (*see Figure 7.9*).

Metacarpophalangeal joint

Open injuries here are human tooth injuries until a different mechanism is proven beyond doubt. This said, the surgeon will not find himself in the unenviable position of having closed a human bite. These wounds are commonly sustained with the hand in a clenched fist posture as the patient strikes another in the mouth. Patients are reluctant to identify this mechanism of injury even when directly questioned, and this often prevents them from seeking early treatment (Goldstein *et al.*, 1978; Goldstein, Barones and Miller, 1983). The later treatment is instituted, the more likely complications will develop. Appropriately selected antibiotics are always begun preoperatively (following cultures) when the patient is seen in the emergency room.

When a clenched fist injury occurs, the skin, tendon, joint capsule and metacarpal head are in a different relationship than during surgical exploration (Lister, 1984; *Figure 7.10*). Injury to each of these structures must be sought in turn and debrided. X-rays may reveal a foreign body if a portion of the tooth has broken free and is in the wound. A chondral fracture of the metacarpal head is the rule, although X-rays will not reveal it. These principles are remembered during preoperative and intraoperative evaluation (Lister, 1984).

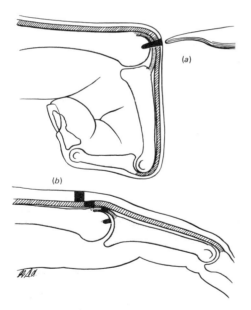

Figure 7.10 The skin, tendon, joint capsule and metacarpal head are at a different level during injury (*a*) than at the time of surgical exploration (*b*). Injury to each structure is particularly sought. (From Lister, 1984)

The wounds are thoroughly lavaged, left open, and a catheter inserted for postoperative irrigation. The wounds are closed in 4–5 days if they are free of infection. These injuries usually only partially lacerate the involved structures (Kleinert and Smith, 1982). The capsule and tendon are repaired at the time of skin closure with 5-0 absorbable and 4-0 non-absorbable suture respectively.

If it can be assured that a relatively clean object caused the injury, primary closure is indicated. All involved structures are repaired, even in partial injuries.

Figure-of-eight 4-0 or 5-0 non-absorbable sutures with the knot placed beneath the tendon are used. The sagittal bands are repaired if injured to prevent subluxation and loss of extension (Kettelkamp, Flat and Moulds, 1971; Smith, 1974; Harvey and Hume, 1980; Iftikhar *et al.*, 1984).

Postoperatively, the hand and wrist are splinted as described for more proximal lesions for 3–5 weeks, followed by gentle active motion.

Proximal phalanx level

Because of the rounded shape of the proximal phalanx (*see Figure 7.8*) and the broad configuration of the extensor mechanism in this region, injuries here are usually incomplete (Kilgore and Graham, 1977; Doyle, 1982; Kleinert and Smith, 1982; Lovett and McCalla, 1983; *Figure 7.11*). Proximal and distal attachments prevent the tendon ends from separating far following division. We believe appropriate treatment includes repair of all injured structures by simple interrupted non-absorbable sutures with buried knots. Uninjured portions of the extensor apparatus are not sutured.

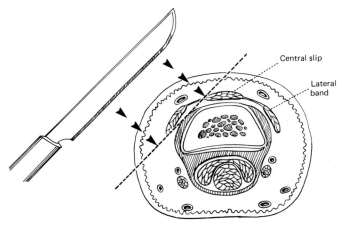

Central slip

Lateral band

Figure 7.11 The broad configuration of the extensor mechanism and the shape of the proximal phalanx make complete tendon injury here uncommon

Postoperatively, the metacarpophalangeal joint is splinted in 20° of flexion with the interphalangeal joints splinted in extension. This is maintained for 4–6 weeks, then progressive gentle active motion is begun. Night splinting may be necessary for an additional 2–3 weeks.

Boutonnière deformity

The extensor mechanism at the proximal interphalangeal joint level is most complex. If the fine balance of this delicate mechanism is interrupted the finger will assume an abnormal posture. Over the proximal phalanx the extensor tendon divides into three slips. The two lateral slips join with the bands from the interossei and lumbrical on either side of the digit and continue distally as conjoined bands (Kaplan, 1959; Tubiana, 1968; Harris and Rutledge, 1972). They unite at their attachment to the proximal dorsal aspect of the distal phalanx. The central slip of the extensor tendon continues distally to its insertion on the proximal dorsal aspect of the middle phalanx. These structures are held in position by retinacular ligaments (Kaplan, 1959; Tubiana and Valentin, 1964). Normally, the lateral bands are dorsal to the axis of rotation of the proximal interphalangeal joint. As this joint is extended, the lateral bands simultaneously extend the distal phalanx (Harris and Rutledge, 1972; *Figure 7.12*).

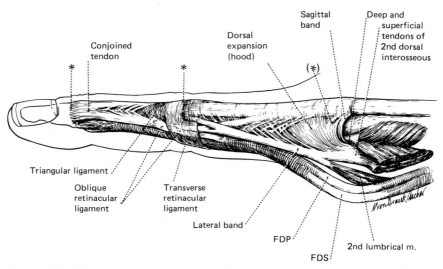

Figure 7.12 The extensor mechanism trifurcates at the proximal joint. The central slip attaches to the middle phalanx and the ulnar and radial slips form the lateral bands. The triangular ligament prevents separation of the lateral bands. The extensor mechanism is secured over the proximal phalanx by the transverse retinacular ligament. The lateral bands are dorsal to the axis of rotation of the proximal interphalangeal joint. * = Bony insertion of tendons. (From Kleinert, Stillwell and Netscher, 1985)

Following laceration of the central slip of the extensor mechanism, the lateral bands may still extend the middle phalanx, but a boutonnière deformity can develop over time (Harris and Rutledge, 1972; Micks and Hager, 1973; Lovett and McCalla, 1983; *Figure 7.13(a)*). Repeated flexion of the proximal interphalangeal joint causes tearing of the triangular ligament, prolapse of the joint through the defect in the extensor apparatus and displacement of the lateral bands volar to the axis of rotation of the joint (Lovett and McCalla, 1983). Here, they flex the middle phalanx, adding to the now unopposed action of the finger flexors (Tubiana, 1968; Elliott, 1970; Harris and Rutledge, 1972; *Figure 7.13(b)*). An undivided central slip checkreins the lateral bands and prevents hyperextension of the distal joint (Harris and Rutledge, 1972). Division increases traction of the terminal tendon on the distal phalanx as the lateral bands are now free and migrate proximally. The

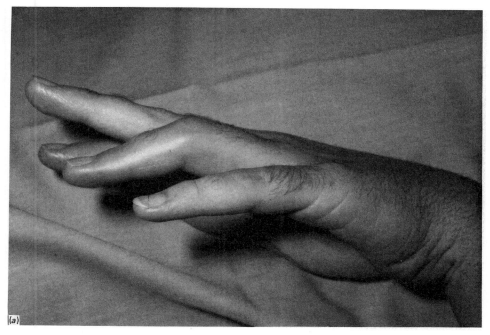

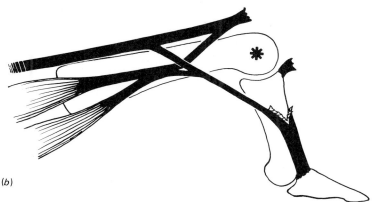

Figure 7.13 (*a*) Patient with chronic boutonnière deformity. (*b*) As the joint prolapses into the defect in the extensor mechanism, the lateral bands are now volar to the axis of rotation of the joint. In this position they flex the proximal joint and extend the distal joint

proximal interphalangeal joint by its herniates between the lateral bands and also increases the tension in the places upon them. Intrinsic pull causes progressive extension at the distal joint and flexion of the proximal joint (Tubiana, 1968).

The retinacular ligaments fix the boutonnière deformity. The transverse retinacular ligaments shorten and maintain the palmar displacement of the lateral bands. The oblique retinacular ligaments contract and maintain the proximal joint in flexion and the distal joint in extension (Zancolli, 1968). Finally, soft tissue changes in the joint occur and the boutonnière deformity is irreducible.

Much evidence supports this mechanism in the production of a boutonnière deformity. Cadaver studies demonstrate that section of the central slip alone will not produce the lesion. Repetitive forced flexion with tension on the extensor mechanism will, however, cause the lateral bands to tear away from the remainder of the extensor mechanism. Then, the condyles may prolapse into the defect (Harris and Rutledge, 1972; Micks and Hager, 1973). Clinically, a Fowler's release for chronic mallet deformity involves careful sectioning of the insertion of the central slip; if no rent is made in the dorsal extensor mechanism prolapse of the joint or luxation of the lateral bands does not occur (Harris and Rutledge, 1972; Bowers and Hurst, 1978). Full extension is still possible.

Injuries may be open or closed. Since an extension deficit may not be present initially, the onus is on the surgeon to suspect central slip involvement with any injury of this area. X-rays are mandatory in all injuries.

Closed injuries without bony involvement are treated conservatively. Pain, tenderness and weakness of extension against resistance with recent trauma are presumptive evidence of injury to the central slip (Lovett and McCalla, 1983). The patient is placed in a static splint immobilizing the proximal interphalangeal joint and allowing active motion of the distal interphalangeal joint for three weeks, and following this is observed for an additional 3-week period. The splint is applied for 6 weeks if an initial extension deficit is noted. The patient is monitored closely after removing the splint and it is reapplied if an extension lag occurs. Excellent results are expected with this protocol.

As Tubiana (1968) and others recommend (Spinner and Choi, 1970; Kleinert and Smith, 1982), we feel that open repair of a closed boutonnière injury is indicated when there is a bone fragment not reduced with the joint in extension or when there is avulsion of the central slip associated with anterior dislocations. Associated injuries to the collateral ligament, volar plate and extensor mechanism are suspected. The avulsed bone fragment with the central slip is secured to bone using a pullout wire technique. An oblique 0.035 K-wire immobilizes the joint in 0° of extension. This is reinforced for 2½ weeks with a volar splint with the wrist in 45° of extension and the metacarpophalangeal joint in 20° of flexion (*Figure 7.14*). At 2½ weeks the wrist and metacarpophalangeal joint are freed and only an alumifoam static splint reinforces the K-wire fixation. Passive flexion of the distal interphalangeal joint is encouraged as this advances the lateral bands and relaxes the repair. At 6 weeks the K-wire and pullout wire are removed. Active exercises in a Capener splint are progressed daily by hourly increments over the next 2 weeks. If an extension lag is noted an additional 2 weeks of static splinting is required.

All open injuries are explored, and injured structures repaired. We feel that identification of the individual components of the extensor mechanism and repair with figure-of-eight 5-0 non-absorbable suture with end-to-end approximation is desirable. Though some authors recommend splinting, we transfix the joint with a 0.035 K-wire. Antibiotics are used with joint injury or wound contamination, preferably commenced before surgery. Thereafter, management is identical to the closed injury except if the lateral bands are lacerated. Then passive flexion of the distal interphalangeal joint is commenced at 4 weeks rather than 2.

Not all injuries are seen early. We attempt a primary repair if a patient is seen within a few weeks of the injury. For closed lesions or older open injuries a trial of static splinting for at least 6 weeks followed by a Capener splint is in order. If the joint has a flexion deformity which is not correctible passively, a joint jack is used to improve mobility. If this fails, a more extensive reconstructive procedure would

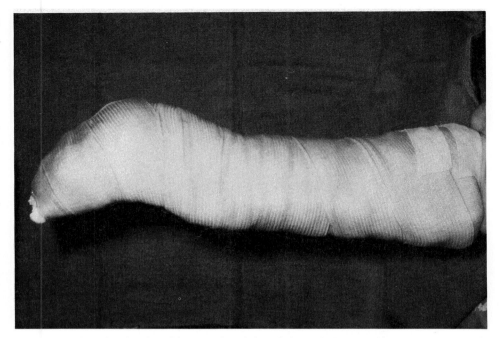

Figure 7.14 Repair of a closed boutonnière injury is immobilized for 2½ weeks with a volar splint with the wrist in 45° of extension and the metacarpophalangeal joint in 20° of flexion

be required. Many procedures have been recommended for the treatment of a chronic deformity with fixed contractures (Tubiana, 1968; Elliott, 1970; McFarlane and Hampole, 1973; Blue, Spira and Hardy, 1976; Sakellarides, 1978; Kleinert and Smith, 1982; Steichen *et al.,* 1982; Curtis, Reid and Provost, 1983). None of these methods are totally satisfactory. As Lovett noted, before reconstructing a chronic boutonnière deformity, several prerequisites should be met; the joint must be supple, X-rays of the proximal interphalangeal joint should be normal, skin coverage must be satisfactory and the patient must be well-motivated. Reconstruction can then be contemplated.

Mallet finger

The conjoined lateral bands of the extensor mechanism continue distally from the proximal phalanx to unite and attach to a broad ridge at the dorsal base of the distal phalanx. The insertion blends into the root of the nail (Kaplan, 1959; *see Figure 7.12*). Division of the structures between the proximal and distal joint results in the same postural defect (Lovett and McCalla, 1983); flexion is unopposed, and a mallet finger deformity results (*Figure 7.15*). Commonly this term applies to loss of continuity of the extensor apparatus at the distal joint, the most common site of injury producing this deformity.

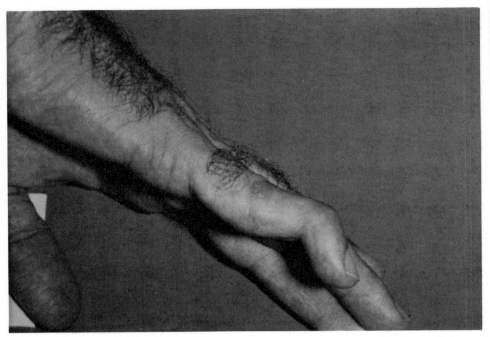

Figure 7.15 Established mallet deformity with loss of extension of the distal interphalangeal joint and compensatory hyperextension of the proximal interphalangeal joint. (From Kleinert, 1978)

Division of the extensor apparatus at the distal joint allows the conjoined lateral bands to displace proximally. As this occurs, an extensive force is applied to the proximal joint through the central slip causing hyperextension and a swan-neck deformity, particularly with relaxation of the volar plate (Elliott, 1970; *Figure 7.16*).

The injuries are either open or closed, but most mallet finger deformities result from closed injuries. A part of the tendon can remain attached to the intact distal plalanx, or the tendon can separate with a portion of the distal phalanx attached. A

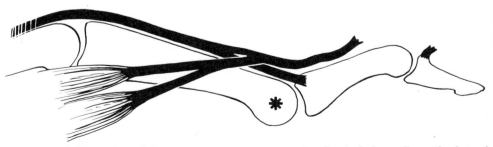

Figure 7.16 Disruption of the extensor apparatus over the distal phalanx allows the lateral band to migrate proximal with volar plate laxity. The proximal interphalangeal joint hyperextends and a swan-neck deformity results

frequent mechanism of injury is sudden forced flexion of an extended finger; this causes a tear of the central tendon or sometimes an avulsion with a flake of bone. A crushing injury can lead to necrosis of the tendon, separation and a mallet deformity. In this case the deformity occurs later. Forced extension injuries can cause intra-articular fractures and subluxation. Mallet finger deformities may also follow epiphyseal injuries in children. These last two injuries should be regarded as a fracture with a secondary mallet deformity. Bone avulsed with the tendon will be visible on a lateral X-ray. Articular surface involvement and joint subluxation should be assessed.

Generally, closed mallet injuries without displaced fractures or subluxation are managed non-operatively for up to six months after the trauma (Doyle, 1982; Crawford, 1984). In a large series, Stark *et al.* found that prognosis and treatment depend upon prior treatment, loss of distal joint extension, functional disability and patient age.

Patient education is paramount in the treatment of a closed mallet deformity. The patient must appreciate that extension of the distal interphalangeal joint is to be continuous until he is instructed to begin motion. Any variance will mean recommencing treatment and possibly an adverse result. If accomplished, the burden of treatment is shared with the patient, and success is more likely.

If no bone is involved or if less than 20% of the articular surface is involved, treatment begins with a well-padded alumifoam splint. The proximal interphalangeal joint is splinted in 45° of flexion for 2–3 weeks, and the distal interphalangeal joint is splinted in 5–10° of hyperextension. The skin over the distal joint is inspected to ensure that there is no blanching with the hyperextension. If there is, then splinting is reduced until good color is noted. Flexion of the proximal joint advances the lateral bands distally and relaxes the repair. The proximal interphalangeal joint is then released at 2–3 weeks to prevent stiffness. There is not a uniform consensus on the validity of this practice, and Kaplan (1959) and others (Pratt, 1964; Abouna and Brown, 1968) have cautioned against it. We believe flexion of the proximal joint for 2–3 weeks relaxes the repair and early mobilization prevents complications.

The patient is seen at weekly intervals for 2–3 weeks. The splint is changed and skin care provided. After release of the proximal interphalangeal joint, an alumifoam splint is constructed for the distal joint only (*Figure 7.17*). A bend is placed at either end of a splint of appropriate length, and a portion of the foam is then cut from the center of the splint where it will overlie the joint. The bend placement and removal of the foam will prevent pressure to the skin over the joint. The joint is hyperextended and checked for blanching (Kleinert and Smith, 1982). The splint is taped so as to compress its width by approximately 50%. Splints are checked weekly; the finger is never flexed during this time. Responsible patients may change their splint, but they must have help. A molded orthoplast splint with a velcro strap can be fashioned if splinting beyond 6 weeks is anticipated. This can be applied by one person. At the end of 6 weeks the splint is removed and the patient gently flexes and extends the finger. If an extension lag is noted the splint is reapplied for 2 more weeks. If none is present, the patient is instructed to remove the splint for increasing periods each day over the next two weeks and gently actively flex the finger. He then reapplies the splint and wears it for the remainder of the time and always at night. By 2 weeks the patient is out of the splint most of the day. The splint is always worn whenever vigorous activity or possible injury may be anticipated. If at two weeks no extensor lag has developed the splint is

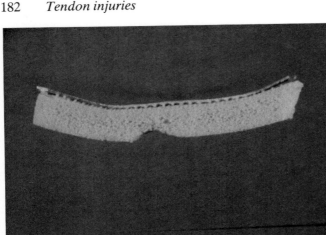

Figure 7.17 An alumifoam splint is fashioned for the distal interphalangeal joint; it is bent at either end and some of the foam removed from the middle to prevent pressure over the joint. (From Kleinert, 1985)

removed and progressive activity encouraged. If a lag occurs, the splint is reapplied for two more weeks continually and this protocol repeated. Old injuries will require longer splinting, up to four months in some instances.

Mallet injuries associated with fractures of more than 20% of the joint surface or joint subluxation are more difficult to treat. Still, closed reduction may be successful and should be attempted. X-rays are obtained following reduction with the joint splinted to ensure accuracy. Some reports contend that the reduction need not be perfect, but we believe to accept much displacement commits the surgeon to a palpable deformity, extension lag, possible late degenerative changes, and a dissatisfied patient. A satisfactory closed reduction should be followed with weekly X-rays in the splint to ensure that it is maintained.

Excellent results have also been reported using the prefabricated Stack finger splint. Doyle (1982) prefers this method for closed mallet injuries. The availability of the splint and ease of application are attractive features. Still close patient follow-up is essential (Stack, 1969; Crawford, 1984).

If reasonable bony alignment is not achieved the mallet fracture is opened. Adequate exposure through a dorsal incision is required. The joint is entered distal to the fracture fragment, unless the fragment has periosteal attachments, then it is recommended that these be undisturbed and the tendon divided proximally for exposure instead (Hamas, Horrell and Pierret, 1978). This certainly has merit, but in our experience in cases requiring open reduction it has not always applied. If the fragment is large enough, a 0.035 K-wire is placed from proximal to distal through the distal phalanx. The fragment is then reduced under direct vision and the K-wire is retrograded across it and the joint (*Figure 7.18*). The K-wire is cut short and bent. A splint is applied and maintained as described for closed treatment and the

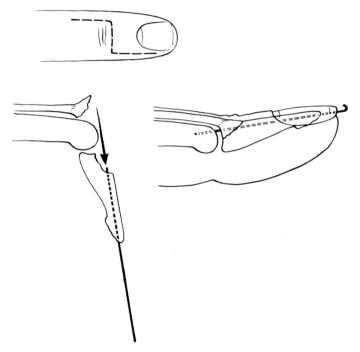

Figure 7.18 With larger fragments, an 0.035 K-wire is placed from proximal to distal through the distal phalanx then retrograded across the fragment at the joint

wire is left for 6 weeks. If the fracture fragment is small or comminuted or is not satisfactorily reduced with this method, the fragment and tendon are secured with a pullout suture of 4-0 prolene. The suture is passed through the distal tendon, around each side of the distal phalanx, brought out through the skin and fixed over a button or dental roll (*Figure 7.19*). The distal joint is immobilized in slight hyperextension by a longitudinal 0.035 K-wire. Smaller wires may fatigue and break. The pullout suture is removed at 4 weeks and the K-wire at 6 weeks. Splinting is maintained as described for closed injuries.

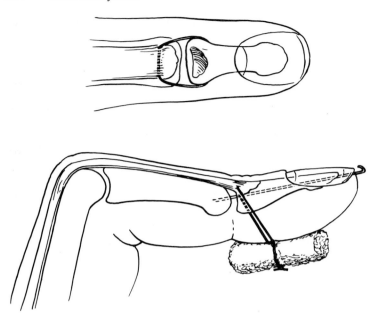

Figure 7.19 A pullout suture of 4-0 prolene immobilizes the fragment and is fixed over a dental roll

Wehbe and Schneider (1984) recently reviewed their experience with 21 cases of mallet fracture. Six were treated surgically and 15 were simply splinted. All but one had a good result. They felt these findings suggested that most mallet fractures could be treated conservatively regardless of joint subluxation and the size and amount of displacement of the bone fragment.

Open mallet injuries are not uncommon. Lacerations over the distal interphalangeal joint will often injure the tendon and enter the joint. A sharp injury often leaves little tendon substance distally to suture, but enough of the distal insertion and periosteum can usually be elevated to hold a few fine braided, non-absorbable figure-of-eight sutures. The proximity and confluence of the nailbed are remembered and avoided. An 0.035 K-wire placed longitudinally across the distal interphalangeal joint and splinting as described is recommended. Open injuries with bony involvement are reduced under direct vision and prophylactic antibiotics are begun preoperatively.

Crush injuries and abrasions with skin loss and loss of tendon substance are not uncommon in this area. Skin loss is replaced appropriately. Loss of tendon substance will require later reconstruction.

References

ABOUNA, J. M. and BROWN, H. (1968) The treatment of mallet finger, the results in a series of 148 consecutive cases and a review of the literature. *British Journal of Surgery,* **55,** 653–667

ARKIN, A. M. and SIFFERT, R. S. (1953) Use of wire in tenoplasty and tenorrhaphy. *American Journal of Surgery,* **85,** 795

BIRDSELL, D. C., TUSTANOFF, E. R. and LINDSAY, W. K. (1966) Collagen production in regenerating tendon. *Plastic and Reconstructive Surgery,* **37,** 504

BLUE, A. I., SPIRA, M. and HARDY, S. B. (1976) Repair of extensor tendon injuries of the hand. *American Journal of Surgery*, **132**, 128–132

BOHLER, J. Cited in Carroll and Metch (1970)

BOWERS, W. H. and HURST, L. C. (1978) Chronic mallet finger: the use of Fowler's central slip release. *Journal of Hand Surgery*, **3**, 373–376

BOYES, J. H. (1950) Flexor tendon grafts in the fingers and thumb. An evaluation of end results. *Journal of Bone and Joint Surgery*, **32A**, 489

BOYES, J. H. (1971) Discussion. In *Symposium on the Hand*, Volume 3, edited by L. M. Cramer and R. A. Chase. St Louis: C. V. Mosby

BOYES, J. H. and STARK, H. H. (1971) Flexor tendon grafts in the finger and thumb. *Journal of Bone and Joint Surgery*, **53A**, 1332

BROCKIS, J. G. (1953) The blood supply of the flexor and extensor tendons of the fingers in man. *Journal of Bone and Joint Surgery*, **35B**, 131

BRUNER, J. M. (1967) The zig-zag volar-digital incision for flexor tendon surgery. *Plastic and Reconstructive Surgery*, **40**, 571

BRUNER, J. M. (1973) Surgical exposure of flexor tendons in the hand. *Annals of the Royal College of Surgeons of England*, **53**, 84

BUNNELL, S. (1922) Repair of tendons in the fingers. *Surgery, Gynecology and Obstetrics*, **35**, 88

BUNNELL, S. (1964) *Surgery of the Hand*, 4th edition. Philadelphia: J. B. Lippincott

CAPLAN, H. S., HUNTER, J. M. and MERKLIN, R. J. (1975) Intrinsic vascularization of flexor tendons. In *American Association of Orthopaedic Surgeons Symposium on Tendon Surgery in the Hand*, Chapter 5. St Louis: C. V. Mosby

CARROLL, R. E. and METCH, R. M. (1970) Avulsion of the flexor profundus tendon insertion. *Journal of Trauma*, **10**, 1109

CARSTAM, N. (1953) The effect of cortisone on the formation of tendon adhesions and on tendon healing: An experimental investigation in the rabbit. *Acta Chirurgica Scandinavica*, Suppl., 182

CARTER, S. J. and MERSHEIMER, W. L. (1966) Deferred primary tendon repair. *Annals of Surgery*, **164**, 913

CHAPLIN, D. M. (1973) The vascular anatomy within normal tendons, divided tendons, free tendon grafts and pedicle tendon grafts in rabbits. *Journal of Bone and Joint Surgery*, **55B**, 369

COOPER, R. R. and MISOL, S. (1970) Tendon and ligament insertion. *Journal of Bone and Joint Surgery*, **52A**, 1

CRAWFORD, G. P. (1984) The molded polythene splint for mallet finger deformities. *Journal of Hand Surgery*, **9**, 231–237

CRONKITE, A. E. (1936) The tensile strength of human tendons. *Anatomy Review*, **64**, 173

CURTIS, R. M., REID, R. L. and PROVOST, J. M. (1983) A staged technique for the repair of the traumatic boutonnière deformity. *Journal of Hand Surgery*, **8**, 167

DeKLERK, A. J. and JONCK, L. M. (1982) Primary tendon healing: an experimental study. *South African Medical Journal*, **62(21)**, 276–280

DOYLE, J. R. (1982) Extensor tendons – acute injuries. In *Operative Hand Surgery*, Chapter 43. Edited by D. P. Green, pp. 1441–1464. Edinburgh: Churchill Livingstone

DURAN, R. J. and HOUSER, R. G. (1975) Controlled passive motion following flexor tendon repair in zones 2 and 3. In *American Association of Orthopaedic Surgeons Symposium on Tendon Surgery In The Hand*, p. 105. St Louis: C. V. Mosby

EARLEY, M. J. and MILWARD, T. M. (1982) The primary repair of digital flexor tendons. *British Journal of Plastic Surgery*, **35**, 133–139

EDWARDS, D. A. W. (1946) The blood supply and lymphatic drainage of tendons. *Journal of Anatomy*, **80**, 147

EIKEN, O., LUNDBORG, G. and RANK, F. (1975) The role of the digital synovial sheath in tendon grafting. *Scandinavian Journal of Plastic Surgery*, **9**, 182

EIKEN, O., HOLMBERG, J., EKEROT, L. and SALGEBACK, S. (1980) Restoration of the digital tendon sheath. *Scandinavian Journal of Plastic and Reconstructive Surgery*, **14**, 89–97

EJESKAR, A. (1980a) Flexor tendon repair in No Man's Land – I. Follow-up study on primary tendon repair ad modum Verdan. *Scandinavian Journal of Plastic and Reconstructive Surgery*, **14**, 273–277

EJESKAR, A. (1980b) Flexor tendon repair in No Man's Land – II. Early versus late secondary tendon repair ad modum Kleinert. *Scandinavian Journal of Plastic and Reconstructive Surgery*, **14**, 279–283

ELLIOTT, D. H. (1965) Structure and function of mammalian tendons. *Biological Review*, **40**, 302

ELLIOTT, R. A. (1970) Injuries to the extensor mechanism of the hand. *Orthopedic Clinics of North America*, **1**, 335–354

ENTIN, M. A. (1960) Repair of the extensor mechanism of the hand. *Surgical Clinics of North America*, **40**, 275–285

FETROW, K. O. (1967) Tenolysis in the hand and wrist. A clinical evaluation of two hundred and twenty flexor and extensor tenolyses. *Journal of Bone and Joint Surgery,* **40A,** 667

FIELD, P. L. (1971) Tendon fibre arrangement and blood supply. *Australian and New Zealand Journal of Surgery,* **40,** 298

FLYNN, J. E. and GRAHAM, J. H. (1962) Healing following tendon suture and tendon transplants. *Surgery, Gynecology and Obstetrics,* **115,** 467

FLYNN, J. E. and GRAHAM, J. H. (1965) Healing of tendon wounds. *American Journal of Surgery,* **109,** 315

FURLOW, L. T. JR (1972) Early active motion in flexor tendon healing. *Journal of Bone and Joint Surgery,* **54A,** 911

GELBERMAN, R. H., MENON, J., GONSALVES, M. *et al.* (1980) The effects of mobilization on the vascularization of healing flexor tendons in dogs. *Clinical Orthopedics,* **153,** 382–389

GELBERMAN, R. H., WOO, S. L. Y., LOTHRINGER, K., AKESON, W. and AMIEL, D. (1982) Effects of early intermittent passive mobilization on healing canine flexor tendons. *Journal of Hand Surgery,* **7(2),** 170–177

GELBERMAN, R. H., VANDE BERG, J. S., LUNDBORG, G. and AKESON, W. H. (1983) Flexor tendon healing and restoration of the gliding surface. *Journal of Bone and Joint Surgery,* **65A,** 75–80

GELBERMAN, R. H., MANSKE, P. R., VANDE BERG, J. S. *et al.* (1984) Flexor tendon healing *in vitro*: comparative histologic study of rabbit, chicken, dog and monkey. *Journal of Orthopedic Research,* **2,** 39–48

GILLARD, G. C., MERRILEES, M. J., BELL-BOOTH, P. G., REILLEY, H. C. and FLINT, M. H. (1977) The proteoglycan content and the axial periodicity of collagen in tendons. *Journal of Biochemistry,* **163,** 145

GOLDSTEIN, E. J. C., BARONES, M. F. and MILLER, T. A. (1983) *Eikenella corrodens* in hand infections. *Journal of Hand Surgery,* **8,** 563–567

GOLDSTEIN, E. J. C., MILLER, T. A., CITRON, D. M. and FINEGOLD, S. M. (1978) Infections following clenched-fist injury: a new prospective. *Journal of Hand Surgery,* **3,** 455–457

GRANT, M. E. and PROCKOP, D. J. (1972) The biosynthesis of collagen. *New England Journal of Medicine,* **286,** 194

GREEN, W. L. and NIEBAUER, J. J. (1974) Results of primary and secondary flexor tendon repairs in No Man's Land. *Journal of Bone and Joint Surgery,* **56A,** 1216

GREENLEE, T. K., BECKHAM, C. and PIKE, D. (1975) A fine structural study of the development of check flexor digital tendon: a model for synovial sheathed tendon healing. *American Journal of Anatomy,* **143,** 303

HAMAS, R. S., HORRELL, E. D. and PIERRET, G. P. (1978) Treatment of mallet finger due to intra-articular fracture of the distal phalanx. *Journal of Hand Surgery,* **3,** 361–363

HARRIS, C. and RUTLEDGE, G. L. JR (1972) The functional anatomy of the extensor mechanism of the finger. *Journal of Bone and Joint Surgery,* **54A,** 713–726

HARVEY, F. J. and HUME, K. F. (1980) Spontaneous recurrent ulnar dislocation of the long extensor tendons of the fingers. *Journal of Hand Surgery,* **5,** 492–494

HERNANDEZ, A., VELASCO, F., RIVAS, R. *et al.* (1967) Preliminary report on early mobilization for the rehabilitation of flexor tendons. *Plastic and Reconstructive Surgery,* **40,** 354

IFTIKHAR, T. B., HALLMANN, B. W., KAMINSKI, R. S. and RAY, A. K. (1984) Spontaneous rupture of the extensor mechanism causing ulnar dislocation of the long extensor tendon of the long finger. *Journal of Bone and Joint Surgery,* **66,** 1108–1109

ISELIN, M. (1958) 'Delayed emergencies' in fresh wounds of the hand. *Proceedings of the Royal Society of Medicine,* **51,** 713

JAMES, J. I. P. (1959) The use of cortisone in tenolysis. *Journal of Bone and Joint Surgery,* **41A,** 209

JENSON, E. G. and WEILBLY, A. (1974) Primary tendon suture in the thumb and fingers. *The Hand,* **6(3),** 208

KAPLAN, E. B. (1959) Anatomy, injuries and treatment of the extensor apparatus of the hand and fingers. *Clinical Orthopedics,* **13,** 24–41

KELLY, A. P. JR (1959) Primary tendon repairs. A study of 789 consecutive tendon severances. *Journal or Bone and Joint Surgery,* **41A,** 581

KESSLER, I. (1973) The grasping technique for tendon repair. *The Hand,* **5,** 253

KESSLER, I. and MISSIM, F. (1969) Primary repair without immobilization of flexor tendon division within the flexor tendon sheath. An experimental and clinical study. *Acta Orthopaedica Scandinavica,* **40,** 587

KETCHUM, L. D. (1971) The effects of triamcinolone on tendon healing and function. *Plastic and Reconstructive Surgery,* **47,** 471

KETTELKAMP, D. B., FLATT, A. E. and MOULDS, R. (1971) Traumatic dislocation of the long finger extensor tendon. *Journal of Bone and Joint Surgery,* **53,** 229–240

KILGORE, E. S. and GRAHAM, W. P. (1977) *The Hand: Surgical and Non-Surgical Management*, p. 192. Philadelphia: Lea and Febiger

KLEINERT, H. E. (1978) Hand surgery for the general surgeon. In *Surgical Medicine*. Smith, Kline and French

KLEINERT, H. E. (1985) Surgery of the hand. In *Textbook of Surgery*, edited by A. P. Monaco. New York: Macmillan

KLEINERT, H. E. and SMITH, D. J. (1982) Primary and secondary repairs of flexor and extensor tendon injuries. In *Hand Surgery*, 3rd edition, edited by J. E. Flynn, pp. 220–242. Baltimore: Williams and Wilkins

KLEINERT, H. E., KUTZ, J. E. and COHEN, M. J. (1975) Primary repair of zone 2 flexor tendon lacerations. In *American Association of Orthopaedic Surgeons Symposium on Tendon Surgery of the Hand*, Chapter 11. St Louis: C. V. Mosby

KLEINERT, H. E., KUTZ, J. E., ASHBELL, T. S. and MARTINEZ, E. (1967) Abstract: primary repair of lacerated flexor tendons in No Man's Land. *Journal of Bone and Joint Surgery*, **49A**, 577

KLEINERT, H. E., KUTZ, J. E., ATASOY, E. A. and STORMO, A. (1973) Primary repair of flexor tendons. *Orthopedic Clinics of North America*, **4**, 865

KLEINERT, H. E., STILLWELL, J. H. and NETSCHER, D. T. (1985) Complications of tendon surgery. In *Current Management of Complications in Orthopedics – The Wrist and the Hand*, edited by S. C. Sandzen, Chapter 12. Philadelphia: Williams and Wilkins

LEFFERT, R. D., WEISS, C. and ATHANASOULIS, C. A. (1974) The vincula, with particular reference to their vessels and nerves. *Journal of Bone and Joint Surgery*, **56A**, 1191

LINDSAY, W. K. and THOMSON, H. G. (1959) Digital flexor tendons: an experimental study (part I). *British Journal of Plastic Surgery*, **12**, 289

LISTER, G. D. (1983) Incision and closure of the flexor sheath during primary tendon repair. *The Hand*, **15(2)**, 123–135

LISTER, G. D., KLEINERT, H. E., KUTZ, J. E. and ATASOY, E. A. (1977) Primary flexor tendon repair followed by immediate controlled mobilization. *Journal of Hand Surgery*, **2**, 441–451

LISTER, G. D. (1984) *The Hand: Diagnosis and Indications*, 2nd edition, pp. 231–232. Edinburgh: Churchill Livingstone

LITTLER, J. W. (1960) Extensor habitus. *Journal of Bone and Joint Surgery*, **42A**, 913

LITTLER, J. W. (1967) The finger extensor mechanism. *Surgical Clinics of North America*, **47**, 415–432

LOVETT, W. L. and McCALLA, M. A. (1983) Management and rehabilitation of extensor tendon injuries. *Orthopedic Clinics of North America*, **14(4)**, 811–826

LOWRY, O. H., GILLIGAN, D. R. and KATERSKY, E. M. (1942) The determination of collagen and elastin in tissues with results obtained in various normal tissues from different species. *Journal of Biological Chemistry*, **143**, 271

LUNDBORG, G. (1976) Experimental flexor tendon healing without adhesion formation – a new concept of tendon nutrition and intrinsic healing mechanisms: a preliminary report. *The Hand*, **8**, 235

LUNDBORG, G. and RANK, F. (1978) Experimental intrinsic healing of flexor tendons based upon synovial fluid nutrition. *Journal of Hand Surgery*, **3**, 21

LUNDBORG, G. and RANK, F. (1980) Experimental studies on cellular mechanisms involved in healing of animal and human flexor tendon in synovial environment. *The Hand*, **12**, 3–11

LUNDBORG, G., MYRHAGE, R. and RYDEVIK, B. (1977) The vascularization of human flexor tendons within the digital synovial sheath region – structure and functional aspects. *Journal of Hand Surgery*, **2**, 417

LUNDBORG, G., HOLM, S. and MYRHAGE, R. (1980) The role of synovial fluid and tendon sheath for flexor tendon nutrition. *Scandinavian Journal of Plastic and Reconstructive Surgery*, **14**, 99–107

LUNDBORG, G., HANSSON, H. A., RANK, F. and RYDEVIK, B. (1980) Superficial repair of severed flexor tendons in synovial environment – an experimental study on cellular mechanisms. *Journal of Hand Surgery*, **5**, 451–461

MADESEN, E. (1970) Delayed primary suture of flexor tendons cut in the digital sheath. *Journal of Bone and Joint Surgery*, **52B**, 264

MANSKE, P. R., WHITESIDE, L. A. and LESKER, P. A. (1978) Nutrient pathways to flexor tendons using hydrogen washout technique. *Journal of Hand Surgery*, **3**, 32

MANSKE, P. R., BIRDWELL, K. and LESKER, P. A. (1978) Nutrient pathways to flexor tendons of chickens using tritiated proline. *Journal of Hand Surgery*, **3**, 352–357

MANSKE, P. R., BIRDWELL, K., WHITESIDE, L. A. and LESKER, P. A. (1978) Nutrition of flexor tendon in monkeys. *Clinical Orthopedics*, **136**, 294

MANSKE, P. R. and LESKER, P. A. (1982) Nutrient pathways of flexor tendons in primates. *Journal of Hand Surgery*, **7**, 436

MANSKE, P. R. and LESKER, P. A. (1983) Caomparative nutrient pathways to the flexor profundus tendons in zone II of various experimental animals. *Journal of Surgical Research*, **34**, 83

MANSKE, P. R., GELBERMAN, R., VANDE BERG, J. *et al.* (1984) Flexor tendon repair: morphological evidence of intrinsic healing *in vitro*. *Journal of Bone and Joint Surgery,* **66A,** 385–396

MANSKE, P. R. and LESKER, P. A. (1984a) Histological evidence of flexor tendon repair in various experimental animals. An *in vitro* study. *Clinical Orthopedics,* **182,** 353–360

MANSKE, P. R. and LESKER, P. A. (1984b) Biochemical evidence of flexor tendon participation in the repair process. An *in vitro* study. *Journal of Hand Surgery,* **9B,** 117–120

MANSKE, P. R., OGATA, K. and LESKER, P. A. (1985) Nutrient pathways to extensor tendons of primates. *Journal of Hand Surgery,* **10B,** 8–10

MASON, M. L. (1940) Primary and secondary tendon suture. *Surgery, Gynecology and Obstetrics,* **70,** 392

MASON, M. L. and SHEARON, C. G. (1932) The process of tendon repair. *Archives of Surgery,* **25,** 615

MASON, M. L. and ALLEN, H. S. (1941) The rate of healing of tendons. *Annals of Surgery,* **113,** 424

MATTHEWS, P. (1976) The fate of isolated segments of flexor tendons within the digital sheath – a study in synovial nutrition. *British Journal of Plastic Surgery,* **29,** 216

MATTHEWS, P. and RICHARDS, H. (1974) The repair potential of digital flexor tendons. *Journal of Bone and Joint Surgery,* **56B,** 618

MATTHEWS, P. and RICHARDS, H. (1975) The repair reaction of flexor tendon within the digital sheath. *The Hand,* **7,** 27

MATTHEWS, P. and RICHARDS, H. (1976) Factors in the adherence of flexor tendon after repair. *Journal of Bone and Joint Surgery,* **58B,** 230–236

MAYER, L. (1916) The physiological method of tendon transplantation – I. Historical: anatomy and physiology of tendons. *Surgery, Gynecology and Obstetrics,* **22,** 182, 298

McDOWELL, C. L. and SNYDER, D. M. (1977) Tendon healing: an experimental model in the dog. *Journal of Hand Surgery,* **2,** 122

McFARLANE, R. M. and HAMPOLE, M. K. (1973) Treatment of extensor tendon injuries of the hand. *Canadian Journal of Surgery,* **16,** 366–375

McFARLANE, R. M., LAMON, F. and JARVIS, G. (1968) Flexor tendon injuries within the finger. A study of the results of tendon suture and tendon graft. *Journal of Trauma,* **8,** 987

MICKS, J. E. and HAGER, D. (1973) Role of the controversial parts of the extensor of the finger. *Journal of Bone and Joint Surgery,* **55A,** 884

PALMER, A. K., SKAHEN, J. R., WERNER, F. W. and GLISSON, R. R. (1985) The extensor retinaculum of the wrist: an anatomical and biomechanical study. *Journal of Hand Surgery,* **10B,** 11–16

PARKES, A. (1971) The 'lumbrical plus' finger. *Journal of Bone and Joint Surgery,* **53B,** 235

PEACOCK, E. E. (1959) A study of the circulation in normal tendons and healing grafts. *Annals of Surgery,* **149,** 415

PEACOCK, E. E. and VAN WINKLE, W. (1970) *Surgery and Biology of Wound Repair.* Philadelphia: W. B. Saunders

POTENZA, A. D. (1962) Tendon healing within the flexor digital sheath in the dog. *Journal of Bone and Joint Surgery,* **44A,** 49

PRATT, D. R. (1964) Follow-up note: internal splint for closed and open treatment of injuries of the extensor tendon at the distal joint of the finger. *Journal of Bone and Joint Surgery,* **46A,** 701

PULVERTAFT, R. G. (1956) Tendon grafts for flexor tendon injuries in the fingers and thumb. A study of technique and results. *Journal of Bone and Joint Surgery,* **38B,** 175

PULVERTAFT, R. G. (1958) Experiences in secondary flexor tendon grafting in the hand. *Acta Orthopaedica Belgica,* **24** (Suppl. 3), 62

RANK, B. K. and WAKEFIELD, A. R. (1950) Flexor tendon injuries in the hand. *Australian and New Zealand Journal of Surgery,* **19,** 232

RANK, B. K. and WAKEFIELD, A. R. (1951) The repair of flexor tendons in the hand. *British Journal of Plastic Surgery,* **4,** 244

ROBINS, P. R. and DOBYNS, J. H. (1975) Avulsion of the insertion of the flexor digitorum profundus tendon associated with fracture of the distal phalanx: A brief review. In *American Association of Orthopaedic Surgeons Symposium on Tendon Surgery of the Hand,* Chapter 17. St Louis: C. V. Mosby

SAKELLARIDES, H. T. (1978) The extensor tendon injuries and the treatment. *Rhode Island Medical Journal,* **61,** 307–313

SALVI, V. (1971) Delayed primary suture in flexor tendon division. *The Hand,* **3,** 181

SCHATZKER, J. and BRANEMARK, P. (1969) Intravital observations on the microvascular anatomy and microcirculation of the tendon. *Acta Orthopaedica Scandinavica,* Supplement 126, 3

SCHNEIDER, L. H. and HUNTER, J. M. (1975) Flexor tendolysis. In *American Association of Orthopaedic Surgeons Symposium on Tendon Surgery of the Hand,* Chapter 18. St Louis: C. V. Mosby

SMITH, J. W. (1965) Blood supply of tendons. *American Journal of Surgery,* **109,** 272

SMITH, R. J. (1974) Balance and kinetics of the fingers under normal and pathological conditions. *Clinical Orthopedics,* **104,** 92–111

SPINNER, M. and CHOI, B. Y. (1970) Anterior dislocation of the proximal interphalangeal joint, a cause of rupture of the central slip of the extensor mechanism. *Journal of Bone and Joint Surgery,* **52A,** 1329–1336

STACK, H. G. (1969) Mallet finger. *The Hand,* **1,** 83–89

STEICHEN, J. B., STRICKLAND, J. W., CALL, W. H. and POWELL, S. G. (1982) Results of surgical treatment of chronic boutonnière deformity: an analysis of prognostic factors. In *Difficult Problems in Hand Surgery,* Chapter 8, edited by J. W. Strickland and J. B. Steichen, pp. 62–69. St Louis: C. V. Mosby

STRICKLAND, J. W. and GLOGOVAC, S. V. (1980) Digital function following flexor tendon repair in zone II: a comparison of immobilization and controlled passive motion techniques. *Journal of Hand Surgery,* **5,** 537–543

TSUGE, J., IKUTA, Y. and MATSUISHI, Y. (1977) Repair of flexor tendons by intratendinous tendon suture. *Journal of Hand Surgery,* **2,** 436

TUBIANA, R. (1968) Surgical repair of the extensor apparatus of the fingers. *Surgical Clinics of North America,* **48,** 1015–1031

TUBIANA, R. and VALENTIN, P. (1964) Anatomy of the extensor apparatus and the physiology of the finger extension. *Surgical Clinics of North America,* **44,** 897–918

URBANIAK, J. R., CAHILL, J. D. and MORTENSON, R. A. (1975) Tendon suturing methods; analysis of tensile strengths. In *American Association of Orthopaedic Surgeons Symposium on Tendon Surgery in the Hand,* Chapter 8. St Louis: C. V. Mosby

VERDAN, C. (1960) Primary repair of flexor tendons. *Journal of Bone and Joint Surgery,* **42A,** 647

VERDAN, C. (1972) Half a century of flexor tendon surgery. *Journal of Bone and Joint Surgery,* **54A,** 472

VERDAN, C. and CRAWFORD, G. (1971) Flexor tendon suture in the digital canal. *Proceedings of the 5th International Congress of Plastic Surgery, Melbourne,* 22/25.2

WEHBE, M. A. and SCHNEIDER, L. H. (1984) Mallet fractures. *Journal of Bone and Joint Surgery,* **66,** 658–669

WEEKS, P. M. and WRAY, R. C. (1976) The rate and extent of functional recovery after flexor tendon grafting with and without silicone rod preparation. *Journal of Hand Surgery,* **1,** 175
Journal of Bone and Joint Surgery, **66,** 658–669

WEEKS, P. M. and WRAY, R. C. (1976) The rate and extent of functional recovery after flexor tendon grafting with and without silicone rod preparation. of rabbit tendon. *Clinical Orthopedics and Related Research,* **81,** 171

WHITAKER, J. H., STRICKLAND, J. W. and ELLIS, R. K. (1977) The use of flexor tenolysis in the palm and digits. *Journal of Hand Surgery,* **2(6),** 462

WHITE, W. L. (1960) Extensor habitus. *Journal of Bone and Joint Surgery,* **42A,** 913

WRENN, R. L., GOLDNER, J. L. and MARKEE, J. L. (1954) An experimental study of the effect of cortisone on the healing process and tensile strength of tendons. *Journal of Bone and Joint Surgery,* **26A,** 558

YOUNG, L. and WEEKS, P. M. (1970) Profundus tendon blood supply within the digital sheath. *Surgical Forum,* **21,** 504

ZANCOLLI, E. (1968) *Structural and Dynamic Bases of Hand Surgery,* pp. 105–106. Philadelphia: J. B. Lippincott

8
Nerve injuries*

Paul M. Weeks

INTRODUCTION: HISTORY

Occasional reports of repair of severed peripheral nerves appeared from the ninth until the eighteenth century (Ochs, 1980). However, it was not until the nineteenth century that significant developments in peripheral nerve surgery were made. Baudens (1836) performed the first brachial plexus repair. Mitchell (1864) published his treatise on peripheral nerve injuries incurred during the American Civil War, including his classic description of causalgia (Mitchell, Morehouse and Keen, 1864). The foundation for our current concepts of nerve response to injury was established by neuropathologists including Ranvier, Purkinje, and Waller. Waller (1850) described distal axonal degeneration after division of the hypoglossal and glossopharyngeal nerves and demonstrated that the axon cylinder was continuous with the cell body cytoplasm.

During the First World War, Tinel (1915) in France and Hoffmann (1915) in Germany described the clinical sign of axonal regeneration that now bears their names. During the Second World War, Sir Herbert Seddon (1947) advanced our understanding of the response of peripheral nerves to trauma and reported the results of nerve grafting. Concomitantly, Barnes Woodhall (1949), an American neurosurgeon, contributed significantly to our understanding of peripheral nerve repair and reconstruction. Sir Sidney Sunderland (1945) provided extensive studies of the internal anatomy of peripheral nerves. A major technical advance occurred when Zeiss produced the first binocular microscope in 1923. However, the development of microsurgery did not occur until the 1960s.

ANATOMY

The neuron is the anatomical and functional unit of the peripheral nervous system. It consists of a nerve cell body, one axon and multiple dendrites. The nerve cell body of a motor neuron is located in the lamina of the anterior horn of the corticospinal tract, whereas the nerve cell body of a sensory neuron is located in the

* With contributions by Keith F. Brewer and Samuel E. Logan

190

dorsal root ganglia (*Figure 8.1*). Each cell body communicates with adjacent nerve cells via dendrites. A neuron may have numerous dendrites but has only one axon. Dendrites are thought to provide afferent impulses to the neuronal body and axons efferent impulses. Histologically and chemically, they are indistinguishable. The axon is an extension of the neuronal cytoplasm from the nerve cell body as a gradually tapering cylinder ending in one or more synapses. It can vary from several millimeters to several meters in length and from less than 1 to approximately 20µ in diameter.

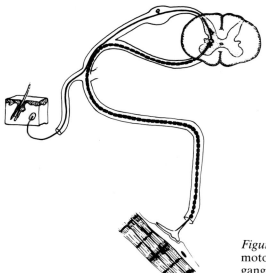

Figure 8.1 The cell bodies of the sensory and motor neurons are located in the dorsal root ganglia and anterior horn of the corticospinal tracts respectively

The surface membrane enveloping the axon is the axolemma. The principal constituents contained within the axonal cylinder are microtubles, neurofilaments, endoplasmic reticulum, and mitochondria. The microtubules and neurofilaments are contained within a thick, viscous axoplasm extending the length of the cylinder, imparting some stiffness to the axonal cylinder. These structures are involved in antegrade and retrograde axonal transport of neurotropic substances. Thus, axons function as transmitters of nerve impulses both centrally and peripherally and act as conduits for substances essential to nerve growth, maintenance and integrity (Sunderland, 1978).

Nerve sheath

The axonal sheath, a connective tissue envelope, surrounds an axon–Schwann cell complex. Each sheath is separated from the rest by a basement membrane, or neurolemma. The connective tissue envelope consists of the outer and inner layer of endoneurium. The Schwann cell layer may or may not contain myelin. The diameter of the axon appears to be dependent upon myelin. Unmyelinated axons tend to be smaller, less than 1–2μ, whereas myelinated axons range from 2 to 20μ. Several authors report that the transition from unmyelinated to myelinated fibers is smooth and progressive, while others note an appreciable overlap.

An unmyelinated axon is enveloped by a Schwann cell early in its development. One Schwann cell will associate with multiple axons and gradually envelop them with separate cytoplasmic extensions. When mature, each axon is separately encased with Schwann cell cytoplasm except for a slender mesoaxon. Schwann cells are arranged in sequence along an axon forming a continuous longitudinal chain. At each cell interface there are interdigitations of numerous cytoplasmic extensions from adjacent Schwann cells (Schmitt and Bear, 1937). They assist in extracellular to intracellular transport of energy-rich compounds and in maintenance of the ionic milieu of axons (*Figure 8.2a*).

Myelinated axons have a more individualized relationship with the Schwann cell (*Figure 8.2b*). Early in the development of the axon a longitudinal strand of Schwann cells align with the axon and envelop it except for the mesoaxon. Each

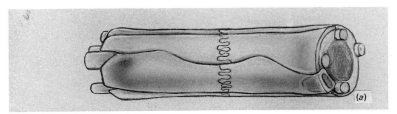

Figure 8.2a Unmyelinated nerve fibers share Schwann cells

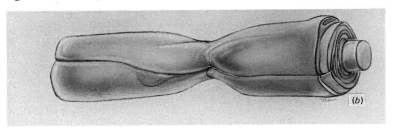

Figure 8.2b Each myelinated nerve fiber is enveloped by a Schwann cell

Schwann cell occupies one internodal space and is associated with only one axon, in contrast to the unmyelinated axon. As the axon grows it is progressively wrapped by Schwann cell cytoplasm, except for the mesoaxon. This results in the development of concentric lamellae of myelin with the potential submicroscopic space being occupied by the mesoaxon. The myelin sheath consists of bimolecular lipid leaflets separated by a thin proteinaceous layer. Myelin, which is produced by the Schwann cells, is composed of phospholipid, cholesterol and cerebroside (Sunderland, 1978). It functions primarily as an insulator, allowing more rapid axonal conduction.

Nodes of Ranvier are unmyelinated areas of axons where Schwann cells abut. The nodes measure from 0.1–0.8μ in length (Bischoff and Thomas, 1975). Internodal distance varies from axon to axon but appears to increase with increasing diameter of the fiber. They function in saltatory conduction as impulses 'jump' from node to node, allowing more rapid transmission of impulses.

Peripheral nerve fiber

The macroscopic unit of a peripheral nerve is the fascicle (also called funiculus), a group of axons surrounded by a thin but durable sheath of perineurium (*Figure 8.3*). Most nerves are composed of several fascicles, but some contain only a single fascicle. The number of fascicles present on cross-sectional study of a nerve varies with level of section. Intercommunication of fascicles leading to plexus formation changes the neural composition of the individual fascicle at each level studied. Fascicles vary from 0.04 to 2 mm in diameter (Sunderland and Bradley, 1952).

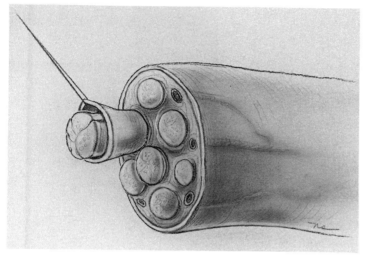

Figure 8.3 Each fascicle consists of a group of axons surrounded by a sheath of perineurium

The fascicular pattern of peripheral nerves in the upper extremity is the source of some controversy. Sunderland (1945), in his classic treatise on the topography of the radial, median and ulnar nerve, noted that in the most proximal portions of the nerves the majority of the fascicles contain axons of most, if not all, of the subsequent peripheral branches (*Figure 8.4a*). At more distal levels a gradual regrouping of fascicles occurs, resulting in individual nerve branches occupying individual fascicles or groups of fascicles. Though there is frequent intercommunication between these fascicles, groups of fascicles can remain in the same quadrant. This interfascicular branching has been quoted frequently as an explanation for the less than optimal results of nerve repair.

Jabaley, Wallace and Heckler (1980) corroborated Sunderland's observation that 'functional units (and often discrete branches) may remain localized in the same quadrants of nerve trunks and were accessible to surgical repair'. Furthermore, they noted 'although internal sectors of a nerve may be changing, other portions may proceed for considerable distances with no major change in position or composition and could be surgically isolated'. They noted, as did Sunderland, that intraneural plexuses were of three types:

(1) those where all the fascicles were derived from one branch and confined to like bundles of origin;

(2) those where fascicles of a bundle or branch blended with fascicles of a nearby but seperate bundle – this implies blending of unlike fascicles; and
(3) those occurring at the most proximal level of the nerve, where bundles contained fibers from diverse sources and divided and combined repeatedly.

Their concept of the fascicular anatomy of the median nerve is shown in *Figure 8.4b*.

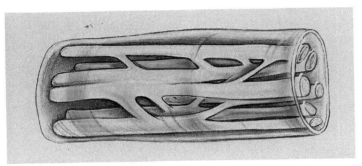

Figure 8.4a Sunderland noted extensive proximal communications among the majority of fascicles

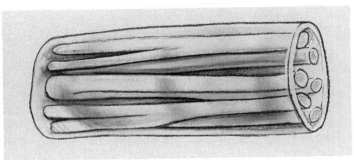

Figure 8.4b Jabaley noted considerable lengths of fascicles with no major change in position or composition

CONNECTIVE TISSUE ELEMENTS OF PERIPHERAL NERVE

Fascicles may contribute from 25 to 75 per cent of the cross-sectional area of a nerve trunk, the remainder being composed of connective tissue (Sunderland and Bradley, 1949). The connective tissue layers include: epineurium, perineurium, and endoneurium – each with a specific function (*Figure 8.5*).

Epineurium

This is the outer investing layer of the peripheral nerve. It consists primarily of collagen fibers and elastin fibers arranged in an irregular fashion. The average

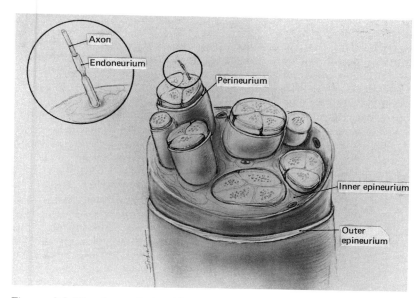

Figure 8.5 The interrelationships of epineurium, perineurium and endoneurium are depicted

thickness is 80 nm (Gamble and Eames, 1964). It can be subdivided into two layers: an outer or extraneural epineurium, which is the looser envelope of the peripheral nerve, and an inner or intraneural epineurium, which separates fascicles. The amount of epineurium in the cross-sectional area of a nerve varies from level to level and from nerve to nerve, ranging between 22 and 80 per cent in humans. Epineurium contributes to elasticity and tortuosity of the nerve, providing protection against tensile loading and cushioning the fascicles against external forces. There is evidence that epineurial fibroblasts contribute extensively to scar formation following nerve repair (Sunderland and Bradley, 1949).

Perineurium

The layer immediately investing the fascicle is the perineurium, which can be subdivided into internal, intermediate and external layers. The internal layer is immediately adjacent to the fascicle and functions as a diffusion barrier. The intermediate zone is a lamellated structure of collagen fibrils which acts as a diffusion barrier helping maintain the chemical integrity of the axon. The external layer is a transition zone between the epineurium and perineurium. Collagen is less well organized in this layer. The primary functions of the perineurium are to:

(1) protect the axon against tensile or elastic stress;
(2) act as a diffusion barrier and maintain intrafascicular pressure; and
(3) serve as a barrier to the spread of infection (Sunderland, 1978).

Endoneurium

The innermost layer of connective tissue is the endoneurium. It envelops and supports the axons within the fascicles. Its outer layer is comprised of longitudinally oriented fibrils of collagen, which envelop each axon to form an endoneurial tube. Its inner layer is adjacent to the Schwann cell basement membrane and is a more delicate structure than the outer layer.

The endoneurium functions are: (1) to resist elongation, (2) to maintain intra-axonal pressure, and (3) to act as an insulator (Sunderland, 1978).

Vascular system

The vascular anatomy of the human nerve consists of an intrinsic and an extrinsic system. The extrinsic vessels accompany the nerve but are not incorporated into the epineurium. Terzis and Breidenback (1984) described five vascular patterns. Pattern I has no dominant extrinsic vessel supplying the nerve; pattern II has one dominant vessel; pattern III has multiple different dominant vessels; pattern IV has one dominant vessel supplying a nerve for only part of its course; and pattern V has multiple dominant vessels with interspaced segments of nerve-free extrinsic vessels. These communicate with intrinsic vessels via vasa nervorum in the mesoneurium.

Lundborg (1979) has contributed to our understanding of the intrinsic vascular anatomy of nerves through his study of the median, ulnar, sensory branch of the ulnar nerve, and digital nerves of the thumb in man. The larger vessels are longitudinally oriented with intricate and frequent anastomoses (*Figure 8.6*). The intrinsic system receives flow from regional extrinsic vessels. All layers of the nerve have an intrinsic vascular plexus. The epineurial plexus consists of large longitudinal vessels which are aligned along the individual fascicles they supply. One vessel will supply numerous smaller vessels throughout its course, and each separate fascicle receives flow from several epineurial vessels.

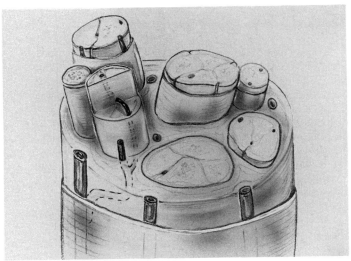

Figure 8.6 The intrinsic vascular system receives flow from the regional extrinsic vessels

The intrafascicular vascular system consists of both a perineurial and endoneurial network. The perineurial network, which is of capillary size, runs longitudinally beneath the external perineurium. These capillaries communicate with a distinct smaller capillary network within the endoneurium of each fascicle. This fascicular plexus is an anatomical vascular unit which is not disturbed when interfascicular dissection is performed. If this intrafascicular plexus is disturbed by dissection, endoneurial edema, scarring and loss of normal nerve function occur. The implication of these observations, as Kline *et al.* (1972) have demonstrated, is that nerves may be mobilized for some distances without jeopardizing nerve function if the epineural plexus is not compromised. Though extraneural fibrosis results from disturbing the epineural vessels, this is not thought to alter long-term function.

Physiological response to injury

The nerve cell body and axonal segments, proximal and distal to the site of injury, undergo a predictable sequence of events following injury (Lehman and Hayer, 1967). Within 6–12 hours the cell begins to swell and the nucleus becomes eccentrically displaced. Chromatolysis or dispersion of Nissl bodies occurs, which represents transformation of the RNA of the endoplasmic reticulum into a more synthetic phase. Protein synthesis is increased after a short period of initial decline and remains increased until recovery or death of the cell occurs. Lysosomal bodies are increased in number and become widely dispersed. There is a marked increase in activity of supporting surrounding glial cells which peaks within the first week of injury. If the nerve cell survives it will enter a recovery phase after 2–3 weeks which can last weeks to months. This is heralded by a reversal of the previously mentioned anatomic changes. If the nerve cell is destined to die, the initial changes are followed by a loss of cellular integrity and degeneration of cellular components. The factors determining neuron survival and response include:

(1) severity of the injury; that is, the greater the trauma, the greater the retrograde reaction;
(2) the proximity of the injury to the nerve cell body; that is, the closer the lesion to the nerve cell body, the greater likelihood of cell death; and
(3) the size of the neuron; that is, larger neurons tolerate the same insult better than smaller ones.

Axon changes proximal to the injury reflect the extent of trauma. A sharp, clean division will produce a small area of change immediately adjacent to the injury, whereas a blunt injury may produce axonal changes several centimeters proximal to the site of the injury. Following transection the axonal stump will swell proximal to the site of the injury, forming a bulb. The cross-sectional area of the bulb may be three or four times larger than that of the normal axon and subsides somewhat over several weeks. There is loss of axonal diameter and myelin thickness between 10 and 21 days in the remaining part of the axon proximal to the bulb.

Distal to the site of injury the axon undergoes Wallerian degeneration (Waller, 1850). Within 1–2 days after transection the neurofilaments and neurotubules in the axons become disorganized. The axonal cylinder progressively deteriorates until only remnants persist. Within 48 hours myelin withdraws from the nodes of Ranvier, leading to a widening of the nodes. Over the subsequent 24–48 hours myelin degeneration occurs, as does phagocytosis of the myelin debris. Individual nerves can be identified by electrical stimulation or histochemical stains up to 72 hours after injury. The Schwann cell undergoes a marked increase in metabolic activity in preparation for its role in Wallerian degeneration. They proliferate and are thought to aid in myelin degradation by development of a phagocytic function. The extent of this activity is proportional to the severity of the injury. From 2–4 weeks after injury the number of cells declines and they align themselves within the empty endoneurial tubes to form bands described by Bungner (1891).

The endoneurial tubes show little, if any, change in the immediate post-injury period. If repair is performed and axonal regrowth occurs, the endoneurial tubes maintain their premorbid character. If repair and reinnervation are delayed, the endoneurial tubes undergo atrophy and collagenization with loss of 80–90 per cent of cross-sectional diameter within three months (Sunderland and Bradley, 1950).

CLASSIFICATION OF NERVE INJURY

The two most commonly used classifications of nerve injury are those of Seddon and Sunderland. The classifications, which are used to predict recovery, are based upon the anatomic derangements caused by the injury.

Seddon (1943) recognized three categories of nerve injury. A neurapraxia, the least severe injury, is characterized by a conduction block. There is no associated Wallerian degeneration, and complete recovery occurs within 3–6 weeks after injury. Axonotmesis describes a more severe injury with loss of anatomic continuity of the axon and endoneurium. The epineurium and perineurium remain intact. Wallerian degeneration occurs and there is a proximal axonal reaction as described above. Yet because of the maintenance of perineurial and epineurial integrity recovery is good, though frequently not complete, and may require 3–6 months. Neurotmesis is the most severe injury, characterized by complete disruption of both the neural and fibrous elements of the nerve fiber. Wallerian degeneration and retrograde fiber reaction occur. Functional recovery requires operative repair and the prognosis is variable, ranging from no return to near complete return of function.

Sunderland's classification

Sunderland (1951) developed a more detailed classification which included five degrees of injury, increasing in severity from one to five. A first-degree injury produces a conduction block without anatomical derangement. Recovery is usually complete, requiring from one week to six months. Sensory tends to precede motor return.

In a second-degree injury axonal continuity is disrupted but the endoneurial tube remains intact. Retrograde fiber changes and Wallerian degeneration occur. Recovery requires axonal growth, thus delaying recovery for months rather than weeks.

Third-degree injury is limited to the fascicle with disruption of the axons and endoneurium, but the epineurium and perineurium remain intact. Axonal growth may be directed into the wrong distal tubules, resulting in incomplete return of function. Recovery is delayed and more incomplete than in the first two degrees of injury.

Fourth-degree injury occurs when the fascicle is entirely disrupted but the nerve is held together by loose epineural tissue. Because of the magnitude of the injury, proximal fiber and cellular reactions are more severe, as is the amount of fascicular disorganization. The chances for spontaneous recovery are minimal, and surgical repair is indicated.

The fifth-degree injury involves complete disruption of neural and fibrous continuity and retraction of the nerve ends. Surgical repair is necessary.

PHYSICAL DIAGNOSIS OF NERVE INJURY

A thorough history and physical examination will lead to the diagnosis of every nerve injury. Historically, determining when, where and how the injury occurred, is the *sine qua non* of a proper evaluation. It is most important to determine how the injury occurred including the exact circumstances and position of the extremity at the time of injury. What object produced the injury? What were the patient's chief complaints after injury? Have they changed? Were there associated injuries? Age, dominant extremity, and occupation may be important in selecting therapy.

Physical examination should begin by simple observation of the extremity. When evaluating an acute injury the nerves at risk are suggested immediately by the site of injury. With a thorough knowledge of the neuroanatomy of the upper extremity, all nerve injuries should be diagnosed without difficulty. Variations in innervation must be appreciated. Partial laceration of a nerve may present difficulty in diagnosis momentarily, but a thorough history and physical examination will clarify the site and extent of injury. Is there muscle atrophy or skin change? Ask the patient what tasks he cannot perform and observe him in action. Sensory and motor function in the median, ulnar and radial in the forearm and hand should be evaluated.

Sensory examination is first conducted by observing the hand. In other than acute injuries the denervated skin can be discolored, dry and scaly. Beads of sweat are absent, usually contrasting with normal innervated areas. Sudomotor (sympathetic) activity is frequently altered after a peripheral nerve injury, producing a dry, scaly appearance to the skin. This is of value in that one can observe it without the time-consuming effort to document it with a ninhydrin print test. The examiner lightly strokes both hands in comparable areas as an initial test for sensory loss. Static and moving two-point discrimination are tested as indicated in areas of suspected sensory deficit. Weber (1835) described the static two-point discrimination test. The test determines the minimum distance between two stimuli that the patient can distinguish. It evaluates the slowly adapting fiber/receptor system.

Although it has been criticized when used as a test for functional recovery, if the contralateral extremity is normal, it is considered the best standard of reference for comparison. Moving two-point discrimination described by Dellon (1978) assesses tactile gnosis by requiring an individual to distinguish between two simultaneously applied stimuli as they are moved in a proximal to distal fashion along the volar aspect of the finger. Normal is 2 mm over the distal phalanx, which is frequently the only area evaluated. Dellon (1980) recommends use of a 256 cps tuning fork. The prong end of the fork is applied to each finger of the injured and normal hand. Diminished perception means there is a loss of nerve conduction. He has never had a false negative or false positive with this single test.

The muscles should be palpated during contraction. The examiner should be aware of supplementary actions of muscles and tendons, depending upon the position of the extremity and joints in question. Children rapidly adapt to nerve deficits and substitute adjacent, synergistic activities to replace lost motion. The combined results of observation, moving light touch, two-point discrimination and motor testing will provide the proper diagnosis without further testing. More sophisticated tests have been developed but are not required in routine practice. A battery of tests may be used in evaluating nerve return.

THE TIMING OF NERVE REPAIR

Primary nerve repair is that which is done prior to the development of scar within the wound; in other words, 5–6 days. This may be further subdivided into immediate, within several hours, or delayed, within several days. Secondary repair is that which is done any time thereafter.

Much experience with nerve repair was obtained during the two world wars. Because of the complexity of the combat injuries most nerve repairs were done secondarily. In the First World War the average time before re-exploration was three months, as that was thought to be the earliest time that previously contaminated wounds could be safely opened. During the Second World War progress in the surgical management of wounds and the understanding of nerve response to injury shortened the delay period, but nearly all injuries continued to be repaired secondarily. It was thought that after 3–5 weeks the metabolic activity in the neuron and axon was optimal for nerve repair and subsequent recovery of function (Jabaley, 1981).

Sunderland (1945), writing after the war, arbitrarily divided nerve injuries associated with wounds into two general categories. Group I consists of those wounds in which extensive soft tissue injury, contamination, and vascular or osseous injuries coexisted with a nerve injury. These are commonly seen in warfare. Group II is the typical civilian injury in which nerve transection has occurred with less associated soft tissue damage or contamination. He felt that because of the associated contamination, devitalized tissue, and inability to ascertain the proximal extent of injury, secondary repair after a wound had healed was preferable in group I. The optimum time for exploration would be 3–5 weeks after wound closure.

In group II injuries he recommended primary repair under the following circumstances:

(1) the nerve was cleanly divided and the wound was such that residual scarring was unlikely;
(2) repair can be done within 36 hours;
(3) surgeons skilled in the techniques of nerve repair are available;
(4) repair can be accomplished without tension; and
(5) there is no evidence of infection.

He noted that secondary repair was indicated if any question exists about the extent of nerve injury, contamination of the wound and ability to coapt the nerve ends without tension. Secondary repair under favourable conditions would be superior to primary repair under unfavorable conditions.

Van Beek and Glover (1975) experimented on rodents, and Kline and Hackett (1975) in reviewing clinical studies have shown that primary repair of civilian-type nerve injuries in wounds converted to surgically clean ones was superior to secondary repair.

Metabolic and structural changes in the neuron proximal and distal to the site of injury influences the decision regarding timing of repair. Ducker, Kempe and Hayes (1969) have suggested that most nerve repairs should be performed 2–3 weeks after injury to take advantage of these metabolic and structural changes. However, no clinical studies are available to support their suggestion.

METHODS OF NERVE REPAIR

End-to-end repair

Epineurial suture

Hueter (1883) introduced the concept of epineurial nerve repair, and until recently it was considered the method of choice for repair of all nerve injuries. Epineurial repair is designed to produce optimum fascicular coaptation and alignment without resorting to perineurial sutures or extensive dissection. It thus avoids distortion of the internal anatomy of the nerve by suture or scarring from suture or dissection of the perineurium. The nerve ends are dissected free from surrounding tissue. The damaged portion of the nerve is resected. The proximal level of resection is determined by gross examination of the bulb and the cross-sectional area (*Figure 8.7*). The neuroma is resected just proximal to the beginning of enlargement of the nerve. The cross-section is inspected under the microscope. If any areas have a

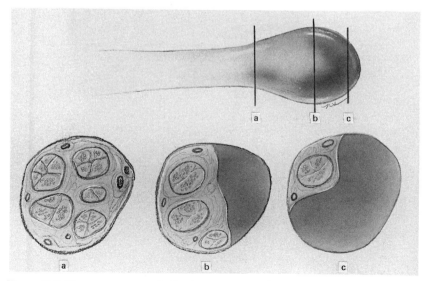

Figure 8.7 The neuroma and glioma are resected until a normal cross-section of nerve is obtained

'ground glass' appearance, more nerve is resected until a normal pattern of fascicles is obtained. Distally, the thickened supporting structures of the axon are resected until all areas of scar are removed and only tubules are present on cross-section. The nerve is inspected to see if prominent vessels in the perineurium are present to help determine proper alignment. The nerve ends are aligned using the outer epineurial vasculature pattern and the fascicular pattern on the inner surface of the nerve to determine correct rotation of the two ends of the nerve (*Figure 8.8*). With the aid of appropriate magnification an epineurial repair is performed with 10–0 nylon. The suture should penetrate the outer epineurium without disturbing the perineurium or fascicular architecture. Care must be taken to avoid: (1) inversion of the perineurium, (2) tension resulting in gaps between the fascicles, and (3) incorporation of too much endoneurium into the suture line, resulting in distortion of fascicular alignment.

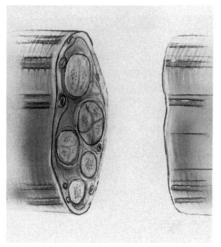

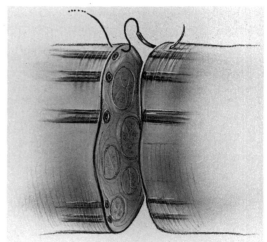

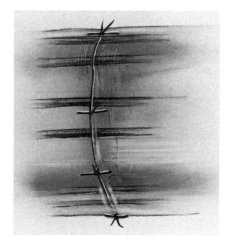

Figure 8.8 Sutures are placed only in the epineurium to provide optimal fascicular coaptation and alignment without distorting the internal anatomy of the nerve

Fascicular suture

Coaptation of individual fascicles using perineurial sutures was attempted by Langley and Hashimoto (1917) before the advent of microsurgery. With the development of microsurgical techniques and the ability to be less traumatic with the handling of tissues, interfascicular nerve repair has been advocated by many surgeons, particularly by Millesi. The cut ends of the nerve are resected back to normal nerve. The cross-sectional pattern is recorded both proximally and distally, as is the vascular pattern. The fascicles are not dissected because orientation is quickly lost. The fascicles are approximated with 10–0 nylon sutures placed through the perineurium of the individual fascicle and interfascicular epineurium (*Figure 8.9*). Tension at the suture line is to be avoided. Fascicular repair is possible only where two to four fascicles are present, for example, the ulnar nerve at the elbow, digital nerves in the fingers and neuromas in continuity. Where there are more fascicles they must be considered in groups.

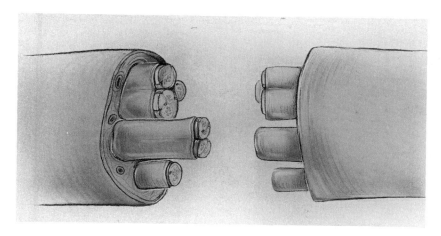

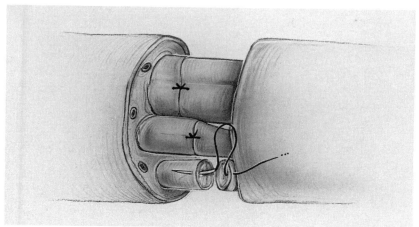

Figure 8.9 Individual fascicles are approximated using sutures in the perineurium

Group fascicular suture

Because of the large number of fascicles in major nerves, group fascicular repair rather than repair of each fascicle is preferred (Millesi, Meissl and Berger, 1976). The technique of group fascicular repair involves interfascicular dissection in the intraepineurial plane under appropriate magnification. The epineurium is gently teased from the surrounding fascicular bundles and each group is transected sharply in a perpendicular plane until normal fascicles are present. One should avoid disruption of the perineurium when dissecting in the inner epineurial plane. Once the corresponding fascicular bundles are identified proximally and distally under magnification, repair is performed by apposing the groups of fascicules with 10–0 nylon stitches catching the inner epineurium (*Figure 8.10*). Care is taken not to disrupt the perineurium because of the deleterious effects.

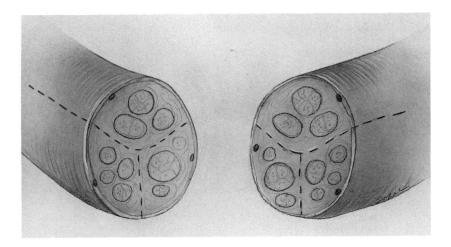

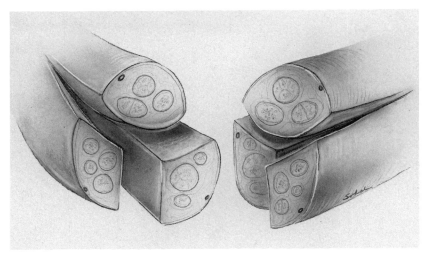

Figure 8.10 Groups of fascicles may be isolated by dissection in the inner epineurium

Identification of corresponding fascicular bundles

Identification of the corresponding proximal and distal fascicular bundles may be done in one of three ways: (1) anatomically, (2) histochemically, or (3) electrophysiologically. Sunderland (1945) has done painstaking dissections with cross-sections of all major peripheral nerves at multiple levels. These studies have explicitly outlined the fascicular pattern in these nerves and may be referred to for guidance in achieving fascicular alignment.

Several histochemical methods have been developed to aid in defining fascicular anatomy. Gruber and Zenker (1973) described staining acetylcholinesterase in nerve endings to distinguish between sensory and motor axons. Unfortunately, this must be performed within 72 hours of injury and a biopsy of the nerve is required for staining. Furthermore, the stain requires 24 hours to be effective. At the moment this method is of no clinical value. Riley and Lang (1984) described a staining technique for detecting carbonic anhydrase activity in debrided nerve endings. This requires 3–4 hours. Myelin is stained in motor axons and axoplasm is stained in sensory axons. Its practical value during nerve repair remains to be demonstrated. Gaul (1983) reported use of electrical stimulation to identify distal motor and proximal sensory branches. Utilizing a wake-up anesthetic technique, the proximal sensory branches are identified after electrical nerve stimulation (by the patient's response). The results were comparable to other series of nerve repair. In summary, the histochemical and electrostimulation have theoretical and experimental merit; but practical considerations limit their applicability in the operating room. The most reliable method of producing fascicular alignment appears to be utilization of the nerve fascicular maps generated by Sunderland's work.

Selection of method of repair based on functional return

Controversy abounds regarding the superiority of epineurial, interfascicular and group fascicular repair. There is evidence supporting each in humans, non-human primates and rodents. Most of the available data is derived from animal studies. These are limited by accurate, meaningful assessment, including return of function, axon counts distal to repair sites, physiological data, muscle weight, and biochemical assays. Cabaud *et al.* (1976) working with cats noted no significant difference between epineurial and group fascicular repair of nerves. Levinthal, Brown and Rand (1977) had similar results using dog peroneal nerves. Bora, Pleasence and Didizian (1976) noted significantly greater distal myelin count with epineurial suture and felt that this technique promoted more rapid nerve regeneration. Orgel and Terzis (1977) reported no significant difference in axonal regrowth when comparing epineurial and fascicular repairs in mice. Kline, Hudson and Bratton (1981) and Cabaud, Rodkey and McCarroll (1980) reported similar results when using perineurial or epineurial suturing of nerve injuries in non-human primates. Young, Wray and Weeks (1981) reported a prospective randomized study in humans of epineurial versus fascicular repair and noted no difference in the return of sensation after repair of digital nerves.

On the other hand, Wise *et al.* (1969), Brushart, Tarlov and Mesulam (1982), Bora (1967) and Grabb *et al.* (1970) report superior results with fascicular versus epineurial repair in laboratory animals.

A cogent analysis and discussion of this controversy is provided by Sunderland (1979) and Jabaley (1981). These authors conclude that epineurial suture is the procedure of choice if:

(1) there is no loss of tissue and fascicular continuity can be restored when the nerve is sutured;
(2) the fascicular patterns of the nerve ends are dissimilar; and
(3) the fascicles are large and closely packed so that a fascicular suture is impractical.

Fascicular repair is advised if:

(1) each fascicle is composed of nerve fibers that are either all sensory or all motor and occupies a constant position; and
(2) fiber composition of the fascicles is such that growth of axons using epineurial repair would result in axons occupying incorrect distal endoneurial tubes.

Jabaley (1981) noted that several areas of the median, ulnar and radial nerves meet the anatomical criteria for fascicular repair. They are as follows:

(1) median nerve – from the distal wrist crease to 5 cm proximally;
(2) median nerve – beginning several centimeters below the elbow and terminating at the origin of the flexor muscles;
(3) ulnar nerve – the area 7–8 cm proximal to the distal wrist crease;
(4) ulnar nerve – in the region of the elbow; and
(5) radial nerve – the area 10–12 cm proximal to the elbow.

Millesi (1980) provides a clearer distinction of indications, recommending that one must adapt surgical techniques to the anatomical peculiarities of the nerve in question. He divides cross-sectional patterns of nerves into four groups – monofascicular, oligofascicular, polyfascicular without grouping, and polyfascicular with grouping (*Figure 8.11*). In monofascicular and oligofascicular patterns the ratio of fascicular tissue to connective tissue is very high; thus, an epineurial nerve repair is indicated. As the number of fascicles increases it becomes more difficult to achieve fascicular alignment by epineurial sutures. Thus, approximation of the individual fascicles by perineurial suture provides better fascicular alignment. When there are many small fascicles, individual fascicular repair is not feasible and group fascicular repair is indicated. Thus, the technique of nerve repair is based on the cross-sectional pattern of the involved nerve.

Use of nerve grafts

Nerve grafting was first performed by Philipeaux and Vulpian (1870). Bunnell (1927) popularized this technique. However, between the wars the accepted standard of therapy was to achieve an end-to-end neurorrhapy if possible by a variety of manoeuvres including: (1) mobilization of the proximal and distal nerve segments; (2) flexion of adjacent joints; (3) transposition of the nerve when anatomically feasible, and (4) bone shortening. The net result of this was that few grafts were done because nearly all gaps were closed using the above manoeuvres.

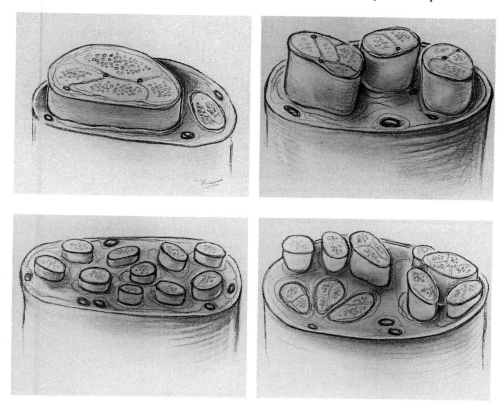

Figure 8.11 Cross-sectional patterns of nerves can be divided into monofascicular (*a*), oligofascicular (*b*), polyfascicular without grouping (*c*), and polyfascicular with grouping (*d*)

Seddon (1947) reported improved results with grafting which encouraged other clinicians to reconsider it as a clinical alternative. It was not until the concept of fascicular repair was applied by Millesi, Meissl and Berger (1972) to interfascicular grafting that results improved enough to make it acceptable as an alternative to end-to-end repair. Clinicians were concerned because the use of nerve grafts introduce a second suture line for the regenerating axons to cross. However, Millesi, Meissl and Berger (1976) and others have shown that the interfascicular grafts under no tension have as good a clinical result and distal axon count as epineurial repairs under mild to moderate tension.

Indications for nerve grafting

Nerve grafts are indicated when the fascicles cannot be approximated without tension using a 10–0 nylon suture to perform either an epineurial, interfascicular or group fascicular repair. The position of involved joints is the main point of controversy. Should the joints be in extension, flexion or neutral? I prefer moderate flexion of the joints to nerve grafting if the nerve ends can be approximated without tension. Some small nerve defects can be overcome to provide nerve repair without tension by (1) moderate joint flexion; (2) nerve mobilization; or (3) bone shortening. The latter is applicable only in amputations, non-unions or acute fractures. The extent of nerve mobilization without affecting functional return has created controversy. Kline *et al.* (1972) demonstrated, in monkeys, that mobilization of a peripheral nerve, even when collateral vessels are sacrificed, has no discernible effect on regeneration and return of function. Transposition of the ulnar nerve at the elbow is an excellent method of gaining length for repair of a severed ulnar nerve near the elbow. Mobilization of the median and radial nerves is rarely used other than soft tissue elevation.

Tension can occur at the site of nerve repair at the time of repair or postoperatively when joint motion is begun. Millesi, Meissl and Berger (1972) showed that tension at the time of repair at the site of neurorraphy increased scarring and epineurial fibrosis. Similar results were reported by Terzis, Fabishoff and Williams (1975), who noted that conduction velocity declined across a repair as it is stretched acutely and that the conduction velocity of a tension-free graft was significantly faster than a stretched repair. Miyamoto (1979) showed that increasing tension affected the vascular supply and resulted in increased fibrosis at the site of repair. In a subsequent experiment he noted that epineurial nerve repairs in dogs performed under 0 g of tension produced the best distal axon counts, whereas epineurial repairs done under 25 g of tension could produce a comparable distal axon count but frequently did not. Grafted nerves were slow to have axonal sprouts migrate distally but by ten months were comparable to the zero tension group.

The effect of joint mobilization postoperatively on nerve regeneration after mild to moderate joint flexion was required at operation to accomplish a tension-free repair has not been demonstrated in man.

Classification of nerve grafts

Free nerve grafts

A variety of nerve graft techniques are available, each with its own set of indications and usefulness in specific situations. Cable grafts popularized by Seddon (1947) consist of donor nerve lengths grouped together to form a bridge between proximal and distal nerve stumps. Use of cable grafts disregards the anatomical alignment of fascicles in the proximal and distal nerve ends. Good results were initially reported, but the technique has been abandoned in favour of interfascicular or group fascicular nerve grafting.

Millesi, Meissl and Berger (1972) popularized interfascicular nerve grafts. They felt that (1) suture line tension was detrimental to nerve growth, (2) the epineurium was a source of scar between the nerve ends and that scar increased with increasing tension, and (3) axons crossing the suture line may be damaged by scar proliferation. By performing an interfascicular graft, tension on the suture line was minimized and an accurate group fascicular alignment was achieved, allowing for optimum axonal growth across the repair site.

This technique consists of meticulous preparation of the proximal and distal stumps. The epineurium is incised and reflected for a distance of 10–12 mm. When they are few, individual fascicles are isolated and continuity restored with nerve grafts (*Figure 8.12*). When there are many fascicles, individual groups are isolated

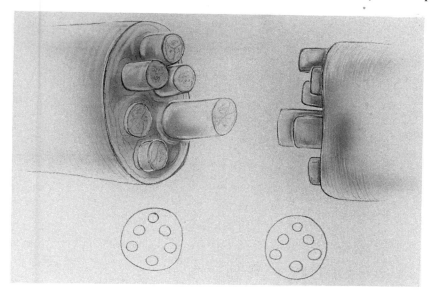

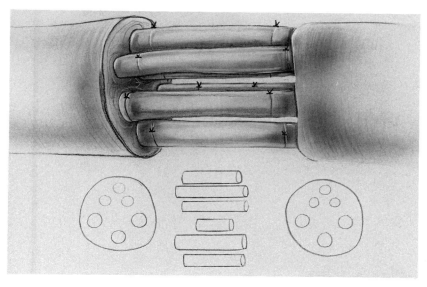

Figure 8.12 Individual fascicles are isolated and continuity restored with appropriate size grafts

by intra-epineurial dissection. Using anatomical maps and comparing the fascicular pattern of the nerve stumps, proximal and distal groups of fascicles are identified and aligned. The group fascicular to graft fascicular alignment is achieved using a minimum of sutures catching the epineurium of the graft and the inner epineurium or epineurium surrounding the group of fascicles (*Figure 8.13*). His results are excellent. For repair of the median nerve, motor function was M5 in 14 out of 20 patients. For the ulnar nerve 33 out of 44 were M3 to M5. Sensory return in the median nerve in 38 of 39 was S3 or better, and in the ulnar nerve 39 out of 44. Young, Weeks and Wray (1980) retrospectively reviewed the literature and compared interfascicular repair to epineurial repair, finding that there was no significant difference between the two methods of graft suture with the exception of the return of the median nerve motor function. Median motor function was significantly better in the epineurial repair group than in the nerve grafting group. When large defects exist there is significant variation in fascicular anatomy between the nerve ends. The use of a group fascicular repair is recommended to reduce error.

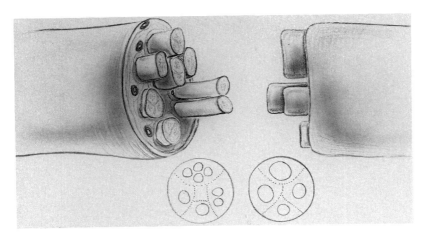

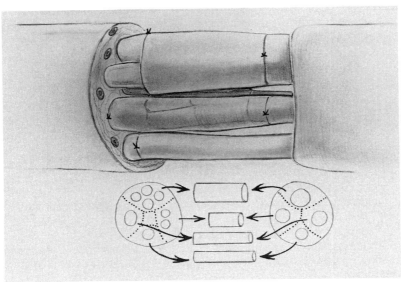

Figure 8.13 Corresponding groups of fascicles matched from anatomic maps of the proximal and distal stumps are connected using free grafts

Source of free nerve grafts

Many nerves have been used as grafts including the sural, medial and lateral antebrachial cutaneous nerves, brachial cutaneous nerves, terminal branch of the posterior interosseous nerve, and superficial branch of the radial nerve. The choice of a nerve graft is dependent upon the deficit it causes and the proportion of neural tissue in the cross-sectional area. More neural and less connective tissue is preferred. The sural nerve is an ideal graft. Proximally, it consists of one to three large fascicles. Distally there are many small fascicles. It can be readily identified beneath the lesser saphenous vein at the lateral malleolus and traced proximally to where it penetrates the fascia between the two heads of the gastrocnemius muscle. It is most easily identified at the ankle and traced proximally through a longitudinal incision. Most patients dislike a longitudinal scar. Multiple transverse incisions may be used. If the latter is used a few small branches 3–4 cm above the lateral malleolus can be a nuisance when retrieving the nerve and care must be taken to divide these branches. About 40 cm of sural nerve can be obtained from one leg.

We avoid using other cutaneous nerves in the upper extremity as grafts because of the occasional patient who develops extreme disability associated with its removal, especially the sensory branch of the radial nerve.

Pedicle nerve graft

Strange (1947) described the pedicle nerve graft for use in isolated and unusual cases in which both the median and ulnar nerve are severely damaged in the same forearm. The technique requires creation of an end-to-end neurorrhapy between the median and the ulnar nerve. The ulnar or the median nerve, depending upon which nerve is to be sacrificed, is then divided proximally to pre-degenerate the endoneurial tissues. At a second stage, the donor nerve is transferred as a vascularized graft to the distal end of the recipient nerve. Indications for its use are rare.

Free vascularized nerve graft

The free vascularized nerve graft was described by Taylor and Hamm (1976). The donor nerve is isolated on its vasculature and transferred as a free graft. Vascularized nerve grafts may be of benefit in the presence of a scarred bed or to bridge large gaps. The authors feel that graft survival is increased significantly when a vascularized graft rather than a free graft is placed in an unfavorable recipient bed. There is evidence to indicate that axonal growth is more rapid in vascularized grafts, thus theoretically decreasing the risk of atrophy at the end organs and fibrosis at the distal suture line (Koshima and Haru, 1985). Terzis and Breidenbach (1984) have suggested that a vascularized graft can act as a carrier for routine nerve grafts over long distances in unfavorable beds.

Six nerves with suitable vascular pedicles have been described: (1) the superficial radial; (2) the medial sural nerve; (3) the anterior tibial nerve; (4) the ulnar nerve; (5) the superficial peroneal; and (6) the saphenous nerve. Use of the superficial radial or anterior tibial nerve requires sacrifice of a major artery in the extremity. Presently there is no evidence that free vascularized nerve grafts give better results than free grafts.

Neuroma in continuity

A neuroma in continuity represents disruption of one or more fascicles with one or more fascicles remaining intact. Comparing the findings of a thorough sensory and motor examination with the known cross-sectional topography of the nerve at the level of injury, one can predict which fascicles will be disrupted. If there is significant functional loss, the nerve is exposed proximal and distal to the neuroma. The nerve is inspected using magnification. Intact fascicles beneath the outer epineurium will be immediately evident. The outer epineurium is opened and the intact fascicles are freed from the scar about the neuroma by dissecting in the inner epineurial plane. If possible, the intact fascicles should be dissected as a group and not as individual fascicles. Once all intact fascicles have been isolated, the neuroma and glioma are resected. The distance between the nerve ends is noted. In the authors' experience a graft has been required in repair of most neuromas in continuity. The cut ends are inspected and a drawing made of the fascicular pattern at both ends. A decision is made to do either an interfascicular repair or a group fascicular repair. This decision is based upon the number and size of fascicles cut, and if this is an area where fascicles are committed to a major functional unit. If one or several large fascicles are present in the neuroma and glioma, then an interfascicular nerve graft is used. If there are many small fascicles a group fascicular repair is performed.

Postoperative management

The rate of tensile strength gain of human nerves following suture after nerve division cannot be studied. Tarlov (1947) and Mukherjee (1953) studied bursting strengths of severed and repaired nerves in rabbits and dogs and found they were equal to that of a normal nerve within 3–4 weeks. Higgs, Wray and Weeks (1979) noted that the bursting strength of repaired severed nerves in rats was only 62 per cent of that of normal rat nerves at 12 weeks after repair. In a similar study using monkey median and ulnar nerves, the average bursting strength four weeks after repair was 77 per cent of normal. Empirically, the nerve repair site is protected for 3–4 weeks by maintaining the extremity in the position in which the nerve was repaired at the operating room table. Initially, this is accomplished by a dressing placed prior to awakening the patient and later by splinting. While immobilized, all joints that safely can be passively manipulated without endangering the repair are ranged to prevent the development of stiff joints and tendon adhesions. After four weeks of protection the repair is gently manipulated first by passive motion about the flexed joints followed by gentle active motion. If a direct repair has been accomplished without joint flexion, the joints are gradually mobilized over 3–4 weeks. If a direct repair has been performed with the joints moderately flexed extensive protection of the nerve repair site must be practised. The involved joints are kept immobile for approximately six weeks. Gradual extension is encouraged, requiring approximately six weeks to regain full extension. When nerve grafts are used, enough length is included to permit full joint extension without tension on the grafts. After three weeks of immobilization the joints are gradually mobilized over 3–4 weeks.

Assessment of nerve recovery

Evaluation of the nerve-injured patient both preoperatively and postoperatively has been standardized by the British Medical Research Council (*Table 8.1*, Highet and Holmes, 1943). Moberg's sensory classification, while simpler, allows that any sensory result with a two-point discrimination on the fingertip of greater than 15 mm is poor.

Table 8.1   Highet's method of end result evaluation

Motor recovery	
M0	No contraction
M1	Return of perceptible contraction in the proximal muscles
M2	Return of perceptible contraction in both proximal and distal muscles
M3	Return of function in both proximal and distal muscles of such a degree that all important muscles are sufficiently powerful to act against resistance
M4	Return of function as in stage 3; in addition, all synergic and independent movements are possible
M5	Complete recovery
Sensory recovery	
S0	Absence of sensibility in the autonomous area
S1	Recovery of deep cutaneous pain sensibility within the autonomous area of the nerve
S2	Return of some degree of superficial cutaneous pain and tactile sensibility within the autonomous area of the nerve
S3	Return of superficial cutaneous pain and tactile sensibility throughout the autonomous area, with disappearance of any previous over-response
S3+	Return of sensibility as in stage 3; in addition, there is some recovery of two-point discrimination within the autonomous area
S4	Complete recovery

A pattern of sensory recovery has been described by Dellon, Curtis and Edgerton (1972). Their evaluation included finger stroking and pressure with the examiner's finger on the patient's finger to stimulate perception of moving touch and constant touch respectively, and tuning forks of 30 and 256 cps to stimulate perception of flutter and vibration. Following recovery of perception of painful stimuli, a constant pattern was found for the touch submodality. Perception that the 30 cps stimuli was first to recover, followed very closely by perception of moving touch, followed in several months by perception of constant touch and finally by perception of 256 cps. Thus, the order of recovery is as follows: recovery of painful stimuli, perception of 30 cps, perception of moving touch, perception of constant touch, and finally perception of 256 cps.

Each patient should be thoroughly evaluated for the modalities of (1) constant touch, (2) moving touch, (3) two-point discrimination, (4) vibration at 30 and 256 cps, (5) ninhydrin printing, and (6) tactile gnosis by the Moberg pickup test at regular intervals with the progress or lack thereof being recorded. The Tinel's sign should be identified initially proximal to the repair and mapped as it progresses. Its maximum is 2.5 mm/day, with an average of 1 mm/day in the adult.

Return of motor function is followed by the reinnervation of the denervated musculature and the return of these muscles toward normal function. The sequence of progress is dictated by the innervation pattern of the involved nerve. Strength, speed and endurance are utilized to arrive at the appropriate evaluation.

Sensory re-education

The first formal program of sensory re-education following nerve repair was published by Wynn-Parry (1966). Sensory re-education has been popularized by Dellon, Curtis and Edgerton (1971) and modified by individual therapy units to reflect their experiences.

Sensory re-education is based upon the concept that no matter how accurate the nerve repair, some of the regenerating axons will enter foreign tubes and be misdirected either into the wrong receptors or into the wrong area, or that the distal tubule which it enters will have degenerated, impairing regeneration, or the distal end organ will have degenerated. In fact, there are a number of axons which never enter the distal endoneurial tubes, no matter how accurate the repair. As a result, the patient's sensory cortex receives foreign neural impulses, that is, ones which are new and unrecognizable. The object of sensory re-education is to educate the patient to correlate these new impulses with what he sees with his eyes. Thus, a correlation is established and he regains fine discrimination.

Essentially the process consists of giving a blindfolded patient a series of familiar large household objects to identify. The time required for object identification is recorded and used as a baseline. Coins, erasers, paper clips, keys, cards and so forth are used for identification purposes. If a patient is unable to recognize an object in 60 seconds, the test on that object ends and he goes to the next object. Objects are found which the patient can identify. If he is unable to identify smaller objects, then he begins with large wooden blocks of varying weight, size and shape covered with different textured materials. If he is still unable to identify the object, he is permitted to visualize the object and study it carefully and then to close his eyes again and try to combine the mental image with the visual picture. The same procedure is carried out with the unaffected hand so that he may compare the sensation on the two sides. Training is given daily, or patients are asked to have someone help them at home daily. After nerve repair one follows Tinel's sign, constant moving touch, and perception of vibration at both 30 and 256 cps. When the 256 cps stimulus is perceived at the fingertips sensory re-education is reintroduced.

Callahan (1984) has developed a very elaborate sensory re-education program. She recognizes two groups of candidates for sensory re-education: (1) those in whom protective sensation is lacking or severely decreased, and (2) those who have the ability to perceive pinprick, temperature and touch but lack localization, two-point discrimination and tactile gnosis. Thus, the sensory re-education program is divided into two phases: a protective sensory re-education, and a discriminative sensory re-education program.

Protective sensory education teaches the patient to protect the hand from exposure to excessively hot or cold or sharp objects, to avoid excessive gripping force, and to utilize low-grade repetitive pressure, low-grade repetitive grip and pinch in performing activities. The dangers of dry, cracked skin associated with denervation are stressed.

Sensory re-education is a more elaborate program. Patients entering the program are limited to those who (1) have regained protective sensation in the fingertips; (2) are intelligent and able to concentrate; (3) can devote time daily to re-education; and (4) are willing to incorporate the hand consciously into daily activities. The program is divided into tasks that require localization and graded discrimination. The result is that patients who have been followed for several years after sensory re-education have been observed to maintain and increase their functional gains if they continue using the hand activity for fine activities.

Onne (1962) and others have argued that only after 3–5 years can a satisfactory evaluation of return of nerve function be made. As a consequence, we must await late evaluation to resolve some of the controversial areas of nerve management presented in this chapter.

References

BAUDENS, J. B. L. (1836) *Clinique des Place d'Armes a Feu*. Paris: Baillière

BISCHOFF, A. and THOMAS, P. K. (1975) Microscopic anatomy of myelinated nerve fibers. In *Peripheral Neuropathy*, Chapter 6, 1, 104

BORA, F. W. (1967) Peripheral nerve repair in cats. *Journal of Bone and Joint Surgery*, **49A(4)**, 659–666

BORA, F. W., PLEASENCE, D. and DIDIZIAN, N. (1976) A study of nerve regeneration and neuroma formation after nerve suture by various techniques. *Journal of Hand Surgery*, **1(2)**, 138–143

BRUSHART, T., TARLOV, E. C. and MESULAM, M. M. (1982) Specificity of muscle reinnervation after epineurial and individual fascicular suture in the rat sciatic nerve. *Journal of Hand Surgery*, **8(3)**, 248–253

BUNGNER, O. (1891) Von uber die degenerations – regenerations – vorgange am nerven nach verletzengen beitr. *Pathologie und Anatomie*, **10**, 321

BUNNELL, S. (1927) Surgery of the nerves of the hand. *Surgery, Gynecology and Obstetrics*, **44**, 145–

CABAUD, H. E., RODKEY, W. G. and McCARROLL, H. R. (1980) Peripheral nerve injuries: studies in higher nonhuman primates. *Journal of Hand Surgery*, **5(3)**, 201–206

CABAUD, H. E., RODKEY, W. G., McCARROLL, Jr., H. R., MUTZ, S. B. and NIEBAUER, J. J. (1976) Epineurial and perineurial nerve repairs: a critical comparison. *Journal of Hand Surgery*, **1(2)**, 131–137

CALLAHAN, A. D. (1984) *Methods of Compensation and Reeducation for Sensory Dysfunction in Rehabilitation of the Hand*, 2nd edition, edited by Hunter, Schneider, Mackin and Callahan, pp. 432–442. St Louis: C. V. Mosby

DELLON, A. L. (1978) The moving two-point discrimination test: clinical evaluation of the quickly-adapting fiber/receptor system. *Journal of Hand Surgery*, **3**, 474–481

DELLON, A. L. (1980) Clinical use of vibratory stimuli to evaluate peripheral nerve injury and compressive neuropathy. *Plastic and Reconstructive Surgery*, **65**, 466–476

DELLON, A. L., CURTIS, R. M. and EDGERTON, M. T. (1971) Re-education of sensation in the hand following nerve injury (abstract). *Journal of Bone and Joint Surgery*, **53A**, 813

DELLON, A. L., CURTIS, R. M. and EDGERTON, M. T. (1972) Evaluating recovery of sensation in the hand following nerve injury. *Johns Hopkins Medical Journal*, **130**, 235–245

DUCKER, T. B., KEMPE, L. G. and HAYES, G. J. (1969) The metabolic background for peripheral nerve surgery. *Journal of Neurosurgery*, **30**, 270

GAMBLE, H. J. and EAMES, R. A. (1964) An electron microscope study of connective tissue of human peripheral nerve. *Journal of Anatomy*, **98**, 655

GAUL, J. S. (1983) Electrical fascicle identification as an adjunct to nerve repair. *Journal of Hand Surgery*, **8**, 289–296

GRABB, W. C., BEMENT, S. L., KOEPKE, G. H. and GREEN, R. A. (1970) Comparison of peripheral nerve suturing in monkeys. *Plastic and Reconstructive Surgery,* **46 (1)**, 31–37

GRUBER, H. and ZENKER (1973) Acetylcholinesterase: histochemical differentiation between motor and sensory nerve fibers. *Brain Research,* **51**, 207–214

HIGGS, P., WRAY, R. C. and WEEKS, P. M. (1979) Rate of bursting strength gain in repaired nerves. *Annals of Plastic Surgery,* **3**, 338–340

HIGHET, W. B. and HOLMES, W. (1943) Traction injuries to the lateral popliteal nerve and traction injuries to peripheral nerves after suture. *British Journal of Surgery,* **30**, 212

HOFFMANN, P. (1915) Ueber eine methode, den erfolg einer nervennaht zu beurteilen. *Medizinische Klinische,* **11**, 359

HUETER, K. (1883) *Die Allgemeine Chirurgie.* Leipzig: Vogel Verlag

JABALEY, MICHAEL (1981) Current concepts of nerve repair. *Clinics in Plastic Surgery,* **8**, 33–44

JABALEY, M. E., WALLACE, W. H. and HECKLER, F. R. (1980) Internal topography of major nerves of the forearm and hand: a current view. *Journal of Hand Surgery,* **5**, 1–19

KLINE, D. G. and HACKETT, E. (1975) Reappraisal of timing for exploration of civilian peripheral nerve injuries. *Surgery,* **78(1)**, 54–65

KLINE, D. G., HUDSON, A. R. and BRATTON, B. R. (1981) An experimental study of fascicular repair with and without epineurial closure. *Journal of Neurosurgery,* **54**, 513–520

KLINE, D. G., HACKETT, E. R., DAVIS, G. D. and MYERS, M. B. (1972) Effect of mobilization on nerve blood supply. *Journal of Surgical Research,* **12**, 254–266

KOSHIMA, I. and HARU, K. (1985) Experimental study of vascularized nerve grafts: multifactorial analyses of axonal regeneration of nerves transplanted into an acute burn wound. *Journal of Hand Surgery,* **10A(1)**, 64–72

LANGLEY, J. N. and HASHIMOTO, M. (1917) On the suture of separate nerve bundles in a nerve trunk and on internal nerve plexus. *Journal of Physiology, London,* **51**, 318

LEHMAN, R. A. and HAYER, G. J. (1967) Degeneration and regeneration in peripheral nerve. *Brain,* **90**, 285

LEVINTHAL, R. W., BROWN, W. J. and RAND, R. W. (1977) A comparison of fascicular, interfascicular and epineural suture techniques in repair of simple nerve lacerations. *Journal of Neurosurgery,* **47**, 744–750

LUNDBORG, G. (1979) The intrinsic vascularization of human peripheral nerves: structural and functional aspects. *Journal of Hand Surgery,* **4(1)**, 34–41

MILLESI, H. (1980) Interfascicular nerve repair and secondary repair with nerve grafts. In *Nerve Repair and Regeneration,* edited by D. L. Jewett and H. R. McCarroll, Jr. St Louis: C. V. Mosby

MILLESI, H., MEISSL, G. and BERGER, A. (1972) Interfascicular nerve grafting of median and ulnar nerves. *Journal of Bone and Joint Surgery,* **54A**, 727

MILLESI, H., MEISSL, G. and BERGER, A. (1976) Further experience with interfascicular grafting of the median, ulnar and radial nerves. *Journal of Bone and Joint Surgery,* **58A**, 209–

MITCHELL, S. W., MOREHOUSE, G. R. and KEEN, W. W. (1864) *Gunshot Wounds and Other Injuries of Nerves,* pp. 110–111. Philadelphia: J. B. Lippincott

MIYAMOTO, Y. (1979) Experimental study of results of nerve suture under tension vs. nerve grafting. *Plastic and Reconstructive Surgery,* **64(4)**, 540–549

MUKHERJEE, S. R. (1953) Tensile strength of nerves during healing. *British Journal of Surgery,* **1192**, 192

OCHS, S. (1980) A brief history of nerve repair. In *Nerve Repair and Regeneration,* edited by D. L. Jewett and H. R. McCarroll. St Louis: C. V. Mosby

ONNE, L. (1962) Recovery of sensibility and sudomotor activity in the hand after nerve suture. *Acta Chirurgica Scandinavica,* Suppl 300

ORGEL, M. and TERZIS, J. (1977) Epineurial vs. perineurial repair. *Plastic and Reconstructive Surgery,* **60(1)**, 80–91

PHILIPEAUX, J. M. and VULPIAN, A. (1870) Note sur les essais de greffe d'un troncon du nerf lingual des deux bouts du nerf hypnoglosse, après excision d'un segment de cet dernier nerf. *Archives du Physiologie et Normale Pathologie,* **3**, 618

RILEY, D. and LANG, D. (1984) Carbonic anhydrase activity of human peripheral nerves: a possible histochemical aid to nerve repair. *Journal of Hand Surgery,* **9A**, 112–120

SCHMITT, F. O. and BEAR, R. S. (1937) The optical properties of vertebrate nerve axons as related to fiber size. *Journal of Cellular Comparative Physiology,* **9**, 261

SEDDON, H. J. (1943) Three types of nerve injury. *Brain,* **66**, 237

SEDDON, H. J. (1947) The use of autogenous grafts for repair of large gaps in peripheral nerves. *British Journal of Surgery,* **35**, 151

STRANGE, F. G. (1947) An operation for nerve pedicle grafting. *British Journal of Surgery,* **34**, 423

SUNDERLAND, S. (1945) The intraneural topography of median, ulnar and radial nerves. *Brain,* **68**, 243–298

SUNDERLAND, S. (1951) A classification of peripheral nerve injuries producing loss of function. *Brain,* **74,** 491

SUNDERLAND, S. (1978) *Nerves and Nerve Injuries,* 2nd edition, pp. 10, 509–514 Edinburgh: Churchill/Livingstone

SUNDERLAND, S. (1979) The pros and cons of funicular nerve repair. *Journal of Hand Surgery,* **4(3),** 201–211

SUNDERLAND, S. and BRADLEY, K. C. (1949) The cross-sectional area of peripheral nerve trunks devoted to nerve fibers. *Brain, 72,* 428

SUNDERLAND, S. and BRADLEY, K. C. (1950) Endoneurial tube shrinkage in the distal segment of the severed nerve. *Journal of Comparative Neurology, 93,* 411

SUNDERLAND, S. and BRADLEY, K. C. (1952) The perineurium of peripheral nerves. *Anatomical Record,* **113,** 125

TARLOV, I. M. (1947) How long should an extremity be immobilized after nerve suture? *Annals of Surgery,* **126,** 366

TAYLOR, G. I. and HAM, F. J. (1976) The free vascularized nerve graft. *Plastic and Reconstructive Surgery,* **57,** 413

TERZIS, J. and BREIDENBACH, W. (1984) The anatomy of free vascularized nerve grafts. *Clinics in Plastic Surgery,* **11(1),** 65–71

TERZIS, J., FABISHOFF, B. and WILLIAMS, H. B. (1975) The nerve gap: suture under tension vs. graft. *Plastic and Reconstructive Surgery,* **56,** 166–170

TINEL, J. (1915) Le signe du fourmillement dans les lesions des nerfs péripheriques. *Presse Médicale,* **47,** 388–389

VAN BEEK, A. and GLOVER, J. (1975) Primary vs. delayed primary neurorrhaphy in rat sciatic nerve. *Journal of Surgical Research,* **18,** 335–339

WALLER, A. V. (1850) *Philosophical Transactions of Royal Society of London,* **140,** 143

WEBER, E. (1835) Ueber den tastsinn. *Archiv für Anatomie und Physiologie, Wissenschaftliche Medizin (Muller's Archives),* **1,** 152–159

WISE, A. J., Jr., TOPUZLU, C., DAVIS, P. and KAYE, I. S. (1969) A comparative analysis of microsurgical neurorrhaphy technique. *American Journal of Surgery,* **117(6),** 566–572

WOODHALL, B. (1949) A modern history of peripheral nerve surgery. World War II and the postwar study of peripheral nerve regeneration. *Journal of the American Medical Association,* **139,** 564

WYNN-PARRY, C. B. (1966) *Rehabilitation of the Hand,* pp. 92, 107–109, 112–113. London: Butterworths

YOUNG, V. L., WEEKS, P. M. and WRAY, R. C. (1980) The results of nerve grafting in the wrist and hand. *Annals of Plastic Surgery,* **5(3),** 210–214

YOUNG, V. L., WRAY, R. C. and WEEKS, P. M. (1981) A randomized prospective comparison of fascicular and epineurial digital nerve repairs. *Plastic and Reconstructive Surgery,* **68(1),** 89–93.

9
Joint injuries of the hand

James B. Bennett

INTRODUCTION

Joint injuries may result in significant disability initially as well as producing residual long-term impairment. Many of these injuries are missed because of a more noticeable fracture or may be totally ignored if X-rays are interpreted as normal. Discussion in this chapter will include injuries to the interphalangeal joints, metacarpophalangeal joints, carpometacarpal joints, intercarpal joints, radiocarpal joints, and the radio-ulnar joint. The discussion will include associated fractures, either intra-articular or periarticular, to the involved joints. The residual disabilities of instability, stiffness and pain will be considered along with the various modalities of treatment.

The literature is replete with the anatomy, biomechanics, and pathophysiology of bone and joint injuries and therefore will not be discussed in any general measure by this review (Bradford and Dolphin, 1975; Green and Rowland, 1975; Sandzen, 1979; Weeks, 1981; Milford, 1982; Louis and Greene, 1984). Rather, we will discuss those points of anatomy, biomechanics, and pathophysiology as they apply to a specific injury and are utilized in the treatment course of these injuries. Likewise, those fractures dealing with the diaphyseal, metaphyseal and epiphyseal injuries of the phalanx and metacarpals will not be discussed as they are quite adequately and accurately covered in many articles and texts in orthopedic surgery and surgery of the hand (von Raffler, 1964b; Narakas, 1972; Bora, Ignatius and Nissenbaum, 1976; Wood, 1976; Barton, 1979).

Specific attention will be less on the bony anatomy, which is generally well known to the surgeon, and more attention will be given to the ligamentous, tendinous and articular components of the joint. Complications of joint injuries and treatment alternatives will be discussed (Butler, Neviaser and Adams, 1978; Dobyns and Linscheid, 1978).

DISTAL INTERPHALANGEAL JOINT (DIP) INJURIES

The interphalangeal joints of the hand are stable due to their bicondylar configuration and dorsal tongue-in-groove articulation. The interphalangeal joints allow only flexion and extension as with the true hinged or ginglymus joint.

Collateral ligament position is similar at the interphalangeal joints and the metacarpophalangeal joints. The shape of the head of the middle phalanx and proximal phalanx is less eccentric than that of the metacarpal head, the volar plate less mobile in the interphalangeal joints than the metacarpophalangeal joints, and inherently the interphalangeal joints present a much more stable joint than the metacarpophalangeal joints. If dislocation of the distal interphalangeal joints without fracture or concomitant tendon injury is reduced, it is stable. With satisfactory reduction and splinting resultant deformity and late restriction of motion is uncommon. Irreducible dislocation of the distal interphalangeal joint has been reported in association with interposition of the volar plate, flexor tendon, or osteochondral fracture (Milford, 1982; Stripling, 1982). Epiphyseal fracture dislocation and malrotation may also cause irreducible distal interphalangeal joint injuries in children (Narakas, 1972; Barton, 1979; *Figure 9.1*).

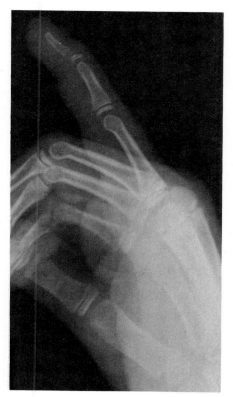

Figure 9.1 Mallet finger deformity secondary to epiphyseal Salter II fracture of the distal phalanx

Extensor tendon avulsion injuries, with minimal or no fracture fragment, are best managed conservatively with extension splinting or, on occasion, percutaneous K-pin fixation of the distal phalangeal joint in extension for 4–6 weeks. Extensor tendon disruption with intra-articular fractures, from 30 to 50% articular surface, have been managed both conservatively and operatively with varying results (Moss and Steingold, 1983; Wehbe and Schneider, 1984; *Figure 9.2*). The ultimate goal is joint preservation and congruency when the fracture is healed. Without a fracture, the goal is prevention of a mallet finger or drop finger deformity of the distal interphalangeal joint and a secondary hyperextension deformity with residual stiffness of the proximal interphalangeal joint. Many surgeons prefer to treat both the proximal interphalangeal joint and distal interphalangeal joint in patients with mallet finger deformities. The distal interphalangeal joint is placed in neutral or slight hyperextension, while the proximal interphalangeal joint is allowed to assume a position of flexion. This position advances the central slip and the lateral bands to allow relative lengthening of the shortened terminal extensor tendon at the distal interphalangeal joint.

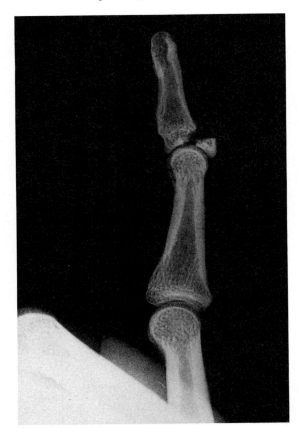

Figure 9.2 Mallet finger fracture with 50% articular cartilage surface involvement and displacement

The deformity of the mallet finger may be relatively mild with little or no impairment of function. In some cases deformity can be severe with secondary proximal swan-neck hyperextension deformity and stiffness of the finger. Bony union may occur in an elongated position, to leave a residual dorsal prominence and a mild mallet deformity. However, the joint surfaces are generally contoured and the incidence of traumatic arthritis is relatively low. Operative procedures which realign the joint and reconstruct the extensor tendon of the joint require K-pin bony fixation and often pull-out wire tendon fixation. Secondary traumatic arthritic changes resulting in pain with a restricted range of motion in the distal interphalangeal joint may be observed. Arthrodesis of the distal interphalangeal joint is, therefore, recommended for the late complaints of persistent pain.

A large fracture fragment may also be associated with volar subluxation of the distal phalanx at the interphalangeal joint level and subsequent deformity with restricted or painful range of motion. Attention must be focused on the accurate reduction of the distal interphalangeal joint. Joint reduction and pinning in extension is critical in the operative intervention of these injuries. A small fracture fragment may be excised and the extensor mechanism advanced into the dorsal raw bony surface with either suture through drill holes in bone or pull-out wire technique. The latter must be done carefully to avoid pulp, skin or nail-bed injury. Fragments of one-third to one-half of the articular surface may be secured with an additional small Kirschner wire to the distal phalanx perpendicular to the axis of the distal interphalangeal joint, once the joint has been secured in an extended position with K-wire fixation. If the tension on the distal interphalangeal joint extensor tendon repair prevents reduction, then flexion of the proximal interphalangeal joint to 60° should be maintained for approximately 3–4 weeks. If, however, the repair is satisfactory without tension, and the proximal inter-phalangeal (PIP) joint can be taken through a range of motion without undue tension at the repair site, then the proximal interphalangeal joint may be left free and only the distal interphalangeal joint immobilized. Fracture fragment healing requires 4–6 weeks, while soft tissue extensor tendon healing to bone requires generally eight weeks. The finger is further intermittently protected for an additional four weeks before active unprotected motion in a normal environment is allowed. Active motion is initiated during this time.

Casting may be utilized by the surgeon skilled in this procedure, but this is a meticulous, demanding procedure (in other words, extending the distal interpha-langeal joint, and flexing the proximal interphalangeal joint in plaster).

For those patients who cannot continue with their profession with splint fixation, percutaneous pin fixation in extension with the pin buried may be used. This is particularly advantageous for the physician, dentist or possibly musician. If the pin is buried just below the nail it is protected from trauma and is not in the pulp area.

Late sequelae of treating mallet deformity utilizing open reduction, and internal fixation includes traumatic arthritis, pin tract infections, migration and breakage of pins, and recurrence of original deformity. Ultimate range of motion return may take up to six months.

Flexor tendon avulsion injury with fracture of the distal phalanx is a commonly misdiagnosed injury (*Figure 9.3*). The most common mechanism of injury is a forceful flexion against a resisting force such as seen in football jersey tackling injuries. The patient complains of pain and swelling of the distal interphalangeal joint with inability to flex the distal interphalangeal joint. X-rays are obtained and must be scrutinized closely for small avulsion fractures association with the avulsion of the flexor digitorum profundus tendon. These fractures may be quite obvious and quite large and, therefore, allow reinsertion with either pull-out wires, K-pins, or screw fixation (*Figure 9.4*). At other times these fracture fragments may be quite small and may be observed at the level of the proximal interphalangeal joint at the chiasma of Camper where the profundus is often held in this position of proximal

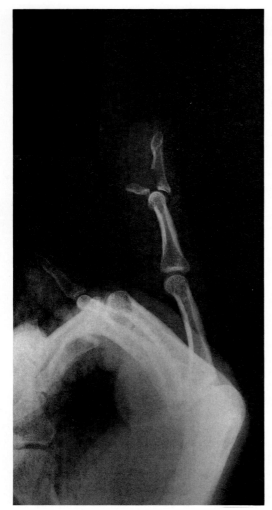

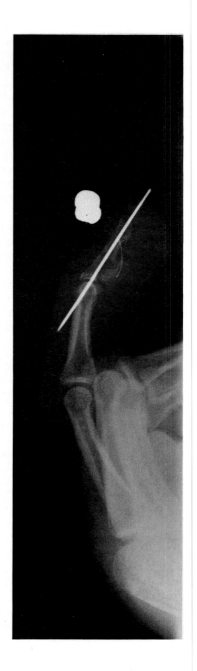

Figure 9.3 Avulsion of the profundus tendon with intra-articular fracture of the volar aspect of the distal phalanx with displacement

Figure 9.4 Reduction of the fracture fragment with profundus tendon avulsion utilizing pull-out wires and K-pin fixation of the distal interphalangeal joint

retraction by the sublimis and vincula system. In more forceful injuries, the profundus may retract well into the palm within the lumbrical musculature and present a painful mass in the hand with inability to flex the distal interphalangeal joint. These injuries must be diagnosed and repaired acutely, as musculotendinous units will shorten and make repair impossible after approximately 2–3 weeks. Repairs performed after that time result in significant flexion contractures of the distal interphalangeal joint and, in fact, arthrodesis of the distal interphalangeal joint is generally the procedure of choice if fixed flexion of the distal joint is required. Tenodesis may also be performed; however, with profundus avulsion injuries this must be performed with either volar plate or tendon graft and may stretch out in the young active individual.

Chronic instability or dislocation of the distal interphalangeal joint is rare in the dorsal and volar planes of flexion/extension. Collateral ligament instability and deviation is seen and is difficult to correct surgically without resulting in a significant decrease in range of motion of the distal interphalangeal joint. The procedure of choice, if chronic instability of the distal interphalangeal joint is present, would be arthrodesis of the distal interphalangeal joint (*Figure 9.5*).

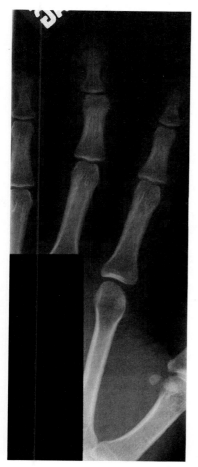

Figure 9.5 Radial collateral ligament laxity with ulnar deviation of the distal interphalangeal joint of the middle finger

Collateral ligament reconstruction, particularly of the radial collateral ligament which is required in pinch of the interphalangeal joint of the fingers, may be corrected with a slip of the volar plate (Faithfull, 1981) or a tendon graft. However, the results are quite tenuous with residual instability or secondary stiffness as a problem as well as swelling and scarring at the reconstruction site. The finger must also be protected for sports. In musicians with an unstable distal interphalangeal joint secondary to trauma or degenerative changes this presents even more of a problem. There is no operative procedure that will give both good motion and stability to the distal interphalangeal joint. Either stability or motion will be sacrificed in these reconstructive procedures. Persistent hyperextension instability may be treated by volar plate capsulodesis or flexor profundus tenodesis.

Comminuted fractures of the distal interphalangeal joint, involving the entire articular surface of either the base of the distal phalanx or the condyles of the middle phalanx, are splinted until the patient is relatively comfortable and free of pain. Early motion is then initiated. These patients usually end up with traumatic arthritis and require joint arthrodesis. Occasionally, comminution is such that intra-articular arthrodesis is performed as the primary procedure of choice. This is accomplished with debridement of the articular surface, coaptation of bony fracture fragment ends and K-pin or wire fixation in slight flexion.

Prosthetic implants at the distal interphalangeal joint have not been used due to instability in pinch activity and are, therefore, not recommended as reconstructive options.

Isolated condylar fractures or base of the distal phalanx fractures, which are intra-articular and displaced, are treated either by pinning percutaneously, if anatomical reduction can be obtained, or as an open operative procedure with anatomical reduction of the articular surface and K-pin or screw fixation. Long oblique fractures that are intra-articular may be held with small screws (Heim, Pfeiffer and Meuli, 1974).

Collateral ligament injury with avulsion fractures that are non-displaced are treated with extension splints until bony healing occurs. Displaced fracture fragments with collateral ligament injury are reduced and either K-pin or pull-out wire fixation are utilized for stability. Small volar plate chip fractures are treated with slight flexion splinting until comfortable, then early range of motion is initiated. Total recovery time from injury to maximum range of motion recovery may require six months.

Epiphyseal plate injuries may result in a mallet type deformity requiring reduction and splinting or pin fixation. Nail growth disturbance may result due to irreparable damage to the germinal matrix secondary to the injury. Growth disturbances with angulation, rotation or partial growth arrest may also occur in epiphyseal fractures about the joints.

PROXIMAL INTERPHALANGEAL (PIP) JOINT INJURIES

The proximal interphalangeal joint is similar in configuration and function to the distal interphalangeal joint. It also is a true hinge joint with volar plate, collateral and accessory collateral ligament configuration. The proximal interphalangeal joint is, however, complicated volarly by both the sublimis and profundus tendons, dorsolaterally by the lateral band mechanism, and dorsally by the central slip mechanism. Any or all of these structures may add to the complexity of fracture dislocations about the proximal interphalangeal joint (Lee, 1963; Wilson and Roland, 1966; Spinner and Choi, 1970; Wiley, 1970; Eaton, 1971; Sprague, 1975; Eaton and Dray, 1982). The neurovascular bundles as well may be compromised with severe injury at the level of the proximal interphalangeal joint. The neurovascular status must be carefully monitored during the management of these injuries. Condylar fractures of the proximal phalanx are anatomically reduced and percutaneously pinned with Kirschner wires or, if reduction is not complete, open reduction and internal fixation with mini-fragment screws is used (Kilbourne and Paul, 1958; Heim and Pfeiffer, 1974; Ikuta and Tsuge, 1974; Crawford, 1976), wire loops (Lister, 1978) or Kirschner wires (Clifford, 1953; Green and Anderson, 1973; Massengill *et al.*, 1979; *Figure 9.6*). This maintains joint integrity and prevents malalignment of the digit. Surgical approach to these joints may be either dorsally through the central slip, dorsolaterally between the lateral band and central slip insertion or lateral and volar to the lateral bands. The finger is splinted in approximately 15° of flexion for approximately two weeks, after which protected motion is begun if no tendon injury exists.

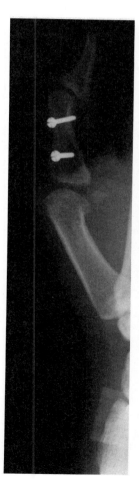
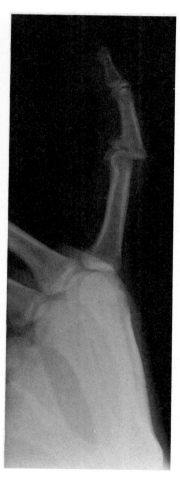

Figure 9.6 (left) Proximal phalanx of thumb with spiral intra-articular fracture internally fixed with mini-fragment screw set

Figure 9.7 (right) Fracture base of middle phalanx with dorsal subluxation

Intra-articular fractures of the base of the middle phalanx are often associated with subluxation or dislocation. These involve the volar bony surface with volar plate and collateral ligament disruption at its insertion, or dorsally at the central slip insertion (*Figure 9.7*). The joint is reduced under metacarpal block anesthetic and the joint is then examined to determine its stability as it is carried through an active and passive arc of motion. X-rays are obtained to assess joint congruency as well as fracture fragment reduction. Displaced fracture fragments, or an incompletely reduced joint, necessitate open reduction and internal fixation (Neviaser and Wilson, 1972; Nathan and Schlein, 1973). Failure to achieve anatomical alignment results in joint incongruity, residual deformity and stiffness, with late traumatic arthritic changes within the proximal interphalangeal joint (*Figure 9.8*).

Irreducible joint dislocations suggest total instability of the joint, which may be due to entrapment of collateral ligament, volar plate, lateral band mechanism, or flexor tendon mechanisms. Central slip rupture or the possibility of an osteochondral interarticular fracture (Milford, 1982) must also be considered.

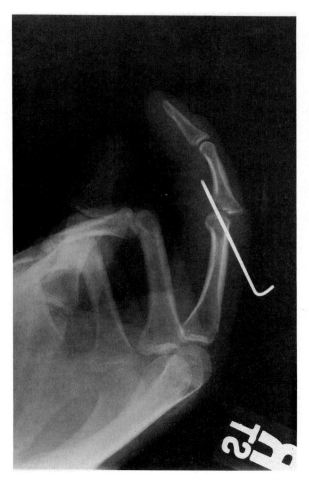

Figure 9.8 Incompletely reduced proximal interphalangeal joint fracture/dislocation with persistence of dorsal subluxation and joint incongruity

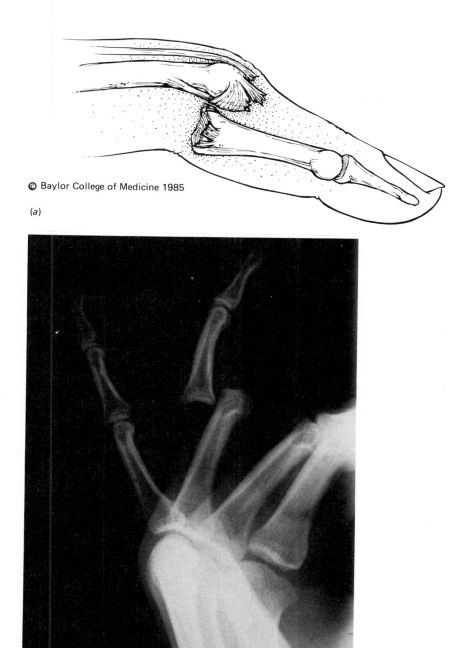

(a)

(b)

Figure 9.9 (a) Proximal interphalangeal dislocation with central slip avulsion secondary to volar position of middle phalanx. (b) Proximal interphalangeal joint dorsal dislocation with colateral ligament and volar plate rupture; however, central slip mechanism should be intact.

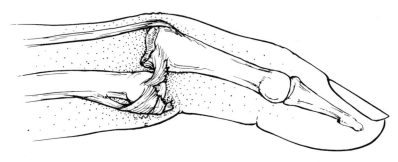

(c)

Figure 9.9 (*c*) Proximal interphalangeal dislocation with central slip intact secondary to dorsal position of middle phalanx

Intra-articular fractures, which are anatomically reduced, are generally splinted for 2–3 weeks and then early protective motion is begun. Those fracture dislocations that require reattachment of central slip mechanism need protection for approximately six weeks with internal Kirschner wire extension splinting until the central slip is healed. Thereafter the patient is treated with protective active and passive motion to regain useful function. An extensive therapy program is required and it may take up to six months before maximal functional range of motion has been achieved. Furthermore, secondary joint release and tenolysis may be required after six months to improve function.

Failure to identify central slip ruptures results in chronic boutonnière deformities of the proximal interphalangeal joint. The most common cause of central slip rupture is dislocation of the middle phalanx volar to the proximal phalanx with tearing of the extensor insertion (*Figure 9.9a*). Dorsal dislocation of the proximal interphalangeal joint, with the proximal phalanx volar to the middle phalanx, does not usually disrupt the central slip insertion (*Figure 9.9(b)* and (*c*)). The volar plate collateral ligament complex structures afford stability to the proximal interphalangeal joint. Volar fracture with dorsal subluxation or dislocation of the joint requires manipulation and pin fixation (*Figure 9.10*) or extension blocking techniques to prevent recurrent subluxation dislocation (McElfresh, Dobyns and O'Brien, 1972). If a 30–50% fracture of the base of the middle phalanx exists and the reduction is unstable, open reduction, K-pin fixation and volar plate arthroplasty, as described by Eaton and Malerich (1980), is performed. This is a very exacting procedure and at times difficult to perform, particularly in the late or chronic dorsal subluxated proximal interphalangeal joint. Reduction of these chronically dislocated joints requires accurate assessment of the joint surfaces to determine whether traumatic arthritis is present. If, in fact, significant traumatic arthritis is present, the procedures of choice would be either arthrodesis (Curtis, 1966) or arthroplasty (Swanson, 1973). If the cartilage coverage and bony contour have been preserved then dorsal capsulectomy, extensor tenolysis, reduction and pinning of the joint in approximately 15–30° of flexion, with volar plate advancement into the volar bony defect, as described by Eaton and Malerich (1980), is performed. A mild flexion contracture is created from this procedure;

however, a satisfactory resurfacing with the volar plate can correct the incongruency of the proximal interphalangeal joint and the patient can regain a useful arc of motion.

Chronic hyperextension deformities of the proximal interphalangeal joint (swan-neck deformity), secondary to traumatic disruption or stretching of the volar plate and accessory collateral ligaments, are less common disabling injuries except

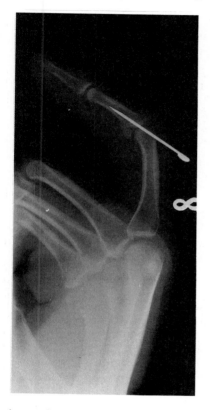

Figure 9.10 Reduced proximal interphalangeal joint fracture/dislocation with reduction of fracture fragments and pinning of the proximal interphalangeal joint in flexion to maintain reduction

in patients with rheumatoid arthritis. When present, however, they may be corrected through volar plate capsulodesis or a sublimis slip check reign ligament into the distal portion of the proximal phalanx (Curtis, 1966). Tendon grafting procedures as a volar ligament may also be performed.

Isolated collateral ligament instability is rare. However, if the volar plate is also involved then recurrent lateral dislocations may occur (*Figure 9.11*). Reconstructive surgery, in those cases which present a significant disability, consists of volar plate reconstruction as well as collateral ligament reconstruction. This has been performed acutely by reattachment of the collateral ligament with a pull-out wire, or in late cases with a free tendon graft or with a sublimis slip stabilization (Palmer and Linscheid, 1978). Significant scarring and stiffness may result from this reconstruction. Prolonged splinting to the adjacent finger is required. If instability is a significant disability despite reconstructive procedures, arthrodesis is the treatment of choice. Replacement arthroplasty may be used; however, instability is not significantly corrected by arthroplasty alone.

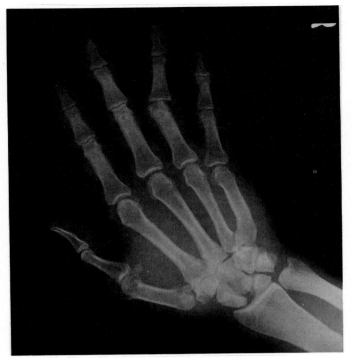

Figure 9.11 Chronic lateral dislocation of proximal interphalangeal joint, with radial collateral ligament insufficiency and ulnar deviation

Severely comminuted proximal interphalangeal joint fractures, which preclude internal fixation techniques, may be treated using a distraction technique requiring distal pin fixation and dynamic traction with early range of motion (Quigley and Urist, 1947; Moberg, 1949–50; *Figure 9.12(a)* and (*b*)). This technique will allow joint mobilization and contouring of the fracture fragments and can produce an acceptable result which is relatively pain-free and has a functional arc of motion for many years. A complication of this injury is traumatic arthritis, which may require secondary procedures such as arthrodesis or arthroplasty.

Hemijoint injury, whether it is the base of the middle phalanx or the condyle of the proximal phalanx, may be resurfaced with one-half the volar plate in a similar fashion to the volar plate arthroplasty described by Eaton and Malerich (1980). However, some instability and deviation may occur if these fractures have a significant depression or angulation. Elevation of the fracture with a bone grafting procedure can re-establish the joint surface although residual stiffness is a complicating factor with this procedure.

Partial joint or whole joint transfers have been performed utilizing the metatarsophalangeal joint or the proximal interphalangeal joint of the toes (Mikkelsen, 1984). Previously these had been performed primarily in children and were essentially non-vascular composite tissue transfers. Currently work is being performed on the microsurgical vascularized free joint transfer and it holds some promise for joint reconstruction in these patients (Tsai *et al.*, 1982; Tsai and Singer, 1984; *Figure 9.13(a)* and (*b*)).

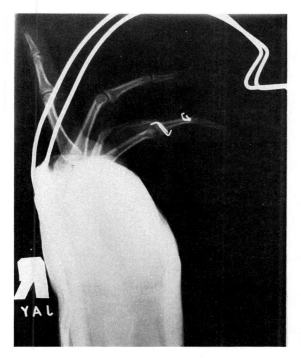

(a)

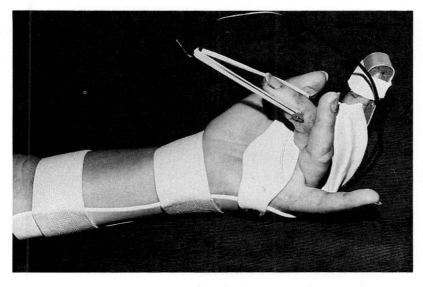

(b)

Figure 9.12 (a) External fixation device for comminuted proximal interphalangeal joint fracture which has been internally fixed with Kirschner B-wires, X-ray lateral. (b) Clinical photograph of external fixation device with dynamic traction and extension block to prevent recurrence of dislocation and allow early motion

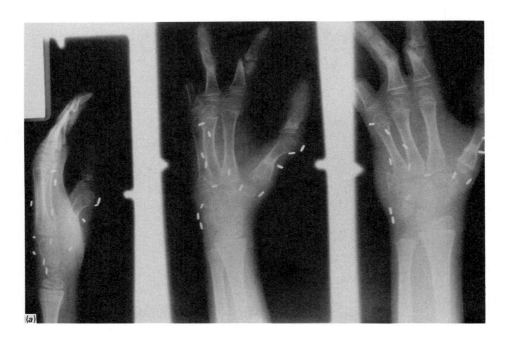

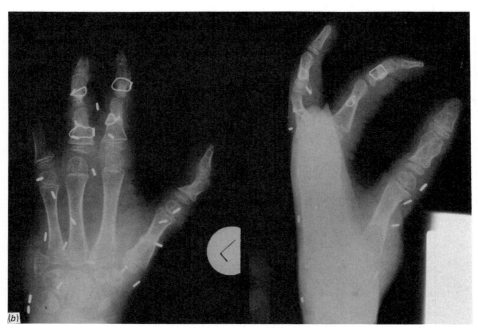

Figure 9.13 Microsurgical free proximal interphalangeal joint transfer (courtesy of Dr Tsu-min Tsai): (*a*) preoperative; (*b*) postoperative

Complications of proximal interphalangeal joint injuries and their treatment require secondary operative procedures, if after extensive therapy, an acceptable range of motion cannot be obtained or pain is a limiting factor in hand function. Extensive joint releases, capsulectomies, and tenolysis have been proposed for stiff proximal interphalangeal joints followed by a prolonged therapy regimen (Curtis, 1966). Prosthetic replacement arthroplasty procedures for traumatic arthritis are rarely indicated at the time of injury, but may yield very satisfactory results for late traumatic arthritis, particularly of the middle and ring fingers which have less stresses applied to them than the border digits. Traditionally, the border digits do not do as well with prosthetic interposition arthroplasty due to instability, and arthrodesis may be the procedure of choice to stabilize these border digits.

METACARPOPHALANGEAL (MCP) JOINT INJURIES

Anatomically the metacarpophalangeal joint provides a greater range of motion than the interphalangeal joints because of its greater condylar articulation. Flexion, extension, abduction, adduction, and circumduction are all part of metacarpophalangeal joint motion. The metacarpophalangeal joint is quite mobile in

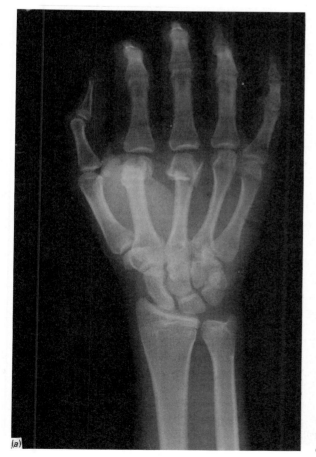

(a)

Figure 9.14 (a) Comminuted metacarpal head fractures with depression of articular surfaces.

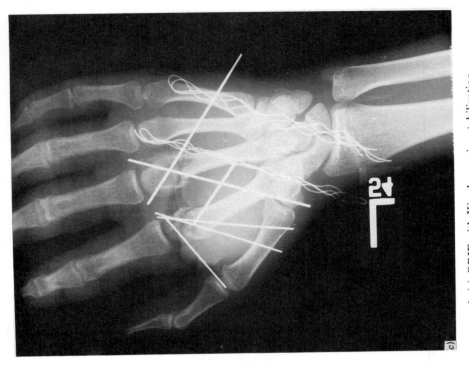

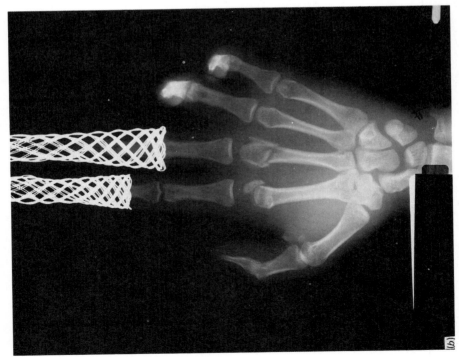

Figure 9.14 (b) Reduction with finger traps, incomplete on the index metacarpal. *(c)* ORIF with Kirschner wire stabilization

extension, but it becomes tight in flexion due to the eccentric shape of the condyle and of the tightened collateral ligaments. It is further stabilized by the interosseous muscles and the transverse metacarpal ligaments.

Intra-articular fractures of the metacarpal head may be vertical, oblique, or transverse, with or without displacement. Displaced fractures, osteochondral fractures with displacement and avulsion fractures through the collateral ligament should be anatomically restored and secured with pin or pull-out wire fixation (O'Brien, 1982; McElfresh and Dobyns, 1983; *Figure 9.14(a)*, *(b)* and *(c)*). Collateral ligament integrity should be evaluated. A Brewerton view on X-ray may locate occult fractures of the metacarpal head (Lane, 1977). Epiphyseal injuries likewise must be treated appropriately with acceptable reduction in alignment and rotation.

Fractures of the base of the proximal phalanx also require anatomical reduction and alignment to prevent malunion and malrotation of the fingers (*Figure 9.15*). Compression fractures of the metacarpal head or oblique fractures into the base of the metacarpal head may result in lax, unstable metacarpophalangeal joints due to the relative lengthening of the collateral ligaments.

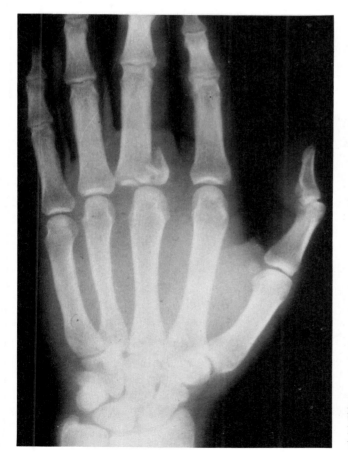

Figure 9.15 Fracture of the base of the proximal phalanx with rotation of fracture fragments

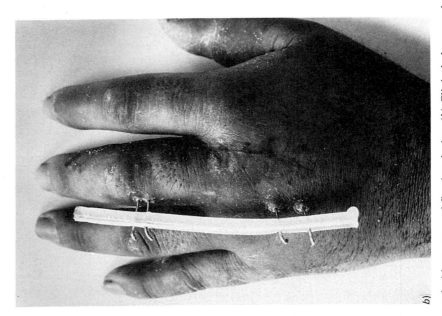

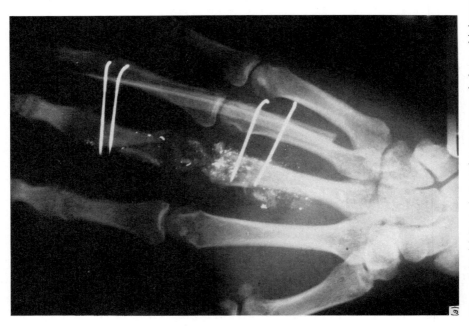

Figure 9.16 (*a*) Bone loss at the metacarpophalangeal joint managed with an external fixation device. (*b*) Clinical photograph of acrylic resin and Kirschner wire external fixation device

Severely comminuted fractures of the metacarpophalangeal joint, involving both sides of the joint surface, may require external stabilization and support until healing occurs (Crockett, 1974; Dickson, 1975; *Figure 9.16(a)* and (*b*)). Secondary arthroplasty procedures or arthrodesis may be required for pain relief when traumatic arthritis develops (Swanson, 1973).

A dislocation of the metacarpophalangeal joint may be irreducible due to the interposition of the volar plate complex within the joint and the entrapment of the metacarpal head by the flexor tendon and lumbrical muscle system (Kaplan, 1957; von Raffler, 1964a; *Figure 9.17*). Failed closed reduction necessitates open reduction and decompression of the metacarpophalangeal joint. Once reduction has been achieved the joint generally is stable and does not require any type of internal fixation. The radial collateral ligament and volar plate may be reattached with a single suture. However, care must be taken not to tighten the volar plate excessively and create a flexion contracture at the metacarpophalangeal joint.

Occasionally, rupture or laxity of the volar plate causes a significant hyperextension deformity of the metacarpophalangeal joint and secondary volar plate capsulodesis may be required. This hyperextension instability can be a significant disability in the thumb metacarpophalangeal joint with power pinch activities. Long-standing dislocations of the metacarpophalangeal joints have

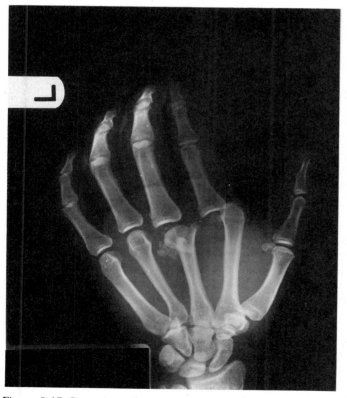

Figure 9.17 Comminuted metacarpal head fracture of the middle finger with irreducible dislocation of the metacarpophalangeal joint of the index finger

complications of traumatic arthritis and open reduction is often unsuccessful due to joint deterioration. Pain is a sequel of the chronic dislocation secondary to traumatic arthritis. Prosthetic replacement (Swanson, 1973), arthrodesis or interpositional perichondrial arthroplasty (Seradge *et al.,* 1984) are currently the treatment options except in the thumb, which is usually stabilized by arthrodesis. Hemiarthroplasty utilizing porous prosthetic material is currently being performed. It may be a very satisfactory way to reconstitute the head of the metacarpal with an intact base of the proximal phalanx. Similarly, disruption of the base of the proximal phalanx may be resurfaced with a silastic, pyrolytic carbon, cemented or porous coated hemiarthroplasty with an intact metacarpal head. Arthrodesis impairs the functional range of motion of the digit, but will create a very stable joint and may be indicated for either the index finger or the little finger border digits to produce a strong stable working hand.

Collateral ligament disruption of the metacarpophalangeal joints of the fingers is generally managed conservatively, except in the radial collateral ligament of the little finger often referred to as a reverse 'gamekeeper's' deformity (Bora and Didizian, 1974). An incompetent ligament allows the little finger to remain in an abducted position and is often caught on objects or in pockets and presents a significant impairment to the hand. Acute injuries to the radial collateral ligament, if unstable, are repaired surgically by reattachment of the radial collateral ligament to the base of the proximal phalanx, or to the metacarpal head, depending on the site of lesion, usually with a pull-out wire. Similarly, complete disruption of the radial collateral ligament of the index finger may present as a disability in certain working people. If strong index finger abduction is required, reattachment of the collateral ligament, a tendon grafting procedure, or transfer of the extensor indicis proprius into the first dorsal interosseous to act as a dynamic transfer to restore abduction for pinch power may be performed.

The thumb

The interphalangeal joint of the thumb is a hinged joint and is treated similarly to the distal interphalangeal joint of the fingers. The injuries are the same and treatment with anatomical restoration, extensor and flexor tendon evaluation remains the same. Interphalangeal joint anatomic reduction with K-pin fixation for displaced fractures is recommended. The development of traumatic arthritis after severe comminuted interphalangeal joint fractures responds satisfactorily to arthrodesis of the thumb interphalangeal joint in slight flexion. Implant arthroplasty lacks stability and is therefore not recommended.

The metacarpophalangeal joint of the thumb is similar in anatomical configuration to the metacarpophalangeal joint of the fingers. The problem of the thumb metacarpophalangeal joint is likewise similar to the finger metacarpophalangeal joints with irreducible dislocations requiring an open reduction with removal of the interposed volar plate from the metacarpophalangeal joint. A dorsal or volar approach may be used. Chronic instability and hyperextension of the metacarpophalangeal joint with dorsal subluxation may occur. Volar capsulodesis will correct this instability.

Collateral ligament disruption, particularly the ulnar collateral ligament of the thumb, presents a significant disability to pinch and grasp. A 'gamekeeper's' thumb is well described and warrants acute surgical repair in those instances of disrupted ulnar collateral ligament or displaced fracture fragment (Moberg, 1960; Stener, 1972; Sakellarides and DeWeese, 1976; Smith, 1977; *Figure 9.18*). On X-rays these may be identified with a displaced flake of bone or by arthrogram and stress X-rays in selected cases (Linscheid, 1974; Bowers and Hurst, 1977). Tendon transfer of the adductor pollicis or extensor pollicis brevis may be performed at the time of injury to give dynamic strength to the repair or as a late procedure for chronic instability

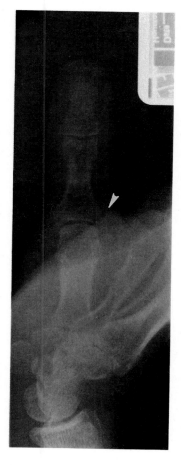

Figure 9.18 Gamekeeper's thumb injury with avulsion fracture fragment

(Moberg and Stener, 1953; Neviaser, Wilson and Lievano, 1971; Sakellarides and DeWeese, 1976). Tendon graft procedures are also successful, but laxity may recur. Similarly, late instability of the radial aspect of the thumb and the radial collateral ligament may be reconstructed with the abductor pollicis brevis advancement transfer. Thumb metacarpophalangeal arthrodesis in approximately 10–15% of flexion presents a very stable, strong, workable thumb and is the treatment of choice for traumatic arthritis, or failed ligament reconstruction of this joint. Prosthetic arthroplasty of this joint is often unstable, and is not recommended for strong working hands, but may be quite satisfactory in the older patient who requires lighter work activity of the hand or in the patient with rheumatoid arthritis.

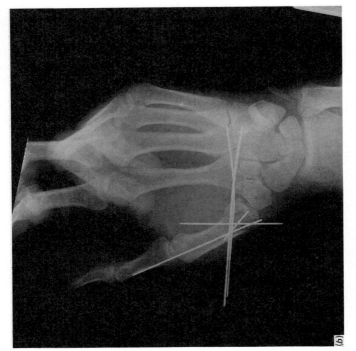

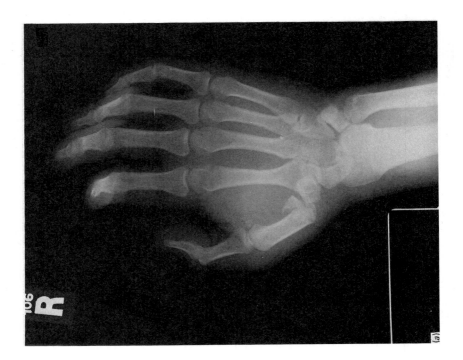

Figure 9.19 (*a*) Bennett's fracture/dislocation of metacarpal trapezial joint. (*b*) ORIF with multiple Kirschner wires the carpometacarpal joint of the thumb

Metacarpal-trapezial fracture and/or dislocation should be reduced anatomically, pinned for stability to allow ligament or fracture fragment healing if the fragment is of significant size. Both Bennett and Rolando fractures are well described and treatment consists of accurate reduction, often open reduction and internal fixation (*Figure 9.19(a)* and (*b*)). Conservative treatment with closed reduction and plaster immobilization may lead to subluxation and subsequent bone and joint deformities resulting in traumatic arthritis.

Dislocation, without fracture of the metacarpal-trapezial joint of the thumb, may be reduced and pinned but often requires late ligament reconstruction for stabilization with a slip of the flexor carpi radialis, extensor carpi radialis longus or abductor pollicis longus (Eaton and Littler, 1969, 1973). Late subluxation or arthritic changes require arthrodesis of the thumb carpometacarpal joint, prosthetic replacement or excision arthroplasty with ligament reconstruction for stabilization.

Sesamoid fractures without displacement are treated with immobilization until healing occurs. Non-unions which are painful, or an arthritic surface on the sesamoids, are treated by excision of the sesamoid bone (Trumble and Watson, 1985), preserving collateral ligament support.

Massive soft tissue injury with bone and joint loss in a thumb with an intact blood supply is treated with external fixation and/or internal fixation to preserve length. This is followed by a bone graft procedure and/or a joint arthrodesis when soft tissue recovery and skin coverage has occurred (*Figure 9.20(a)*, (*b*) and (*c*)).

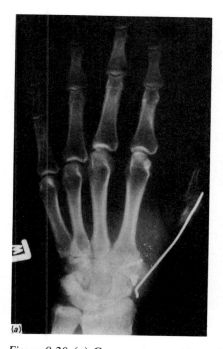
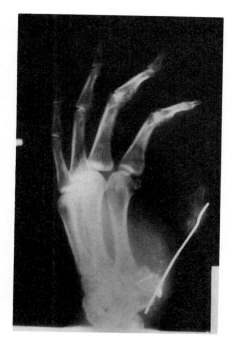

Figure 9.20 (*a*) Carpometacarpal bone loss managed with internal wire splinting.

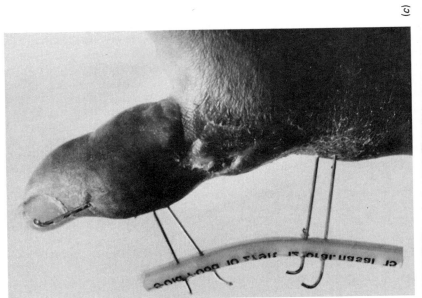

(c)

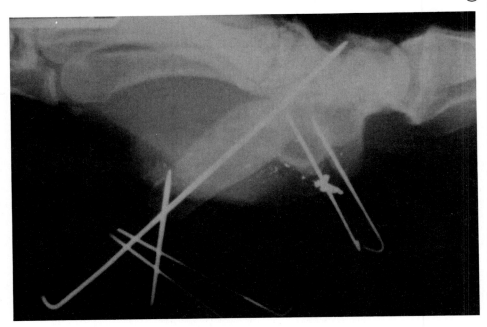

(b)

Figure 9.20 (*b*) X-ray of subsequent bone graft managed with internal wire fixation and external fixation device. (*c*) The same, clinical photograph

CARPOMETACARPAL JOINT INJURIES OF THE FINGERS

The carpometacarpal joints of the index, middle and ring fingers are stable, fixed joints which allow minimal gliding motion at the joint and are classified as arthrodial diarthroses. The fifth carpometacarpal joint is more mobile and is similar to the thumb carpometacarpal joint. As a saddle joint it allows motion, not only in gliding, but also in rotation to allow its opposability to the thumb. These joints are stabilized by very strong intermetacarpal and carpometacarpal ligaments which support the joints both dorsal and volarward.

Injury to these joints occurs with severe force and dislocation is generally dorsal. It may be associated with a fracture (*Figure 9.21*). Volar dislocations are much rarer, being more common in the fifth metacarpal because of its increased mobility. Because of the overlap of the adjacent bone structure, X-ray interpretation is often difficult and various views are required for an accurate interpretation. Tomograms may be indicated to isolate these fracture dislocations. CAT scans may be indicated for more difficult diagnostic problems.

Closed reduction and percutaneous pinning may stabilize the third and fourth carpometacarpal joints. However, redislocation or incomplete reduction often occurs in both the index and the little finger metacarpal due to the pull of the

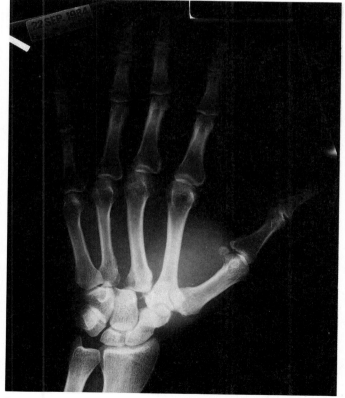

Figure 9.21 Dislocation of index and middle carpometacarpal joint with small avulsion fractures

extensor carpi radialis longus tendon to the second metacarpal, and of the extensor carpi ulnaris to the fifth metacarpal (Hsu and Curtis, 1970; Bora and Didizian, 1974). Spiral fractures with intra-articular components may be reduced and fixed with K-wires, mini-fragment screws or A-O plates (Simonetta, 1970; Steel, 1978).

Closed reduction and cast immobilization often results in the recurrence of carpometacarpal dislocation due to the instability with significant swelling that occurs with these injuries. Percutaneous pinning is therefore indicated and if anatomical reduction cannot be obtained, open reduction and pinning is the treatment of choice (*Figure 9.22*). Late changes of carpometacarpal arthritis or missed dislocation which is painful is treated by arthrodesis of the carpometacarpal joint.

Hemiarthroplasty has been proposed with either resection of metacarpal base and fascial interposition (Milford, 1982) or silastic interposition (Swanson, 1973); however, we have found this somewhat limited in the individual who requires strength and force from his hand, and prefer arthrodesis. In those patients who require a lighter activity of the hand, arthroplasty may serve the purpose of relieving the pain from the arthrosis and decreasing the time of immobilization. The loss of function secondary to arthrodesis is relatively minimal in these patients.

Crush injuries without displacement result in late arthritic changes and may require arthrodesis. If severe bone loss is present (*Figure 9.23(a)*), length is maintained by external fixation or transverse K-wires, followed by bone grafting procedures when soft tissue healing is complete (*Figure 9.23(b)*).

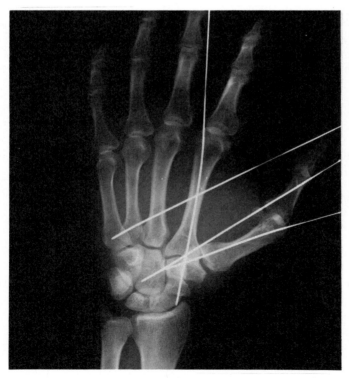

Figure 9.22 Multiple Kirschner wire fixation after open reduction of dislocation

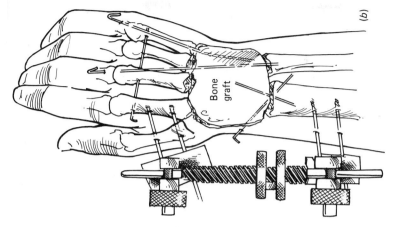

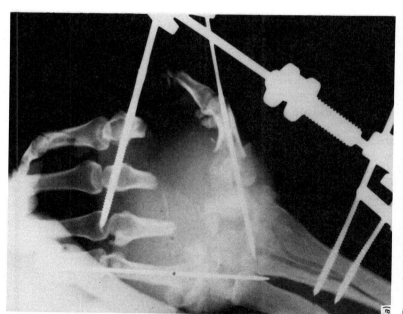

Figure 9.23 (*a*) Massive bone loss at the carpometacarpal articulation managed initially with external fixation to allow soft tissue coverage and pedicle flap coverage. (*b*) Schematic representation of bone grafting for massive carpometacarpal and radiocarpal bone loss

CARPAL DISLOCATIONS

Increasing awareness and controversy have developed in the last few years in regard to the carpus and its relationship to wrist alignment, motion and subsequent instabilities associated with injuries to the wrist. The carpal bones are arranged in transverse rows, excluding the pisiform which is functionally a sesamoid bone. The scaphoid translates both the proximal and distal carpal row in its functional and anatomical alignment. The lateral linkage system of the carpus as well as dorsal/volar relationships have been described in detail by many authors (Taleisnik, 1982; Taleisnik and Watson, 1984; Mayfield, Johnson and Kilcoyne, 1976; and Linscheid *et al.*, 1972).

Taleisnik described the carpus as vertical columns. The central column consists of the trapezium, trapezoid, capitate, hamate and lunate which allows flexion/extension along the radius, lunate, and capitate axes. The lateral rotation column contains the scaphoid while the medial rotation column contains the triquetrum. The pisiform is excluded as it does not participate in carpal rotation or motion.

Ligamentous support of the carpus is primarily intracapsular short fibers connecting carpal bones and is covered dorsally and volarly with a capsular confluence of ligament support. Volar ligaments are stronger than the dorsal ligaments. Radial carpal and ulnar carpal collateral ligaments are less substantial. Potential weakness volarly exists at the capitolunate articulation without capsular or ligament support. The axis of rotation about the wrist lies at the head of the capitate (Taleisnik, 1976, 1978).

Wrist injury and subsequent carpal dislocation are generally secondary to severe acute dorsiflexion or hyperextension injuries. Volar or palmar flexion are less common, as are translocation rotation injuries to the wrist.

Stability must be evaluated radiologically with the wrist in a neutral position in the lateral view. Dorsiflexion instability may produce a collapse pattern in the proximal carpal row (Sebald, Dobyns and Linscheid, 1974). Dorsal intercalary segment instability (DISI) is noted in the lateral X-rays with the capitate dorsal to the center of the lunate (*Figure 9.24a*), (*b*) and (*c*)). Normally the capitolunate angle is 0° with the wrist in neutral. The scapholunate angle is normally between 30° and 60°. With scapholunate dissociation this angle is greater than 80°. Volar intercalary segment instability (VISI) exists when the capitate is volar to the lunate in the lateral view. The radiolunate angle establishes the lunate alignment to the radius and should be 0° in the normal wrist.

Classification of carpal dislocation as described by Green (Green and O'Brien, 1978, 1980; Green, 1982) cover a variety of carpal and intercarpal dislocation patterns, all of which must be carefully identified in the injured wrist:

(1) dorsal perilunate/volar lunate dissociation:
    (a) isolated rotatory subluxation of the scaphoid;
(2) dorsal transcaphoid perilunate dislocation;
(3) volar perilunate/dorsal lunate dislocation;
(4) variance:
    (a) transradial styloid perilunate dislocation;
    (b) naviculocapitate syndrome;
    (c) transtriquetral perilunate fracture dislocation;

247

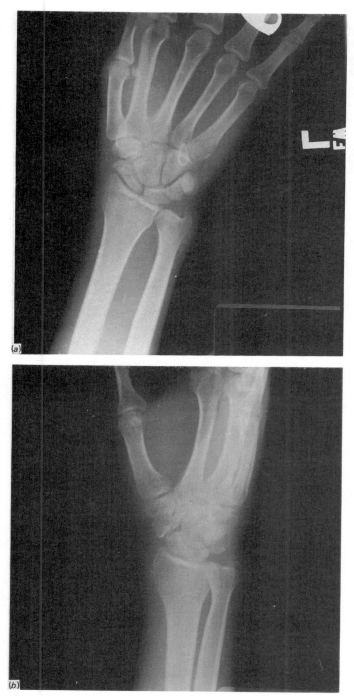

Figure 9.24 (a) Non-union scaphoid fracture with dorsal intercalary segmental instability pattern, anteroposterior view. (b) The same, oblique view.

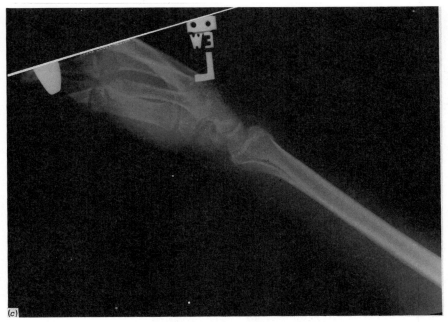

Figure 9.24 (c) The same, lateral view

(5) complete dislocation of the scaphoid;
(6) late post-traumatic carpal instability (*Figure 9.25*);
(7) snapping wrist syndrome.

Clinically pain, restriction of motion, and swelling are the most common complaints related to the wrist. The carpal relationship must be carefully documented by X-rays which would initially include an anterior posterior, a lateral and an oblique view. The lateral view must be a true lateral with the wrist in neutral. The anterior posterior view is taken in supination and if scapholunate dissociation is suspected, a clenched fist view increases the forces across the carpus and demonstrate the dissociation pattern more clearly. Additional views will include a carpal tunnel view, a distraction view utilizing finger traps, and both radial and ulnar deviation views. Cineradiography may be of benefit with fluoroscopy to demonstrate the snapping wrist syndrome or intermittent dislocation patterns. Trispiral tomography and polydirectional computerized tomography may prove useful. Accurate reduction of all dislocations is mandatory, often requiring internal fixation if unstable or recurrent, once anatomical realignment has been established. Ligament repair has been described for scapholunate dissociations (Palmer, Dobyns and Linscheid, 1978). Careful attention must be directed towards fracture dislocation with management of the fracture and the dislocation concomitantly.

Transcaphoid-perilunate fracture dislocation or trans-scaphoid-lunate fracture dislocation must have anatomical reduction of the scaphoid fracture for maximal healing potential (*Figure 9.26*). Open reduction, internal fixation with or without bone grafting, is indicated if any displacement of the scaphoid is present following closed reduction.

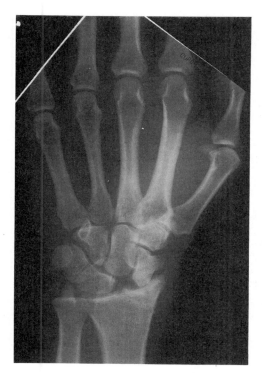

Figure 9.25 Old scapholunate dissociation with radioscaphoid arthrosis

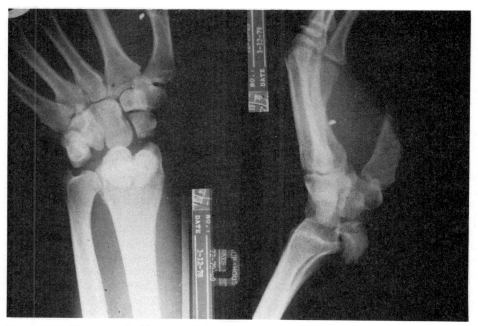

Figure 9.26 Trans-scaphoid lunate dislocation

Both dorsal and volar approaches may be necessary for adequate exposure in complex carpal dislocations. Reduction, pin fixation if unstable and ligament or capsule repair is indicated (Green and O'Brien, 1978). If sensory impairment is present carpal tunnel decompression is performed.

Late sequelae of malreduced dislocations or missed fracture dislocations result in chronic painful instability patterns to the wrist or intercarpal arthrosis (Palmer, Dobyns and Linscheid, 1980; Watson and Ballet, 1984). Intercarpal arthrodesis (Watson, 1980; Faithfull and Herbert, 1984) for rotatory subluxation of the scaphoid or scapholunatocapitate degenerative arthritis offers stability and strength to the wrist with some restriction of motion. Midcarpal instability patterns, if painful and symptomatic, may also be managed with midcarpal arthrodesis at the expense of range of motion for relief of pain and improvement of strength activities. Both dorsal intercalated and volar intercalary segment instabilities have been treated with either ligament reconstruction or intercarpal arthrodesis. Finally, proximal row carpectomy (Inglis and Jones, 1977), total wrist arthroplasty, and wrist arthrodesis may all be alternative procedures when pain persists after ligament reconstruction or intercarpal arthrodesis.

Carpal bone injuries

All of the carpal bones of the wrist have at one time or another been associated with fracture or dislocations (Fish, 1966; Dobyns and Linscheid, 1975, 1978, 1980; Bryan and Dobyns, 1980; Taleisnik, 1982). All are involved in an intra-articular relationship with an adjacent carpal bone, metacarpal or distal radio-ulnar joint. Scaphoid fractures are well recognized in the literature and are initially treated with a high index of suspicion in the patient who has a jammed or traumatized wrist with pain in the anatomical 'snuffbox' and equivocal X-rays. Displaced scaphoid fractures are anatomically reduced and pinned or internal screw fixation utilized (Maudsley and Chen, 1972; Herbert, 1982). If bone loss is present bone grafting is performed acutely. Prolonged immobilization is required until healing and revascularization are obtained. Secondary bone grafting procedures may be indicated for an established non-union of the carpal scaphoid. Electrical stimulation is also advocated in the healing of scaphoid fractures.

Scaphoid fractures associated with comminuted distal radius fractures should not be treated with external fixation devices. Distraction of the scaphoid fracture occurs as well as loss of ligament support if disruption has occurred. Proper treatment is directed at the internal fixation of the scaphoid as well as the comminuted distal radius (*Figure 9.27(a)*, (*b*), (*c*) and (*d*)).

Lunate fractures are uncommonly identified as an isolated injury but may be the etiology of Kienbock's disease (Kienbock, 1910) with recurrent microfractures of the lunate and subsequent avascular necrosis and collapse (Beckenhaugh *et al.*, 1980). Acute fractures of the lunate are immobilized until fracture healing occurs. Kienbock's disease (lunate avascular necrosis) with minimal or no collapse is treated with a variety of procedures. If a negative ulnar variance is associated with the avascular lunate then radial shortening (Gelberman *et al.*, 1975) or ulnar lengthening (Persson, 1950; Armistead *et al.*, 1982) may be combined with a synovectomy of the radiolunate joint to decompress and decrease the stress forces across the lunate (*Figure 9.28(a)* and (*b*)). If collapse has occurred then silicone replacement (Swanson, 1973) or fascial arthroplasty (Nahigian *et al.*, 1970) may be

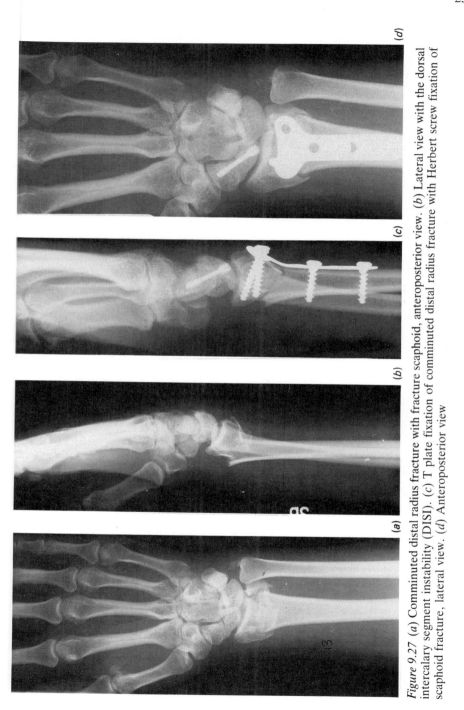

Figure 9.27 (*a*) Comminuted distal radius fracture with fracture scaphoid, anteroposterior view. (*b*) Lateral view with the dorsal intercalary segment instability (DISI). (*c*) T plate fixation of comminuted distal radius fracture with Herbert screw fixation of scaphoid fracture, lateral view. (*d*) Anteroposterior view

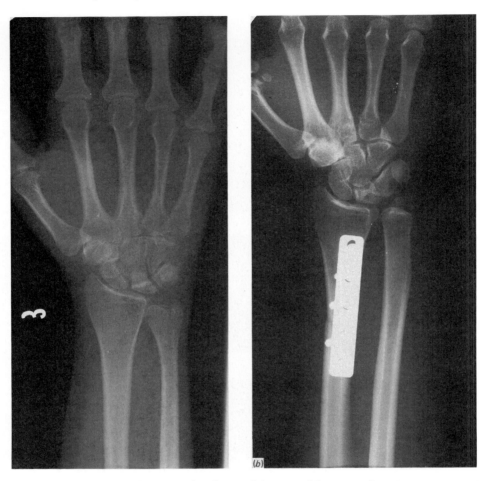

Figure 9.28 (*a*) Avascular necrosis of carpal lunate with a negative ulna variance. (*b*) Avascular necrosis of carpal lunate treated with radial shortening to alter forces across the lunate articulation and prevention of further collapse of the lunate

indicated, and associated capitohamate arthrodesis (Chiunard and Zeman, 1980) or triscaphoid arthrodesis (Watson, 1980; Watson and Ballet, 1984) to prevent collapse and migration of the capitate into the lunate defect.

A vascular pedicle utilizing the terminal portion of the posterior interosseous artery into bone (Hori *et al.*, 1979) or a musculopedicle bone graft with the pronator quadratus (Braun, 1983) have been advocated to revascularize the lunate.

Fractures of the triquetrum may represent a more significant ulnar carpal instability or dislocation pattern. The possibility of a late pisiform/triquetral arthritis is a cause for persistent pain and discomfort in this area. Carpal tunnel views specifically for fractures of the pisiform and pisiform/triquetral arthritis may be useful in making this diagnosis. Excision of the pisiform for treatment of patients with persistent pain is indicated.

Fractures of the trapezium and trapezoid can be identified with oblique views of the thumb carpometacarpal joint to include the trapezium and trapezoid as well as carpal tunnel views which can identify the trapezial ridge fractures (Palmer, 1981). Similar X-rays will identify fractures of the hook of the hamate (*Figure 9.29*). Generally, if non-displaced, these are treated with cast immobilization. Displacement of hook of the hamate fractures, and non-union of the hook of the hamate which is painful, necessitate surgical removal (Carter, Eaton and Littler, 1977).

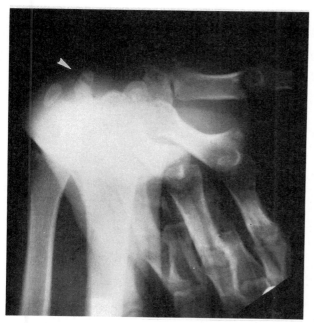

Figure 9.29 Fracture of the hook of the hamate

Fractures of the capitate, usually through the dome, are often associated with trans-scaphoid fractures (Vance, Gelberman and Evans, 1980). The capitate fragment is rotated volarward and is often missed on routine X-ray evaluation. Specific attention is required when observing films with the loss of the dome or a flat proximal capitate identifying fractures of the dome of the capitate (*Figure 9.30(a)* and (*b*)). Carpal tunnel views may show the displaced dome of the capitate within the carpal canal. Open reduction and internal fixation is indicated for acute capitate dome fractures with displacement. Late diagnosis of displaced fractures of the capitate dome are treated by excision of the fragment and interposition arthroplasty or midcarpal arthrodesis (Lowry and Cord, 1981; Kinmel and O'Brien, 1982). If a large avascular proximal dome is present with satisfactory cartilage coverage, a bone grafting procedure with K-wire fixation may be utilized.

Figure 9.31(a), (*b*), (*c*), (*d*) and (*e*) shows severe wrist injury with dislocation/translocation of the carpus, rotatory dislocation of the scaphoid, comminuted dislocated lunate, triquetrum fracture, and radial and ulnar styloid fractures inadequately treated with closed reduction and K-pin fixation of the radial

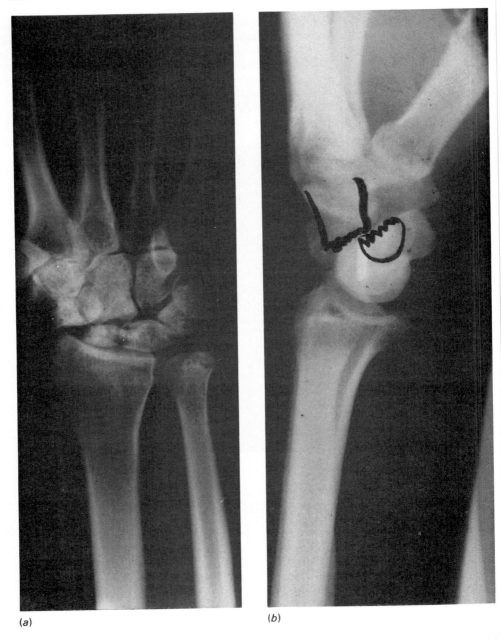

Figure 9.30 (a) Trans-scaphoid transcapitate fracture. (b) Lateral view drawing interposed showing the difficulty in detecting transcapitate fracture on the lateral view

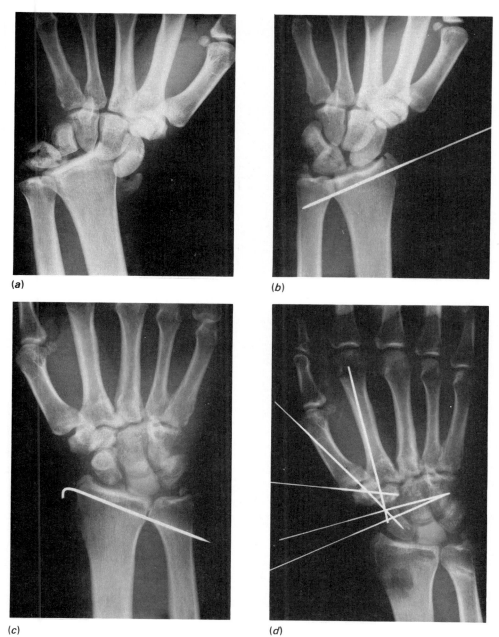

Figure 9.31 (*a*) Severe wrist dislocation with comminuted lunate fracture and rotatory dislocation of scaphoid, triquetrum fracture, radial and ulnar styloid fracture. (*b*) Reduction and pinning of radial styloid fracture, however inadequate reduction of lunate and scaphoid. (*c*) Excision of comminuted lunate fracture and silicone lunate implant, persistence of rotatory scaphoid deformity. (*d*) Triscaphoid arthrodesis accompanying lunate replacement to ultimately stabilize the wrist and restore the anatomical alignment of the wrist.

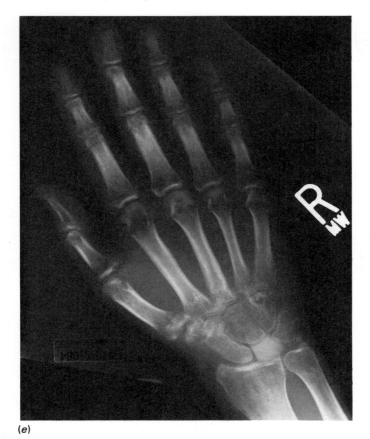

(e)

Figure 9.31 (*e*) Triscaphoid arthrodesis complete, lunate prosthesis, healed styloid fractures

styloid fracture. The comminuted lunate was then treated by excision and replacement with lunate prosthesis. Rotation of the scaphoid was treated by triscaphoid arthrodesis in an effort to preserve wrist stability and alignment (*Figure 9.31(a)–(e)*).

DISTAL RADIAL FRACTURES

Distal radius fractures will not be discussed in any depth. The diagnosis and treatment of the various distal radius fractures, such as Colles', Smith's, Barton's (volar and dorsal) and chauffeur's are well known to the orthopedist and hand surgeon. Closed reduction, open reduction, internal fixation and external fixation devices (Green, 1975; Cooney, Linscheid and Dobyns, 1979) can be utilized in an effort to restore anatomy and congruency of the articular surfaces (*Figure 9.32(a)*, (*b*), (*c*), (*d*) and (*e*)). Fractures of the distal radius which are intra-articular and displaced are disposed to radiocarpal arthritis if not anatomically reduced (Frykman, 1967; Dobyns and Linscheid, 1978). Great attention is directed at

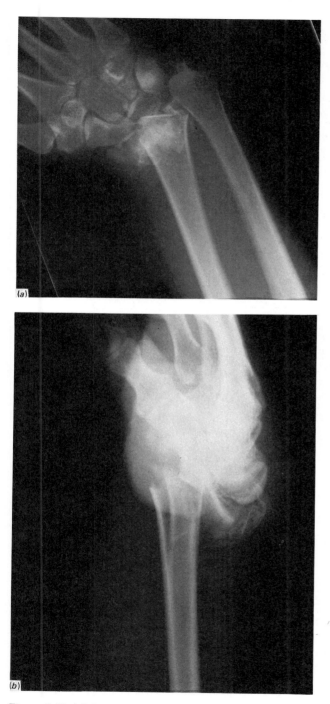

Figure 9.32 (*a*) Severe displaced comminuted distal radius fractures, anteroposterior view. (*b*) Lateral view.

258

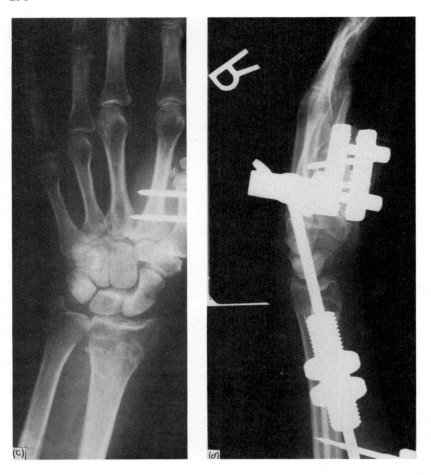

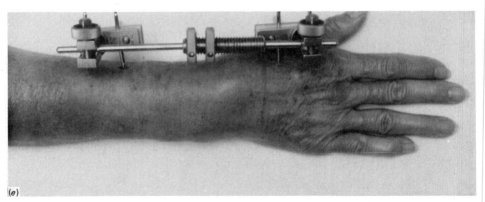

Figure 9.32 (*c*) Hoffmann external fixation device for severe displaced comminuted distal radius fractures (X-ray), anteroposterior view. (*d*) Lateral view. (*e*) Clinical photo of Hoffmann external fixation device for severe displaced comminuted distal radius fractures

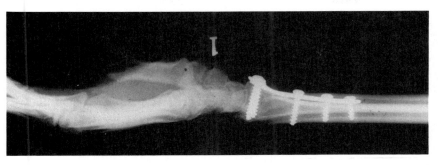

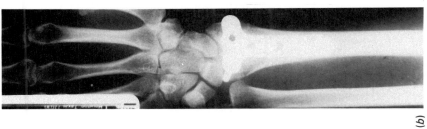

(b)

(a)

Figure 9.33 (a) Distal radius fracture with dye punch fracture fragment and lunate migration into radial lunate fossa. (b) T plate fixation of dye punch fracture fragment with fragment elevation and bone grafting procedures

re-establishing the congruency of the distal radius in these fractures. Displaced radial styloid fractures are reduced and pinned with Kirschner wire fixation. Die punch fractures of the lunate fossa, if depressed, generally cannot be reduced and maintained with closed methods or with external fixation methods. Open reduction, elevation of the central depressed fragment, pin or plate fixation and bone grafting is the procedure of choice (*Figure 9.33(a)* and (*b*)). Even with anatomical alignment, significant radiocarpal arthrosis may develop when extensive cartilage damage exists.

Large distal ulnar styloid fractures, triangular fibrocartilage damage, ulnar carpal complex damage with instability or distal radio-ulnar dislocation should be identified and reconstructed. Large ulnar styloid fractures may be secured with pin fixation or screw fixation. Distal ulnar osteotomy with recession and plate fixation is utilized in cases of ulnar impingement syndrome secondary to healed collapsed radius fractures (*Figure 9.34(a)* and (*b*)). Small styloid fractures may be excised and reattachment of ulnar carpal complex or triangular fibrocartilage to distal ulna is performed, in late cases of instability, pain or impingement syndrome.

Midcarpal instability patterns secondary to fractures of the distal radius may occur (Lichtman *et al.*, 1981; Taleisnik and Watson, 1984). Care is taken on the lateral X-ray to observe alignment between the radius, lunate, capitate and metacarpal. If volar or dorsal angulation of the distal radius is present and there is midcarpal malalignment, realignment with closed reduction and pin fixation or T-plate fixation following upon reduction is indicated.

Late collapse of distal radius fractures with secondary malalignment of the carpus should be reconstituted by anatomical realignment of the distal radius. Osteotomy, plating and bone grafting is often necessary to realign the carpus and distal radius (*Figure 9.35(a)*, (*b*) and (*c*)). Late arthritic deformities of midcarpal instability secondary to malunion or proximal carpal malalignment with pain are managed surgically by proximal row carpectomy, interpositional fascial or silastic arthroplasty or wrist arthrodesis.

Distal radio-ulnar joint

The distal radio-ulnar joint and its importance to the wrist and distal radius biomechanics have been brought to our attention through the work of Bowers (1982) and Palmer and Werner (1981). Derangement of the distal radio-ulnar joint through either fracture, fracture/dislocation or dislocation may cause significant restriction in motion, ulnar wrist pain and disability. Similarly, tears or disruption of the triangular fibrocartilage complex or the ulnar carpal ligament complex may produce an instability pattern exhibited by a painful wrist or clicking wrist. Impingement syndrome from the distal ulna is also a cause of pain at the wrist, with either a positive ulnar variance primarily or secondarily to fractured radius with collapse and shortening. The ulnar carpal ligament complex and the triangular fibrocartilage complex may be evaluated through cineradiography motion studies, arthroscopic and arthrogram examination (*Figure 9.36*). Dorsal dislocations of the distal ulna must be reduced and stabilized in supination, often utilizing K-pin fixation. Volar dislocations reduce in pronation. Open injuries to the ulnar complex are reconstructed anatomically. Chondromalacia changes of the distal ulna if persistently painful may also respond to ulna decompression by shortening or recession procedures which decompress the distal ulnar-carpal joint and tighten the ulnar carpal complex (Milch, 1941).

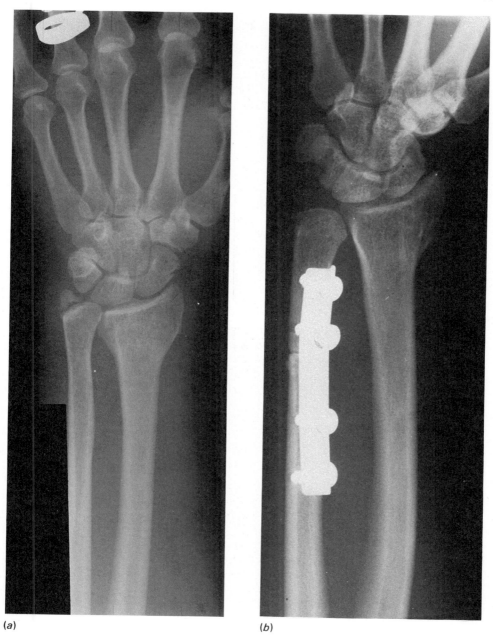

(a)

(b)

Figure 9.34 (a) Ulnar styloid fracture with secondary impingement syndrome due to old radius fracture and collapse. (b) Ulnar shortening to decompress impingement and reattachment of ulnar carpal complex after styloid excision

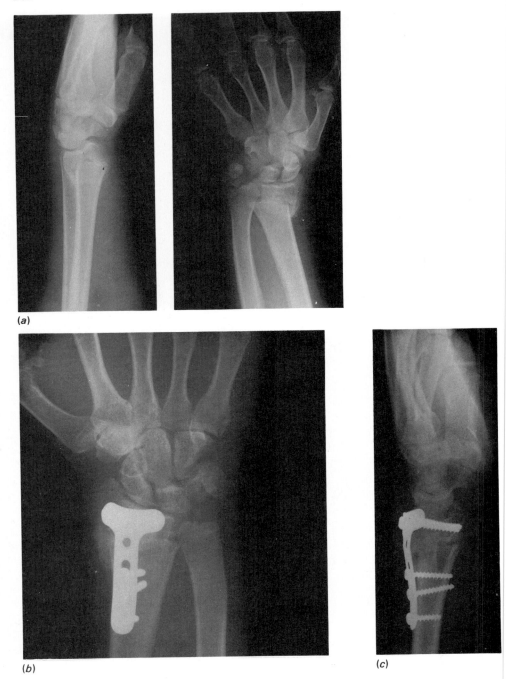

(a)

(b)

(c)

Figure 9.35 (a) Malunion of the distal radius fracture with dorsal instability pattern of the carpus. (b) Correction of malunion through osteotomy, realignment, bone grafting and T-plating to correct dorsal instability pattern, anteroposterior view. (c) Lateral view, postoperative

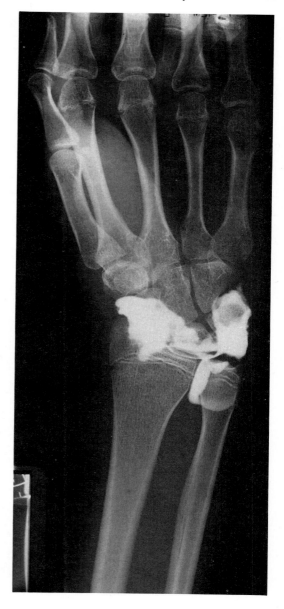

Figure 9.36 Wrist arthrogram showing disruption of triangular fibrocartilage complex

Distal ulna resections (Darrach procedure; Darrach, 1913) for distal radio-ulnar joint arthritis, secondary to fracture or dislocation pathology, are associated with complications of instability, chronic pain and deformity. Great care must be taken in reconstruction and stabilization of the distal ulna complex secondary to distal ulna resection.

Chronic dorsal or volar dislocations of the distal ulna are associated with restriction of motion and pain. Late reduction is unsuccessful and resection or recession arthroplasty may be indicated. Satisfactory results may be obtained by distal radio-ulnar arthrodesis with ulnar resection osteotomy (Baldwin or Lauenstein procedure) (Goncalves, 1974). Silicone interposition arthroplasty has mixed results and is often associated with prosthetic fracture and dislocation. Silicone synovitis and cystic bone changes, particularly in association with silicone carpal prosthesis, have been reported (Gordon and Bullough, 1982; Smith, Atkinson and Jupiter, 1985).

Isolated rupture of the triangular fibrocartilage, if incomplete, may be corrected by partial excision of the flap tear. If complete, then reattachment may resurface the distal ulna and re-establish the triangular fibrocartilage. Attritional changes with perforation of the triangular fibrocartilage complex are noted in the middle-age group patient. Symptoms of 'snapping' or dislocation may also be associated with extensor retinaculum tear and tendonitis of the extensor carpi ulnaris. Stabilization of the extensor carpi ulnaris may be performed. Distal ulnar arthritis at the radioulnar joint may be treated with oblique resection and fascial arthroplasty (Bowers, 1982). Immobilization for 4–6 weeks in a neutral position is followed by pronation supination activity and strengthening over the next three months.

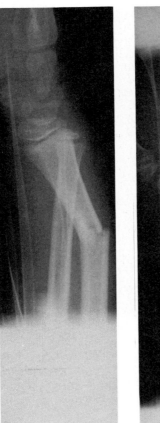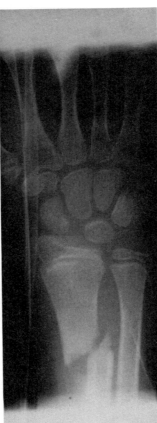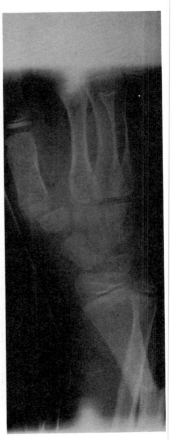

Figure 9.37 Galeazzi fracture with dislocation of distal radio-ulnar joint and fractured radius

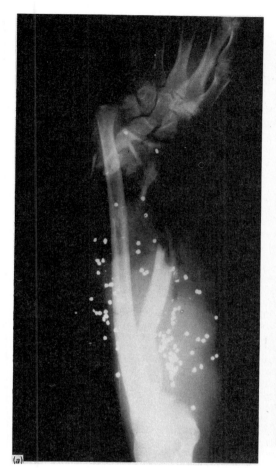 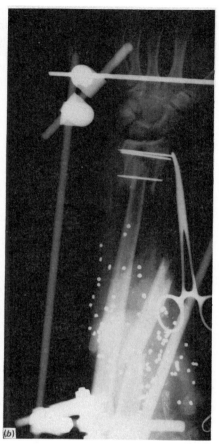

Figure 9.38 (*a*) Complex open injury with bone loss of mid-radius and intact ulna with radio-ulnar dislocation. (*b*) Complex injury managed by creation of single bone forearm with distal radius arthrodesed to distal ulna, utilizing both internal and external fixation due to soft tissue loss and subsequent skin coverage procedures

Galleazzi and Essex-Lopresti fractures involve distal ulna dislocation with radius fracture (*Figure 9.37*). Both dislocation and fracture must be reduced for treatment. Distal radius or ulna bone loss may be reconstructed as a single bone forearm if both bone salvage is not possible. If open injury with soft tissue loss in addition to bone loss is present, external fixation in conjunction with internal skeletal stabilization can salvage and reconstitute the extremity (*Figure 38(a)* and (*b*)).

SUMMARY

Management of joint injuries in the hand requires a thorough knowledge of the normal anatomy and biomechanics and the results of pathological forces from injury to the joints. Treatment of these injuries acutely, require anatomical reconstruction of displaced or disrupted bone, cartilage, ligament, tendon and capsular structures. Appropriate time for healing must occur, followed by a structured rehabilitation program and progressive analysis of return of functional range of motion. Secondary reconstructive procedures are indicated after therapy has plateaued and impairment exists beyond that expected for the injury. The ultimate goal in treatment is the achievement of a maximum functional range of motion with little or no pain while maintaining joint stability.

References

ARMISTEAD, R. B., LINSCHEID, R. L., DOBYNS, J. H. and BECKENBAUGH, R. D. (1982) Ulnar lengthening in the treatment of Kienbock's disease. *Journal of Bone and Joint Surgery,* **64A,** 170–178

BARTON, N. J. (1979) Fractures of the phalanges of the hand in children. *The Hand,* **11,** 134–143

BECKENBAUGH, R. D., SCHIVES, T. C., DOBYNS, J. H. and LINSCHEID, R. L. (1980) Kienbock's disease: the natural history of Kienbock's disease in consideration of lunate fractures. *Clinical Orthopaedics and Related Research,* **149,** 98–106

BORA, F. W. and DIDIZIAN, N. H. (1974) The treatment of injuries to the carpometacarpal joint of the little finger. *Journal of Bone and Joint Surgery,* **56A,** 1459–1463

BORA, F. W., IGNATIUS, P. and NISSENBAUM, M. (1976) Treatment of epiphyseal fractures of the hand. *Journal of Bone and Joint Surgery,* **58A,** 286

BOWERS, W. H. (1982) Distal radioulnar joint. In *Operative Hand Surgery,* Volume 1, edited by D. P. Green, pp. 743–769. New York: Churchill Livingstone

BOWERS, W. H. and HURST, L. C. (1977) Gamekeeper's thumb. Evaluation by arthrography and stress roentgenography. *Journal of Bone and Joint Surgery,* **59A,** 519

BRADFORD, C. H. and DOBYNS, J. A. (1975) Fractures of the hand and wrist. In *Hand Surgery,* edited by J. E. Flynn, pp. 88–115. Baltimore: Williams and Wilkins

BRAUN, R. (1983) The pronator pedicle bone grafting in the forearm and proximal carpal row. *Presented at the Annual Meeting of the American Society for Surgery of the Hand.* California: Anaheim

BRYAN, R. S. and DOBYNS, J. H. (1980) Fractures of the carpal bones other than lunate or navicular. *Clinical Orthopaedics and Related Research,* **149,** 107–111

BUTLER, B. JR., NEVIASER, R. J. and ADAMS, J. P. (1978) Complications of treatment of injuries to the hand. In *Complications of Orthopedic Surgery,* edited by C. H. Epps, Jr, pp. 353–401. Philadelphia: J. B. Lippincott

CARTER, P. R., EATON, R. G. and LITTLER, J. W. (1977) Ununited fracture of the hook of the hamate. *Journal of Bone and Joint Surgery,* **59A,** 583–588

CHUINARD, R. G. and ZEMAN, S. C. (1980) Kienbock's disease: an analysis and rationale for treatment by capitate–hamate fusion. *Orthopaedic Transactions,* **4,** 18

CLIFFORD, R. H. (1953) Intramedullary wire fixation of hand fractures. *Plastic and Reconstructive Surgery,* **11,** 366–371

COONEY, W. P., LINSCHEID, R. L. and DOBYNS, J. H. (1979) External pin fixation for unstable Colles' fracture. *Journal of Bone and Joint Surgery,* **61A,** 840–845

CRAWFORD, G. P. (1976) Screw fixation for certain fractures of the phalanges and metacarpals. *Journal of Bone and Joint Surgery,* **58A,** 487–492

CROCKETT, D. J. (1974) Rigid fixation of bones of the hand using K-wires bounded with acrylic resin. *The Hand,* **6,** 106–107

CURTIS, R. M. (1966) Joints of the hand. In *Hand Surgery,* edited by J. E. Flynn, p. 368. Baltimore: Williams and Wilkins

DARRACH, W. (1913) Habitual forward dislocation of the head of the ulna. *Annals of Surgery,* **57,** 928–930

DICKSON, R. A. (1975) Rigid fixation of unstable metacarpal fractures using transverse K-wires bonded with acrylic resin. *The Hand,* **7,** 284–286

DOBYNS, J. H. and LINSCHEID, R. L. (1975) Fractures and dislocations of the wrist. In *Fractures,* Volume 1, edited by C. A. Rockwood Jr. and D. P. Green, pp. 345–440. Philadelphia: J. B. Lippincott

DOBYNS, J. H. and LINSCHEID, R. L. (1978) Complications of treatment of fracture dislocations of the wrist. In *Complications of Orthopaedic Surgery,* edited by C. H. Epps, Jr, pp. 271–352. Philadelphia: J. B. Lippincott

DOBYNS, J. H. and LINSCHEID, R. L. (1980) Carpal bone injuries. *Symposium: Clinical Orthopaedics and Related Research*, **149**, 1–144

EATON, R. G. (1971) *Joint Injuries of the Hand*. Springfield, Illinois: Charles C. Thomas

EATON, R. G. and DRAY, G. J. (1982) Dislocations and ligament injuries of the digits. In *Operative Hand Surgery*, Volume 1, edited by D. P. Green, pp. 637–666. New York: Churchill Livingstone

EATON, R. G. and LITTLER, J. W. (1969) A study of the basal joint of the thumb. Treatment of its disabilities by fusion. *Journal of Bone and Joint Surgery*, **51A**, 661

EATON, R. G. and LITTLER, J. W. (1973) Ligament reconstruction for the painful thumb carpometacarpal joint. *Journal of Bone and Joint Surgery*, **55A**, 1655

EATON, R. G. and MALERICH, M. M. (1980) Volar plate arthroplasty for the proximal interphalangeal joint: a ten year review. *Journal of Hand Surgery*, **5**, 260

FAITHFULL, D. K. (1981) Treatment of chronic instability of the distal joints using a strip of volar plate. *The Hand*, **13**, 36–38

FAITHFULL, D. K. and HERBERT, T. J. (1984) Small joint fusions of the hand using the Herbert bone screw. *Journal of Hand Surgery*, **9B**, 167–168

FISK, G. (1966) Carpal injuries. In *Clinical Surgery: The Hand*, edited by R. G. Pulvertaft, p. 101. Washington: Butterworths

FRYKMAN, G. (1967) Fracture of the distal radius including sequelae–shoulder–hand–finger syndrome, disturbance in the distal radioulnar joint and impairment of nerve function. *Acta Orthopaedica Scandinavica*, Supplement 108, 27

GELBERMAN, R. H., SALAMON, P. W., JURIST, J. M. and POSCH, J. L. (1975) Ulnar variance in Kienbock's disease. *Journal of Bone and Joint Surgery*, **57A**, 674–676

GONCALVES, D. (1974) Correction of disorders of the distal radio-ulnar joint by artificial pseudarthrosis of the ulna. *Journal of Bone and Joint Surgery*, **56B**, 462–463

GORDON, M. G. and BULLOUGH, P. E. (1982) Synovial and osseous inflammations in failed silicone-rubber prosthesis. *Journal of Bone and Joint Surgery*, **64A**, 574–580

GREEN, D. P. (1975) Pins and plaster treatment of comminuted fractures of the distal end of the radius. *Journal of Bone and Joint Surgery*, **57A**, 304–310

GREEN, D. P. (1982) Carpal dislocations. In *Operative Hand Surgery*, Volume 1, edited by D. P. Green, pp. 703–742. New York: Churchill Livingstone

GREEN, D. P. and ANDERSON, J. R. (1973) Closed reduction and percutaneous pin fixation of fractured phalanges. *Journal of Bone and Joint Surgery*, **55A**, 1651–1653

GREEN, D. P. and ROWLAND, S. A. (1975) Fractures and dislocations in the hand. In *Fractures*, Volume 1, edited by C. A. Rockwood, Jr and D. P. Green, pp. 265–343. Philadelphia: J. B. Lippincott

GREEN, D. P. and O'BRIEN, E. T. (1978) Open reduction of carpal dislocations: indications and operative techniques. *Journal of Hand Surgery*, **3**, 250–265

GREEN, D. P. and O'BRIEN, E. T. (1980) Classification and management of carpal dislocations. *Clinical Orthopaedics and Related Research*, **149**, 55–72

HEIM, U., PFEIFFER, K. M. and MEULI, H. C. (1974) Small fragment set manual. *Technique Recommended by the ASIF Group* (Swiss Association for Study of Internal Fixation). New York: Springer-Verlag

HERBERT, T. J. (1982) Management of the fractured scaphoid bone using a new surgical technique. *Journal of Bone and Joint Surgery*, **64B**, 633

HORI, Y., TAMAI, S., OKUDA, H., SAKAMOTO, H., TAKITA, T. and MASUHARA, K. (1979) Blood vessel transplantation to bone. *Journal of Hand Surgery*, **4**, 23–33

HSU, J. D. and CURTIS, R. M. (1970) Carpometacarpal dislocations on the ulnar side of the hand. *Journal of Bone and Joint Surgery*, **52A**, 927–930

IKUTA, K. and TSUGE, K. (1974) Microbolts and microscrews for fixation of small bones in the hand. *The Hand*, **6**, 261–263

INGLIS, A. E. and JONES, E. C. (1977) Proximal row carpectomy for diseases of the proximal row. *Journal of Bone and Joint Surgery*, **59A**, 460–463

KAPLAN, E. B. (1957) Dorsal dislocation of the metacarpal joint of the index finger. *Journal of Bone and Joint Surgery*, **39A**, 1081–1086

KIENBOCK, R. (1910) Uber Traumatische Malazie des Mondbeins und ihre Folgezustande: Entartungsformen und Kompression Fracturen. *Fortschritte auf dem Gebiete der Rontgenstrahlen*, **16**, 78

KILBOURNE, B. C. and PAUL, E. G. (1958) The use of small bone screws in the treatment of metacarpal, metatarsal and phalangeal fractures. *Journal of Bone and Joint Surgery*, **40A**, 375–383

KINMEL, R. B. and O'BRIEN, E. T. (1982) Surgical treatment of avascular necrosis of the proximal pole of the capitate – case report. *Journal of Hand Surgery*, **7**, 284–286

LANE, C. S. (1977) Detecting occult fractures of the metacarpal head: the Brewerton view. *Journal of Hand Surgery*, **2**, 131–133

LEE, M. L. H. (1963) Intra-articular and peri-articular fractures of the phalanges. *Journal of Bone and Joint Surgery,* **45B,** 103–109

LICHTMAN, D. M., SCHNEIDER, J. R., SWAFFORD, A. A. and MACK, G. R. (1981) Ulnar mid-carpal instability – clinical and laboratory analysis. *Journal of Hand Surgery,* **6,** 515–523

LINSCHEID, R. L. (1974) Arthrography of the metacarpal phalangeal joint. *Clinical Orthopaedics and Related Research,* **103,** 91

LINSCHEID, R. L., DOBYNS, J. H., BEABOUT, J. W. and BRYAN, R. S. (1972) Traumatic instability of the wrist; diagnosis, classification and pathomechanics. *Journal of Bone and Joint Surgery,* **54A,** 1612–1632

LISTER, G. (1978) Intraosseous wiring of the digital skeleton. *Journal of Hand Surgery,* **3,** 427–435

LOUIS, D. and GREENE, T. L. (1984) Fractures and dislocations of the hand. In *The Hand in Radiologic Diagnosis,* Volume 2, edited by Andrew K. Poznanski, pp. 677–707. Philadelphia: W. B. Saunders

LOWRY, W. E. and CORD, S. A. (1981) Traumatic avascular necrosis of the capitate bone – case report. *Journal of Hand Surgery,* **6,** 245–248

MASSENGILL, J. B., ALEXANDER, H., PARSON, J. R. and SCHECTER, M. J. (1979) Mechanical analysis of Kirschner wire fixation in a phalangeal model. *Journal of Hand Surgery,* **4,** 351–356

MAUDSLEY, R. H. and CHEN, S. C. (1972) Screw fixation in the management of the fractured carpal scaphoid. *Journal of Bone and Joint Surgery,* **54B,** 432–441

MAYFIELD, J. K., JOHNSON, R. P. and KILCOYNE, R. F. (1976) The ligaments of the human wrist and their functional significance. *Anatomical Records,* **186,** 417–428

McELFRESH, E. C. and DOBYNS, J. H. (1983) Intra-articular metacarpal head fractures. *Journal of Hand Surgery,* **8,** 383–393

McELFRESH, E. C., DOBYNS, J. H. and O'BRIEN, E. T. (1972) Management of fracture-dislocation of the proximal interphalangeal joints by extension-block splinting. *Journal of Bone and Joint Surgery,* **54A,** 1705

MIKKELSEN, O. A. (1984) Replacement of destroyed metacarpal heads by autografting metatarsal heads. *Journal of Hand Surgery,* **9B,** 337–339

MILCH, H. (1941) Cuff resection of the ulna for mal-united Colles' fracture. *Journal of Bone and Joint Surgery,* **23,** 311–313

MILFORD, L. (1982) Closed hand injuries. In *The Hand,* 2nd edition, edited by A. S. Edmonson and A. H. Crenshaw, pp. 46–88. St Louis: C. V. Mosby

MOBERG, E. (1949–50) The use of traction treatment for fractures of phalanges and metacarpals. *Acta Chirurgica Scandinavica,* **99,** 341–352

MOBERG, E. (1960) Fractures and ligamentous injuries of the thumb and fingers. *Surgical Clinics of North America,* **40,** 297

MOBERG, E. and STENER, B. (1953) Injuries to the ligaments of the thumb and fingers. Diagnosis, treatment, and prognosis. *Acta Chirurgica Scandinavica,* **106,** 166

MOSS, J. G. and STEINGOLD, R. F. (1983) The long-term results of mallet finger injury: a retrospective study of 100 cases. *The Hand,* **15,** 151–154

NAHIGIAN, S. H., LI, C. S., RICHEY, D. G. and SHAW, D. T. (1970) The dorsal flap arthroplasty in the treatment of Kienbock's disease. *Journal of Bone and Joint Surgery,* **52A,** 245–252

NARAKAS, A. (1972) Interphalangeal joint injuries in children. *The Hand,* **4,** 163–167

NATHAN, F. F. and SCHLEIN, A. P. (1973) Multiple dislocations of a single finger. *The Hand,* **5,** 52–54

NEVIASER, J. and WILSON, J. N. (1972) In a position of the extensor tendon resulting in persistent subluxation of the proximal interphalangeal joint of the finger. *Clinical Orthopaedics and Related Research,* **83,** 118–120

NEVIASER, R. M., WILSON, J. N. and LIEVANO, A. (1971) Rupture of the ulnar collateral ligament of the thumb (gamekeeper's thumb). Correction by dynamic repair. *Journal of Bone and Joint Surgery,* **53A,** 1357

O'BRIEN, E. T. (1982) Fractures of the metacarpals and phalanges. In *Operative Hand Surgery,* Volume 1, edited by D. P. Green, pp. 583–635. New York: Churchill Livingstone

PALMER, A. K. (1981) Trapezial ridge fractures. *Journal of Hand Surgery,* **6,** 561–564

PALMER, A. K. and LINSCHEID, R. L. (1978) Chronic recurrent dislocation of the proximal interphalangeal joint of the finger. *Journal of Hand Surgery,* **3,** 95

PALMER, A. K. and WERNER, G. W. (1981) The triangular fibrocartilage complex of the wrist – anatomy and function. *Journal of Hand Surgery,* **6,** 153–162

PALMER, A. K., DOBYNS, J. H. and LINSCHEID, R. L. (1978) Management of post-traumatic instability of the wrist secondary to ligament rupture. *Journal of Hand Surgery,* **3,** 507–532

PERSSON, M. (1950) Causal treatment of lunatomalacies. Further experiences of operative ulna lengthening. *Acta Chirurgica Scandinavica,* **100,** 531–544

QUIGLEY, T. B. and URIST, M. R. (1947) Interphalangeal joints – a method of digital skeletal traction which permits active motion. *American Journal of Surgery,* **73,** 175–183

SAKELLARIDES, H. T. and DeWEESE, J. W. (1976) Instability of the metacarpophalangeal joint of the thumb. Reconstruction of the collateral ligaments using the extensor pollicis brevis tendon. *Journal of Bone and Joint Surgery*, **58A**, 106

SANDZEN, SIGURD, C. JR (1979) *Atlas of Wrist and Hand Fractures*. Littleton, Massachusetts: PSG, Inc.

SEBALD, J. R., DOBYNS, J. H. and LINSCHEID, R. L. (1974) The natural history of collapse deformities of the wrist. *Clinical Orthopaedics and Related Research*, **104**, 140–148

SERADGE, H., KUTZ, J. E., KLEINERT, H. E., LISTER, G. D., WOLFF, T. W. and ATASOY, E. (1984) Perichondrial resurfacing arthroplasty in the hand. *Journal of Hand Surgery*, **9A**, 880–886

SIMONETTA, C. (1970) The use of 'AO' plates in the hand. *The Hand*, **2**, 43–45

SMITH, R. J. (1977) Post-traumatic instability of the metacarpophalangeal joint of the thumb. *Journal of Bone and Joint Surgery*, **59A**, 14

SMITH, R. J., ATKINSON, R. E. and JUPITER, J. B. (1985) Silicone synovitis of the wrist. *Journal of Hand Surgery*, **10A**, 47–60

SPINNER, M. and CHOI, B. Y. (1970) Anterior dislocation of proximal interphalangeal joint. *Journal of Bone and Joint Surgery*, **52A**, 1329–1336

SPRAGUE, B. L. (1975) Proximal interphalangeal joint injuries and their treatment. *Journal of Trauma*, **15**, 380

STEEL, W. M. (1978) The AO small fragment set in hand fractures. *The Hand*, **10**, 246–253

STENER, B. (1962) Displacement of the ruptured ulnar collateral ligament of the metacarpophalangeal joint of the thumb. A clinical and anatomical study. *Journal of Bone and Joint Surgery*, **44B**, 869

STRIPLING, W. D. (1982) Displaced interarticular osteochrondral fracture – cause for irreducible dislocation of the distal interphalangeal joint. *Journal of Hand Surgery*, **7**, 77–78

SWANSON, A. B. (1973) *Flexible Implant Resection Arthroplasty in the Hand and Extremities*. St. Louis: C. V. Mosby

TALEISNIK, J. (1976) The ligaments of the wrist. *Journal of Hand Surgery*, **1**, 110–118

TALEISNIK, J. (1978) Wrist: anatomy, function and injury. *AAOS Instructional Course Lectures*, **27**, 61–87. St Louis: C. V. Mosby

TALEISNIK, J. (1982) Fractures of the carpal bones. In *Operative Hand Surgery*, Volume 1, edited by D. P. Green, pp. 669–702. New York: Churchill Livingstone

TALEISNIK, J. and WATSON, H. (1984) Mid-carpal instability caused by malunited fractures of the radius. *Journal of Hand Surgery*, **9A**, 350–357

TRUMBLE, T. E. and WATSON, H. K. (1985) Post-traumatic sesamoid arthritis of the metacarpophalangeal joint of the thumb. *Journal of Hand Surgery*, **10A**, 94–100

TSAI, T. M. and SINGER, R. (1984) Elective free vascularized double transfer of toe joint from second toe to proximal interphalangeal joint of index finger. *Journal of Hand Surgery*, **9A**, 816–820

TSAI, T. M., JUPITER, J. B., KUTZ, J. E., KLEINERT, H. E. (1982) Vascularized autogenous whole joint transfer in the hand: a clinical study. *Journal of Hand Surgery*, **7**, 335–342

VANCE, R. M., GELBERMAN, R. H. and EVANS, E. F. (1980) Scaphocapitate fractures. *Journal of Bone and Joint Surgery*, **62A**, 271–276

VON RAFFLER, W. (1964a) Irreducible dislocations of the metacarpophalangeal joint of the finger. *Clinical Orthopaedics and Related Research*, **35**, 171

VON RAFFLER, W. (1964b) Irreducible juxta-epiphyseal fracture of a finger. *Journal of Bone and Joint Surgery*, **46B**, 229

WATSON, H. K. (1980) Limited wrist arthrodesis. *Clinical Orthopaedics and Related Research*, **149**, 126–136

WATSON, H. K. and BALLET, F. L. (1984) The SLAC wrist: scapholunate advanced collapse pattern of degenerative arthritis. *Journal of Hand Surgery*, **9A**, 358–365

WEEKS, P. M. (1981) *Acute Bone and Joint Injuries of the Hand and Wrist*. St Louis: C. V. Mosby

WEHBE, M. A. and SCHNEIDER, L. H. (1984) Mallet fractures. *Journal of Bone and Joint Surgery*, **66A**, 658–669

WILEY, A. M. (1970) Instability of the proximal interphalangeal joint following dislocation and fracture dislocation: surgical repair. *The Hand*, **2**, 185–191

WILSON, J. N. and ROLAND, S. A. (1966) Fracture dislocation of proximal interphalangeal joint of the finger. *Journal of Bone and Joint Surgery*, **48A**, 493–502

WOOD, V. E. (1976) Fractures of the hand in children. *Orthopaedic Clinics of North America*, **7**, 527–542

10
Replantation
Jesse B. Jupiter

INTRODUCTION AND HISTORY

The replantation of severed limbs or parts has attracted the interest of surgeons throughout recorded history (Gibson, 1965). While modern surgical investigation began with Halstead in 1887, these early efforts did not involve vascular anastomoses (Halstead, Reichert and Reid, 1922). As techniques of vascular suture developed the experimental limb replantation soon proved an excellent model to assess vascular patency. Höpfner (1903) reported experimental canine hindlimb replantations with one surviving nine days. Carrel and Guthrie (1906) performed similar work in canine replantation and transplantation, once again in the context of research into vascular suture techniques. Insurmountable problems with sepsis and anesthesia in the canine model prevented major developments over the succeeding decades, although Hall (1944) actually established a protocol for clinical upper extremity replantation should a suitable clinical situation arise.

A high rate of failure in experimental replantations continued into the 1960s with some authors reporting a fatal toxemia or 'toxic shock' attendant to these experimental extremity replantations (MacDonald, Tose and Deterling, 1962; Eiken et al., 1964; Mehl et al., 1964). However, Lapchinsky's (1960) presentation of a long-term follow-up of functional canine hindlimb replantations demonstrated the beneficial effects of limb preservation with hypothermia and pump oxygenation and restimulated investigators and clinicians. Similar success in dog limb replantation was soon reported by Snyder et al. (1960), also using preservation with pump oxygenation and thus avoiding the development of fatal toxemia.

It was within this setting that the first successful replantation of the traumatically severed arm of a 12-year-old boy by Malt and McKhann (1964) evoked such worldwide acclaim and rekindled interest in clinical replantation. Reports of successful extremity replantation soon followed from a number of centers led by the Sixth People's Hospital in Shanghai (Williams et al., 1966; Inoue et al., 1967; Ramirez et al., 1967; Sixth People's Hospital, 1967; Christeas, Balas and Giannikas, 1969). In these early successes the replantations were all proximal to the wrist. As noted by Malt and Smith (1977) 'the surgical techniques for these replantation efforts had been available for some time and it required only a synthesizing of the efforts of the general, orthopaedic, and vascular surgeons'.

It remained for Jacobsen and Suarez (1960) and Buncke *et al.* (1965) to develop the techniques of microvascular surgery in the laboratory and enable surgeons to predictably restore blood supply through small blood vessels, and tremendously expand the scope of clinical revascularization, replantation, and tissue salvage in upper extremity trauma. Clinical success in small vessel surgery by Kleinert and Kasdan (1963a, 1963b) and Jacobsen (1963) soon led to the successful replantation of a completely severed digit, first reported by Komatsu and Tamai (1968) who successfully reported replanting the thumb of a 28-year-old machinist. These reports were followed by many reports of successful replantations using microvascular surgical techniques.

Initial efforts centered primarily on revascularizing the amputated parts and early series reflected success solely in terms of survival (Lendvay, 1973; O'Brien, MacLeod and Miller, 1973; O'Brien, 1974; Tsai, 1975). As experience has developed it has become quite clear that survival alone is not a measure of function, and a successful replantation must be equated with a functional and aesthetic restoration (Malt, Remensnyder and Harris, 1972; Weiland *et al.*, 1977; Tamai, 1978; Schlenker, Kleinert and Tsai, 1980; Jones, Schenk and Chesney, 1982; May, Toth and Gardner, 1982).

INDICATIONS

In the practice and evaluation of replantation surgery the term *replantation* must be reserved for those limbs or parts that are completely severed without any residual attachment, whereas *revascularization* is more suitable for those parts incompletely amputated but whose circulation has been so disrupted that immediate vascular repair is necessary for the survival of the part.

Table 10.1 Replantation selection amputations – distal to wrist

---

Indications
Thumb
Multiple digits
Single digit distal to sublimis insertion
Children
Wrist
Transmetacarpal

Relative indications
Multiple level injuries
Mental instability
Nerve avulsion
Favorable amputation in patient of more than 60 years
Ring avulsion

Contraindications
Systemic illness
Associated life-threatening injuries
Mangled parts
Single digit proximal to sublimis insertion?

Table 10.2 Replantation selection amputations – proximal to the wrist

Indications
Forearm
Sharp amputation at elbow
Upper arm in child
Bilateral amputations

Relative indications
Upper arm in young adult
Multiple level injury
Mental instability
Nerve avulsion in child

Contraindications
Brachial plexus avulsion (Horner's sign)
Mangled part
Other severe injuries
Warm ischemia: more than six hours
Systemic illness

Most experienced replantation centers report viability in 80–90% of replantation efforts (Berger *et al.,* 1978; Morrison, O'Brien and MacLeod, 1978; Zhong-Wei *et al.,* 1981; Tamai, 1982); yet a successful replantation must be measured in terms of the ultimate function of the replanted part. It is in this light that the patient selection becomes critical (*Tables 10.1* and *10.2*). The patient's age, occupation, hand dominance, the level of the amputation, the condition of the amputated part, and associated injuries are all determining factors in the decision to attempt a replantation. Although a replantation effort may be technically more difficult in children, their unique regenerative capacity, in particular with neural repair, the inherent supple nature of their joints, and the generally favorable response to rehabilitation all lead to greater chances of functional success (Van Beek, Warak and Zook, 1979; Jaeger, Tsai and Kleinert, 1981). Older individuals, on the contrary, present increased risks as intrinsic vascular disease as well as systemic illnesses are commonplace.

Amputations have been categorized by both level as well as type of injury (*Figure 10.1(a)* to (*c*)). Thumb amputations continue to be considered optimal candidates for replantation, extending out to even the base of the nail. An independent unit, the thumb replant proves exceptionally functional if sensibility and vascularity are restored. Even in the setting of irreparable nerve injury a thumb should be replanted, as sensibility can predictably be restored by any number of techniques (*Figure 10.2(a)* to (*c*)).

The functional capability of a digit, however, also requires mobility. While a single finger amputated through 'no-person's zone' rarely will regain sufficient mobility to be a functional asset and, in fact, often has an adverse affect on hand function, a digital amputation distal to the insertion of the superficialis tendon can prove to be exceedingly successful even when a single finger is replanted. These replantations generally maintain proximal interphalangeal joint motion, sensibility is good even in the face of avulsive injury to the digital nerves, and the aesthetic outcome is often excellent (May, Toth and Gardner, 1982). At this level the replantation effort generally takes 4–6h, and additionally can offset painful

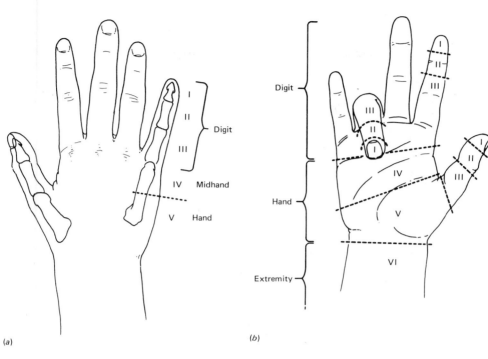

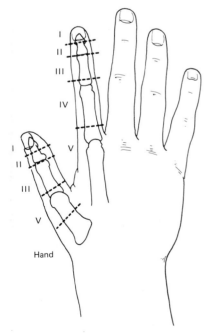

Figure 10.1 Levels of amputation – three separate categories: (*a*) from Biemer, 1980; (*b*) from Daniel and Terzis, 1977; (*c*) from Tamai, 1982. (Modified from Tamai, 1982, by courtesy of the author and publisher)

274

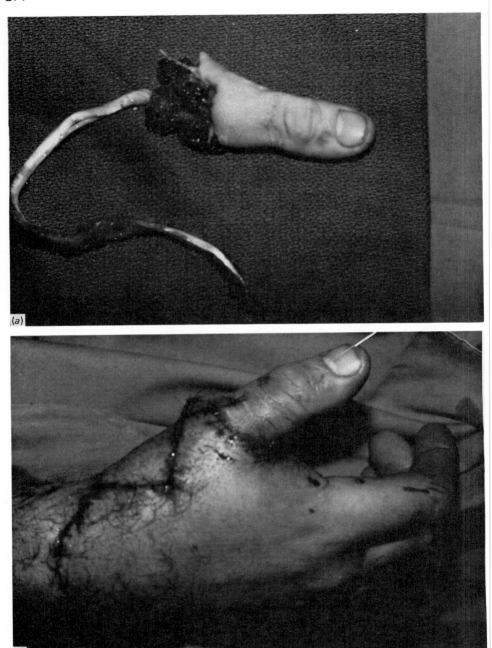

Figure 10.2 Shows a 20-year-old male who sustained an avulsive amputation of his dominant thumb from a rope injury. (*a*) The thumb was traumatically amputated from the hand with the flexor pollicis longus avulsed from its muscle belly. The digital nerves were similarly avulsed. (*b*) Following skeletal, tendon, and venous reconstruction, the vein graft was anastomosed in an end-to-side manner to the princeps pollicis artery in the first web space

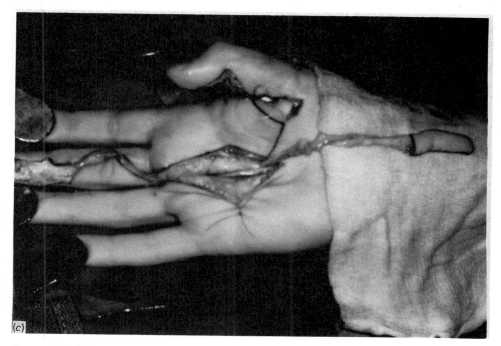

Figure 10.2 (c) At 5 months post-replantation sensibility was provided by a neurovascular island flap taken from the ulnar aspect of the long finger

amputation neuromas (*Figures 10.3(a)* to (*d*)). It should be pointed out, however, that in a laborer with multiple digital amputations distal to the superficialis insertion, the functional results will also be generally good with primary wound closure (Jones, Shenck and Chesney, 1982).

Digital amputations proximal to the superficialis insertion are common. Replantations at this level almost always result in some restriction in proximal interphalangeal joint, and occasionally metacarpophalangeal (MCP) joint mobility. The replantation of a single digit at this level faces the strong likelihood of impeding overall hand function and, in most cases, is not recommended.

Different considerations exist when one is faced with three or more digital amputations proximal to the superficialis insertion. When minimal damage exists to the amputated digits, overall hand performance will be enhanced by the replantation of all the digits. If more severe damage is found, the two best digits are chosen and placed on to the stumps of the index and long finger to enhance pinch function (*Figure 10.4(a)* to (*f*)). While placement of these digits more ulnarward theoretically would better maintain the functional width of the palm, in fact, the limited flexion arc in these digits would negate power grip capabilities.

More difficult is the clinical setting of a two-digit amputation with uninjured adjacent digits. In those cases of avulsive type injuries the patient may be better served by avoiding replantation. Yet, with more sharply divided amputations, replantation can prove to be functionally, psychologically, and aesthetically successful (*Figure 10.5(a)* to (*e*)).

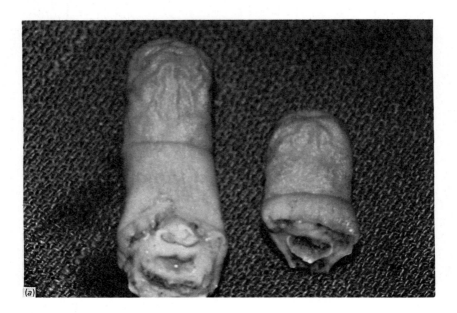

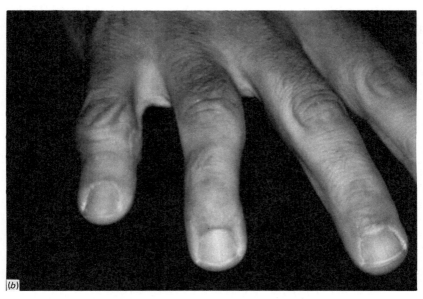

Figure 10.3 Shows a 40-year-old executive who amputated the ring and little fingers of his dominant hand on a home saw. (*a*) The little finger was severed beyond the insertion of the superficialis tendon while the ring finger was amputated at a more proximal level

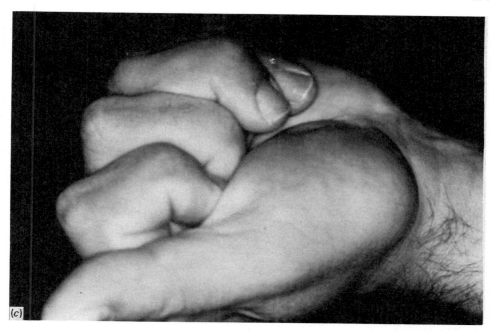

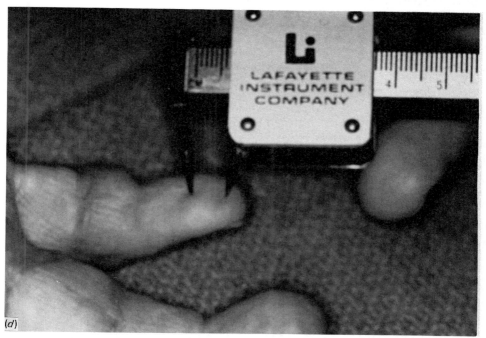

Figure 10.3 (*b*) and (*c*) One digital artery, both digital nerves, three digital veins, and the profundus tendon were repaired in each digit. A flexor tenolysis was later performed on the ring finger; two years post-replantation the patient had an excellent functional outcome. (*d*) Two-point discrimination in both digits was 10 mm

278

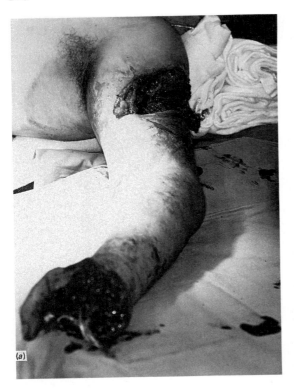

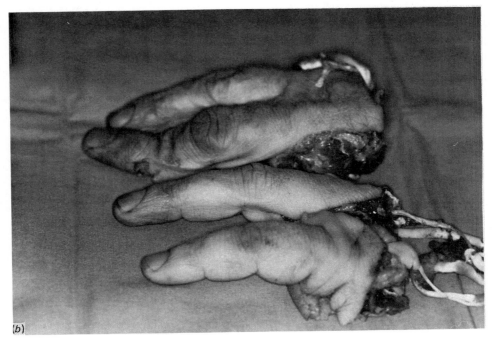

Figure 10.4 Shows a 38-year-old foreman who suffered a severe avulsion injury to his left non-dominant arm on a computerized lathe. (*b*) In addition to an open humerus fracture, crush injury to the elbow and forearm, all four digits were avulsed from the hand

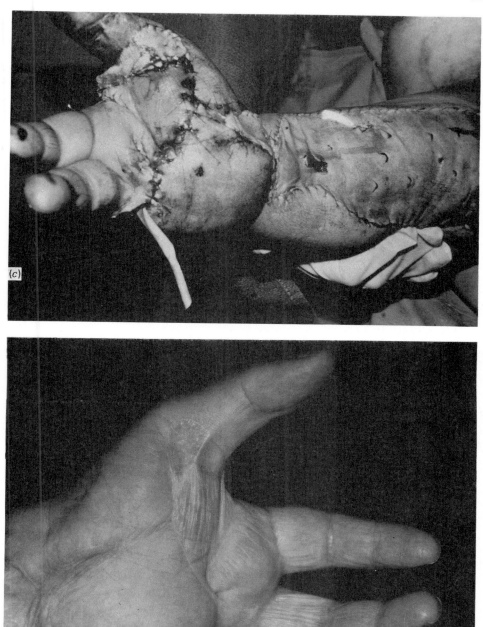

Figure 10.4 (*c*) Following internal fixation of the humerus and forearm fasciotomies, a long vein graft was placed on the common digital artery to the two best digits. These were placed on the index and long metacarpals. The vein graft was sutured end-to-side to the radial artery in the midforearm. The flexor tendons were sutured back into their muscle bellies

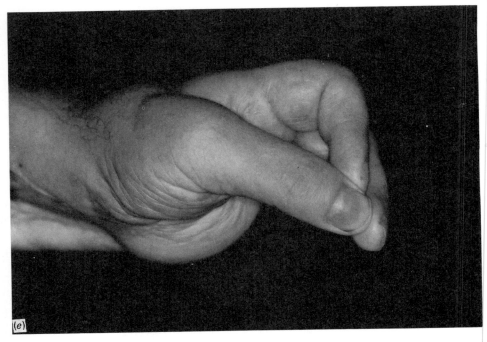

(e)

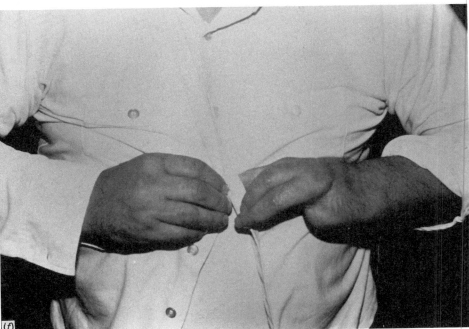

(f)

Figure 10.4 (*d*) and (*e*) At 20 months postreplantation, the hand functions as an assistive hand; flexion proved better in the index finger. (*f*) Two-point discrimination was 15 mm and the patient generated 4.5 kg (10 pounds) on the pinch meter

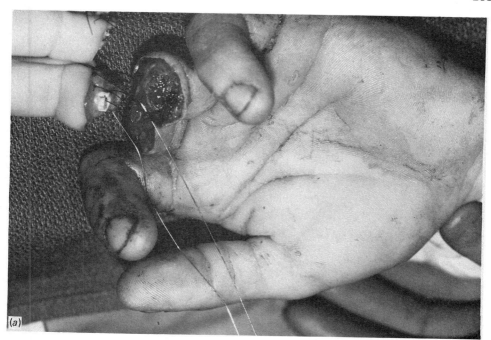

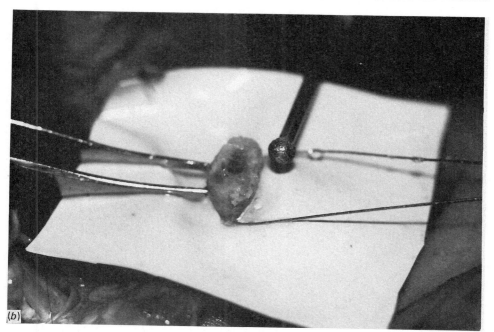

Figure 10.5 Shows a 20-year-old man who sustained sharply divided amputations of his dominant, long and ring fingers on a meat cutter. (*a*) The digits were so sharply divided that minimal skeletal shortening was regained. (*b*) To protect the soft tissue a piece of Esmarch bandage is placed over the bone during debridement with a high speed burr

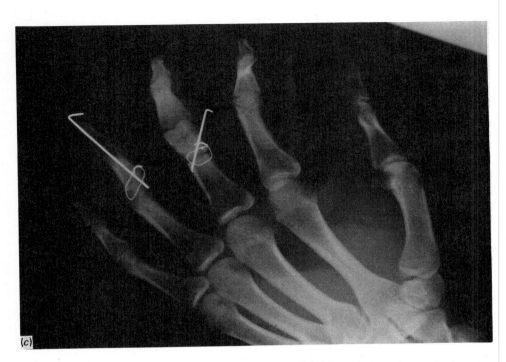

(c)

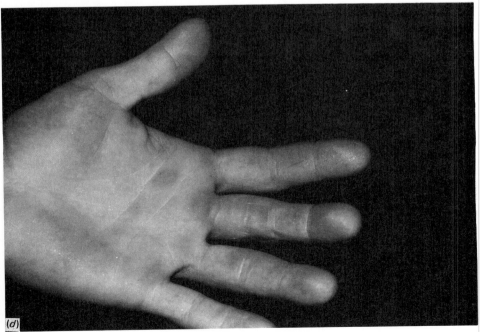

(d)

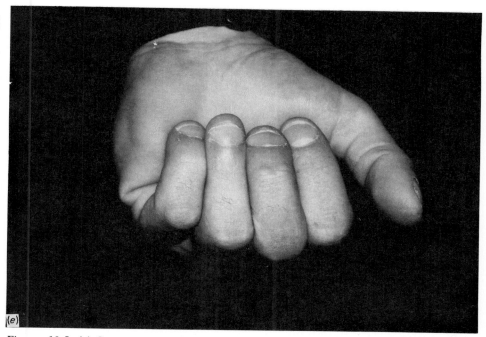

Figure 10.5 (*c*) Interosseous wire fixation plus an oblique Kirschner wire provided satisfactory stabilization. (*d*) and (*e*) At 34 months excellent function resulted; flexion and extension were excellent and two-point discrimination was 8 mm

Probably the most rewarding functional replantations include amputations extending from the transmetacarpal level proximally to the midforearm. Mobility and sensibility is often excellent, the rehabilitation is generally more rapidly accomplished than at the digital level, and the aesthetic outcome is frequently remarkable (*Figure 10.6(a)* to (*e*)).

Controversy continues to surround the replantation of amputations proximal to the elbow despite the fact that these replants frequently receive the most notoriety. The often avulsing nature of these injuries, the long delay and imperfect nerve recovery, and the almost certain need for reconstructive procedures, all present permanent functional liabilities to the patient. Careful considerations of the inherent risks and a fundamental understanding of the prosthetic alternatives must go into any decision regarding a replantation at this level (*Figure 10.7(a)* to (*c*)).

INJURY CLASSIFICATION

The mechanism of injury, the amount and extent of force imparted to both the part and stump, and the individual involved all have a role in the overall ultimate functional outcome of the replanted part.

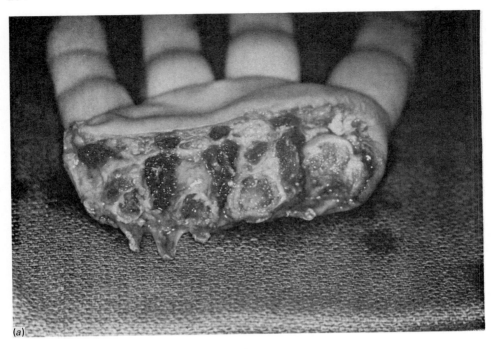

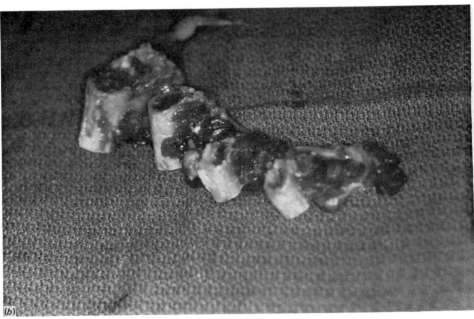

Figure 10.6 Shows a 33-year-old engineer who sustained a transmetacarpal amputation of his right dominant hand on a home table saw. (*a*) The zone of trauma to the hand was limited. (*b*) Debridement consisted of removal of the damaged skeleton and soft tissues, particularly the traumatized intrinsic muscle bellies

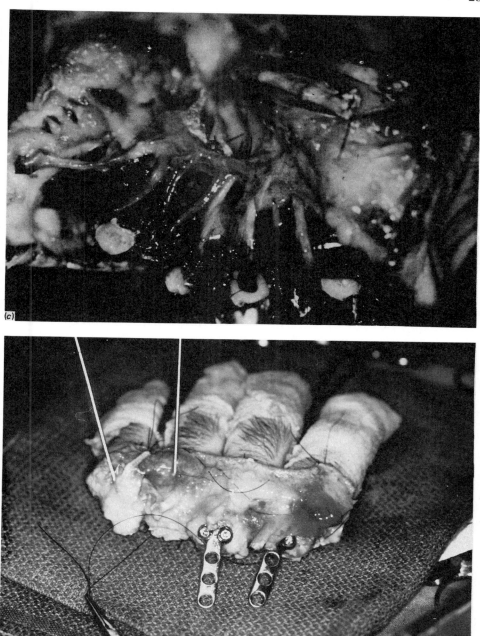

Figure 10.6 (*c*) The carpal tunnel was opened in the stump and the neurovascular structures and flexor tendons identified, debrided, and tagged with marking sutures. (*d*) T plates, 2.7 mm, were placed on the index and long metacarpal heads during the debridement. These were screwed in place on the metacarpal stumps. The ring and little metacarpals were stabilized with an intramedullary Kirschner wire

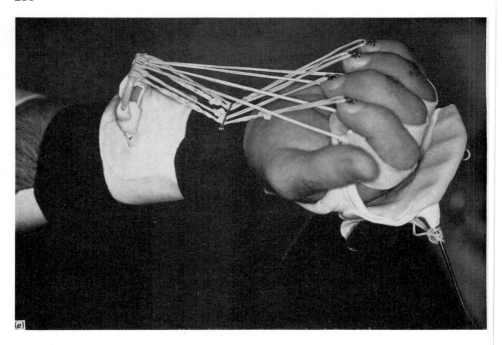

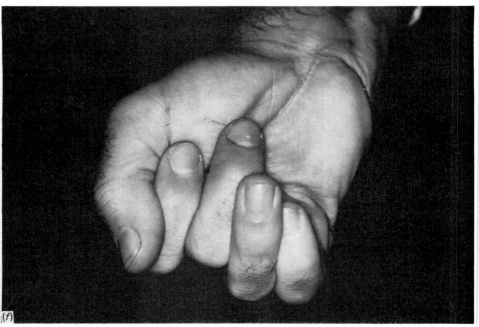

Figure 10.6 (*e*) Once revascularization seemed assured, gentle passive mobilization was begun. Dynamic splints were added about six weeks post-replantation. (*f*) At 30 months post-replantation and post-flexor tenolysis, the patient has regained excellent function. Flexion is noted almost to the midpalmar line. Two-point discrimination was 10 mm

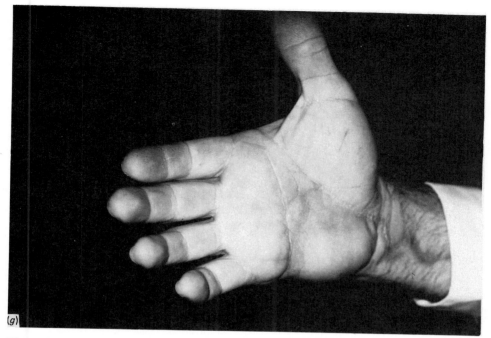

Figure 10.6 (g) Full extension is noted

In general, a standard classification of amputations has been accepted in most centers throughout the world:

(1) *Guillotine:* this is reserved for the sharply divided part with a well-defined and limited zone of trauma. The prognosis for both survival as well as function is best with these injuries (*see Figure 10.5(a)*).
(2) *Crush:* these injuries cover a wider spectrum of soft tissue trauma. When associated with machinery such as a punch press or motor vehicular injury, the zone of trauma may extend considerably beyond the site of amputation and, at times, is not easily defined (*Figure 10.8(a) to (e)*).
(3) *Avulsion:* these amputations reflect a tearing or shearing of tissues rather than a sharp separation. Structures may be injured at different levels and, commonly, the neurovascular structures are injured over a wide zone, necessitating vein and nerve grafts and additional soft tissue coverage (*see Figure 10.4(b)*).

DURATION OF ANOXIA

To achieve success with a replantation effort, measured both by survival as well as function, the restoration of circulation must occur prior to irreversible cellular death (Wilms-Kretschmer and Majno, 1969). Cooling the replanted part in regular ice achieves a temperature of approximately 4°C, which has been shown to be an

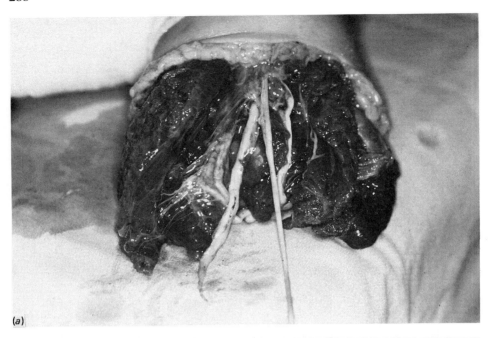

(a)

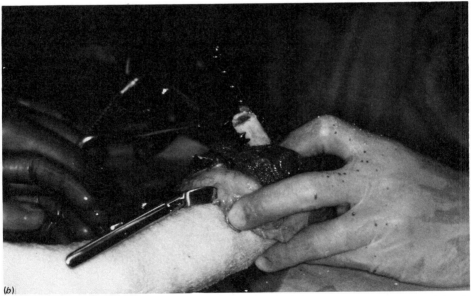

(b)

Figure 10.7 Shows a nine-year-old boy who sustained an avulsive amputation of his left upper extremity at the mid-humeral level from a grain auger. (*a*) Despite the avulsive nature of the injury, replantation was felt indicated because of the patient's age. Note the ulnar nerve avulsed with the amputated part. (*b*) Following extensive debridement of the contaminated skeletal muscle and skeletal shortening, a plate was affixed to the distal humerus to expedite the skeletal fixation. The arm was kept cooled by frequent iced irrigation over the gauze wrapping

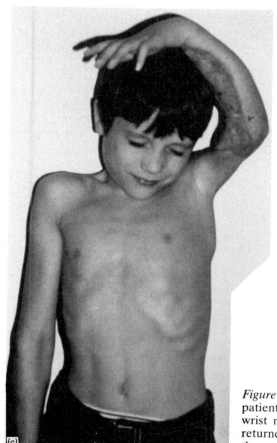

Figure 10.7 (c) At two years post-injury the patient has regained elbow function. Some wrist motion and limited digital motion has returned. Protective sensibility is present in the median nerve distribution

ideal temperature for tissue preservation without freezing (Levy, 1959). Skeletal muscle, in particular, is quite sensitive to ischemia and will undergo irreversible damage after 4–6 hours of warm ischemia (Scully, Shannon and Dickerson, 1961; Solonen and Hjelt, 1978; Jobsis, Boyd and Barwick, 1979). Amputated parts with little skeletal muscle, such as digits, can withstand longer periods of warm anoxia extending upwards of 10 hours (Hayhurst *et al.,* 1974).

It is for these reasons that, in general, an upper limb amputation extending from the wrist proximally should not be considered for replantation if the warm ischemia time has extended beyond 4–6 hours. By the same token, if effectively cooled from the onset, in particular at the digital level, successful replantations have been reported following upwards of 33 hours of ischemia (Chien, Chien and Pao, 1965).

EPIDEMIOLOGY

As experience in microsurgical techniques has grown, 'replantation centers' have developed throughout the world. Although any epidemiological study regarding

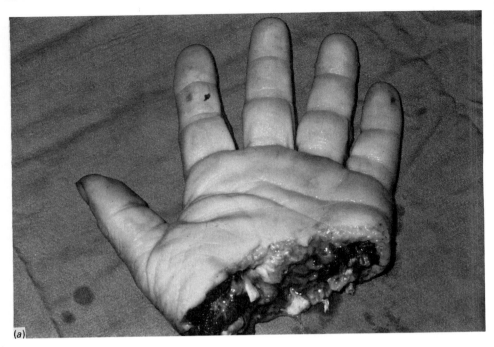

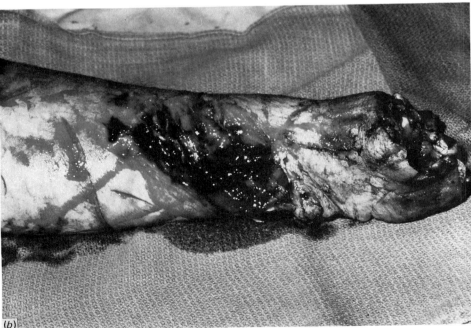

Figure 10.8 (*a*) Shows a 48-year-old truck driver who sustained a complete amputation of his hand at the distal carpus level in a motor vehicle accident. (*b*) In addition, all the soft tissue structures were divided more proximally in the distal forearm

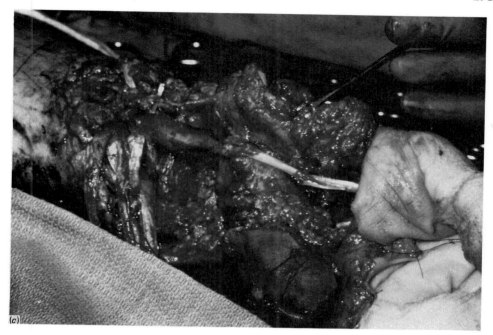

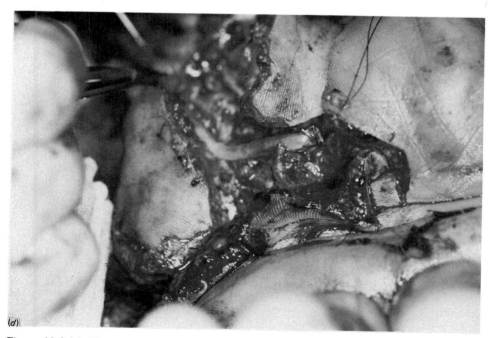

Figure 10.8 (*c*) The sublimus tendons were excised and used as primary intercalary tendon grafts to bridge the tendon gap. (*d*) A long vein graft obtained from the leg was used to reconstruct the superficial palmar arch. The common digital arteries were anastomosed end-to-side on to the vein graft

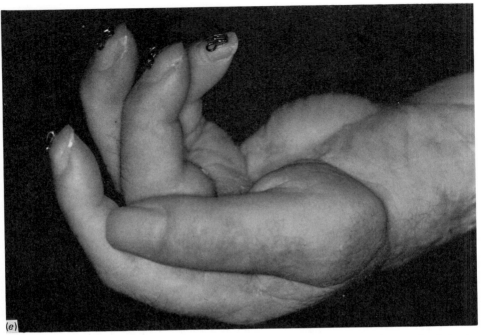

Figure 10.8 (e) Despite subsequent tenolysis, limited mobility and function resulted. In view of the extent of crush, segmental nature of injury and the patient's age, this patient would have better function with a prosthesis

the numbers of amputations suitable for replantation must take into account the degree of industrialization, the extent of industrial and agricultural safety legislation, and the education of the labor force, several studies from Scandinavian countries have suggested upwards of 30 amputations per million population would be replantation candidates (Kiil, 1982; Vilkki and Goransson, 1982; Nylander, Vilkki and Ostrup, 1984).

PREPARATION FOR REPLANTATION

The preparation for any replantation can be divided into three distinct phases: the initial emergency evaluation, transportation to the replantation center, and the evaluation and preparation at the replantation center.

Emergency room physicians who transfer patients for consideration of replantation must be well informed regarding the basic evaluation and stabilization of the patient with a traumatic amputation (Jupiter and Kleinert, 1982). A careful history of associated medical problems and allergies as well as the mechanism of injury – that is, the type of machinery – is frequently most accurately determined at the initial hospital. The patient with major limb trauma must be carefully evaluated for concomitant injury, in particular visceral or spinal trauma. A large-bore intravenous cannula is inserted, tetanus toxoid or Hyper-Tet* and broad-spectrum antibiotics are administered, and a hematocrit and urine analysis obtained as the patient and part are prepared for transportation. The implanted part is rinsed with sterile saline to remove gross debris, wrapped in a sterile sponge which is then placed in a plastic bag, and put into a container of regular ice. The stump is similarly irrigated and wrapped, if necessary with a pressure dressing to contain bleeding. Clamping of neurovascular structures or a proximal tourniquet to contain bleeding from the stump is contraindicated as it will result in extending the zone of trauma. More proximal fractures must be splinted.

During the initial evaluation, arrangements are made with the replantation center regarding the best means of transportation. If possible, beyond a 190 km (120 mile) radius, transportation by air will minimize the ischemic time, in particular with major limb amputations. Trained medical personnel must accompany the patient to monitor vital signs and adjust the intravenous fluids. The patient must be strictly given nothing by mouth.

Upon arrival at the replantation center efforts are made to expedite the evaluation in order to minimize the overall ischemic time. The patient and family are met by a senior member of the replantation team who will not only be able to evaluate the indications for replantation but also begin informing the family of the overall situation. In addition to a careful history and physical examination, radiographs are obtained of the chest, stump, and amputated parts. Blood samples are obtained for CBC, electrolytes, type and crossmatch, and coagulation studies including prothrombin time, partial thromboplastin time, and platelet count. With limb amputations the blood bank should be made aware of the potential need for fresh whole blood transfusions. Evaluation by the anesthesiologist as well as additional medical consultants, if indicated, are best accomplished at this juncture.

REPLANTATION TECHNIQUES

Replantation surgery involves more than just vascular reconstruction and, in reality, is the management of a severe compound upper extremity injury. Basically, five tissues must be identified and reconstructed. These include bone, blood vessels, nerves, musculotendinous units, and skin. An orderly progression of reconstruction should occur in each instance. The type of injury, duration of ischemia, and anticipated functional needs may dictate the specific order and technique of reconstruction. In certain situations, parts may prove more useful if transposed to more functional positions ('transpositional replantation') (*see Figure 10.4*).

Debridement

Success in replantation surgery is contingent upon reuniting non-injured tissues. It is in this light that the initial debridement assumes such a critical role. Despite the extensive degree of tissue contamination, sepsis can be avoided by a thorough debridement of the exposed tissues, in particular skeletal muscle. The latter is of

---

* Tetanus Immune Globulin-Human, Cutter Biological, Div. Miles Laboratories Inc., Emeryville, California 94662.

special importance at the distal forearm and transmetacarpal level where the local skeletal muscle – the pronator quadratus or intrinsics – will be bypassed by the arterial reconstructions.

The debridement is best performed by two surgical teams, one operating on the amputated part(s), the other on the stump. Loupe or microscopic magnification is required in identifying the extent of neurovascular damage and, at times, to establish whether or not a replantation effort should be attempted (*Figure 10.9*).

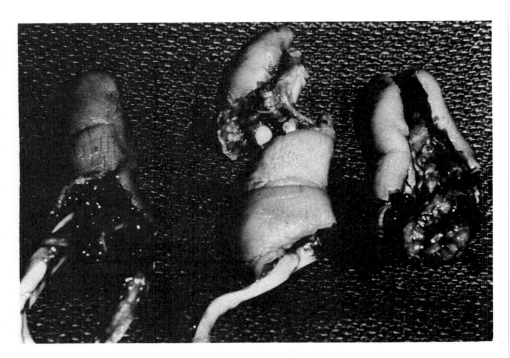

Figure 10.9 Shows a 25-year-old woman who had three digits amputated in a food processor; microscopic examination revealed extensive neurovascular damage rendering these digits unfit for replantation

Sharp dissection and thorough lavage are used to remove foreign matter and traumatized tissue. Pulsed lavage irrigation is also effective in more proximal limb amputations. During the process of debridement, hypothermic support is continued. The amputated part is wrapped in gauze which is frequently irrigated with iced saline (*see Figure 10.7(b)*). With upper arm amputations, hypothermic assistance can be also achieved by irrigation of the arterial tree with iced lactated Ringer's solution.

We generally use mid-axial incisions at the digital and hand levels, permitting a circumferential exposure of all structures. The skin flaps are folded back and the parts to be repaired are identified, debrided, and tagged with color-coded sutures (*Figure 10.10*). Bipolar cautery is required during the mobilization of the vascular structures as it allows local cautery of side branches without injury to the main

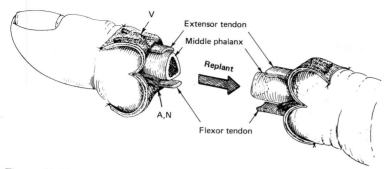

Figure 10.10 Using midaxial incisions, generous skin flaps can be elevated, exposing the underlying neurovascular structures; the digital arteries and veins must be debrided over a wide zone and tagged with color coded sutures to facilitate later microscopic repair

vessel. At the transmetacarpal level the deep palmar arch is identified and coagulated in both the amputated part and the stump to avoid a potentially disastrous hematoma (*see Figure 10.6(c)*).

During the structure labelling it is most important to dissect the structures over a distance to permit exposure and ease of maneuvering during microvascular repair.

Skeletal repair

Skeletal preparation and shortening is a prominent feature of the debridement. In only rare instances involving a joint disarticulation would one not consider skeletal shortening. The extent of skeletal debridement is dependent particularly on the extent of nerve trauma as, optimally, a tension-free neural repair should be achieved.

The periosteum is reflected but preserved, as it can be sutured back over the skeletal junction, enhancing union as well as providing a gliding surface over the internal fixation. During the skeletal debridement the vital soft tissue sutures are protected by placing the skeletal part through a piece of glove rubber or Esmarch bandage (*see Figure 10.5(b)*).

The techniques of internal fixation with replantations vary both with the individual surgeon's preference as well as with the level of the injury. In replantations extending from the upper arm to the transmetacarpal level we prefer rigid internal fixation with plates and screws. These can be initially applied to either the amputated part or the stump following the debridement and shortening (*see Figure 10.6(d)*). Familiarity with the techniques should be a requisite for use of the smaller plates and screws, as undue time must not be spent in the skeletal fixation.

At the phalangeal level interosseous wire fixation, either horizontal or vertical, has proven to be a versatile and reliable form of internal fixation. Additional rotational stability can be gained by step-cutting the bone ends, repairing the fibro-osseous rim of the flexor sheaths, and carefully placing an oblique or longitudinal Kirschner wire (*see Figure 10.5(c)*). Intramedullary screws or pegs have been reported by some authors but have not gained widespread acceptance.

With transarticular amputations a primary arthrodesis is usually indicated. Primary silastic implants have not provided satisfactory motion, likely secondary to the extensive soft tissue injury as well as the limited tendon capabilities early in the postoperative period.

Tendon repair

Tendon debridement and shortening should be consistent with the degree of skeletal shortening. On the flexor side, we tend to repair only the profundus tendon at the digital level. If one should choose to repair both flexor tendons it is advisable to debride the tendons in such a way as to enable the tenorrhaphies to lie at different levels and help offset adhesions arising between the tendons. At the wrist level, however, the repair of both profundus and sublimis tendons can provide additional motors for later tendon transfers.

The same care and precision given to an isolated flexor tendon repair should also be applied in replantation surgery. The modified Kessler suture can be adapted and expedited by placing a 4-0 suture in each trimmed tendon end during the debridement. The tendon can then be approximated by the surgeon and assistant tying each side simultaneously. A circumferential running suture of 6-0 is placed around the tenorrhaphy. As a result of the skeletal shortening the flexor sheath can often be approximated with fine absorbable suture.

On the extensor side the tendons are repaired with 4-0 suture, usually with interrupted mattress sutures. The periosteum is approximated over the bone to aid in restoring a gliding surface under the extensor repair. At the digital level, whenever possible, the lateral bands are included in the extensor reconstruction.

A more difficult problem involves those situations in which the tendon has been avulsed from its muscle. One option to be considered is implanting the tendon back into the muscle belly (Meyer, Zhong-Wei and Beasley, 1981). Adjusting the tension to have the digit in a normal resting position, the tendon is sutured with interrupted mattress sutures into the muscle belly (*Figure 10.11(a) to (c)*).

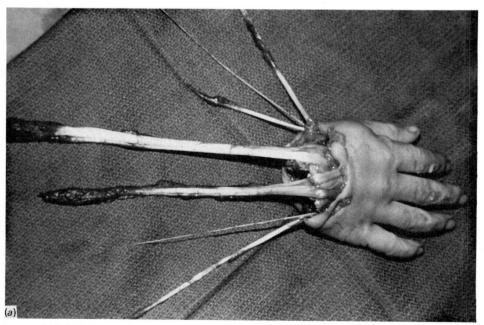

(a)

Figure 10.11 This 9-year-old boy had his hand avulsed in a farming machinery accident; the flexor tendons were avulsed from their muscle bellies

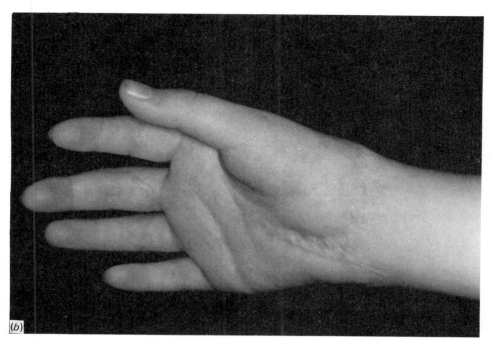

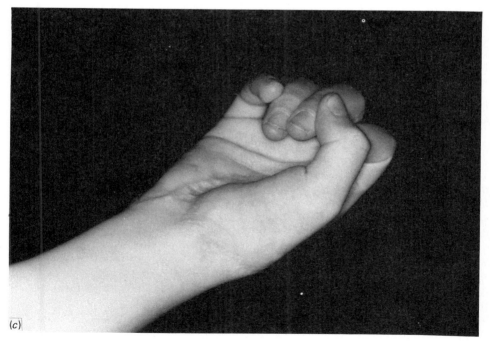

Figure 10.11 (*b*) and (*c*) The flexor tendons were resutured into their muscle bellies with resultant satisfactory flexion and extension. (Case courtesy of Mark Walker, MD)

NEUROVASCULAR REPAIR

A successful vascular repair is fundamental to survival but success in neural repair is critical for a functional outcome. In both instances, the hallmark to success is the precision and care put into the microscopic repairs.

Perhaps the most common error in microvascular surgery is the failure to fully debride the damaged vessels. Under the operating microscope, findings such as separation of the intima and media, persistent fibrin deposition within the vessel lumen, or hemorrhagic discoloration of the vessel wall – all suggest local damage and demand debridement until healthy vessel ends are visible (May and Gallico, 1980). Quite frequently this necessitates interposition vein grafts to reconstruct the ensuing defect. A satisfactory arterial 'spurt test' both in the length as well as the consistency of the arterial inflow from the end of the artery on the stump has been a most helpful guide in assessing the quality of the arterial inflow.

Vasospasm is a common problem encountered in the repair of small vessels. Mechanical dilatation prior to the repair as well as topical application of agents such as 2% lidocaine or papaverine are effective in offsetting local vasospasm. The vessel ends are frequently irrigated with a heparin–saline solution to clear residual debris. We reserve systemic heparin administration only for cases involving extensive soft tissue crush with a 5000 unit parenteral bolus of heparin given just prior to completion of the arterial anastomosis.

Upon completion of any microvascular anastomosis it is necessary to control the vessel patency and the quality of the re-established circulation. A 'patency test' is performed after each vascular anastomosis. Capillary refill is also an excellent early monitor of the circulation. When arteries are repaired first, the capillary refill is generally brisk secondary to associated venous congestion. When the arterial circulation is re-established after a prolonged period of cool ischemia, capillary refill may be delayed. A sponge soaked in warmed saline will frequently help restore a normothermic state to the cooled part and accelerate the opening of microvascular channels.

Venous repair

At the digital level the identification of the dorsal venous anatomy is enhanced by milking the end of the amputated digit, forcing stagnant blood into the venous tree. The fragile dorsal veins are to be found in the subcutaneous fat and must be meticulously isolated and tagged with marking sutures during the debridement. While the optimal ratio of venous repairs to each arterial repair has never been clarified, we generally repair as many veins as possible to ensure adequate venous outflow in the event of an anastomotic failure.

At the digital and metacarpal level we tend to restore the venous anatomy prior to arterial reconstruction. This offsets additional blood loss, in particular with a multiple digital replantation, and permits the nerve and arterial repairs to be achieved in a bloodless field. With more proximal amputations, arterial repair precedes venous repairs in order to re-establish expeditiously arterial inflow to the anoxic skeletal muscle and allow the effluence of the noxious metabolic breakdown by-products to drain into the wound rather than the systemic circulation. Despite this precaution, in major limb replantation, prior to the venous repairs, the patient should be in a well-hydrated state, the blood pH, potassium and PCO_2 monitored, and sodium bicarbonate administered by the anesthesiologist.

Vein grafts

The availability of size-matched donor veins in the forearm or dorsum of the foot has added immeasurably to increased survival rates in replantation efforts. Although the procurement and placement of vein grafts adds to the length of the operative procedure, it is far simpler to do an interpositional vein graft initially than to repeatedly anastomose damaged vessels or return the patient to the operating room for re-exploration and secondary vein grafting (May and Gallico, 1980). Additionally, in certain situations such as thumb amputations at the level of the metacarpophalangeal joint, a vein graft applied directly to the ulnar digital artery permits arterial reconstruction to be accomplished more proximally to the larger and more accessible princeps pollicis artery (*see Figure 10.2*). In certain cases of adjacent digital amputations, a vein graft shaped like a 'Y' with the two shorter limbs anastomosed to the adjacent digital arteries enables both digits to be revascularized with a more proximal anastomosis into a common digital artery (*Figure 10.12*) (Jones and Jupiter, 1985).

At the digital level the distal volar forearm veins or vena comitantes of the radial artery are an ideal size match for the digital arteries or veins. The dorsal veins of the foot are slightly thicker and less distensible. These are ideal for more proximal palmar arch or distal forearm vascular reconstructions. After harvesting the donor veins with meticulous cauterization of side branches with the bipolar microcautery, a suture should be placed at the outflow end in order to maintain the proper orientation with respect to valves.

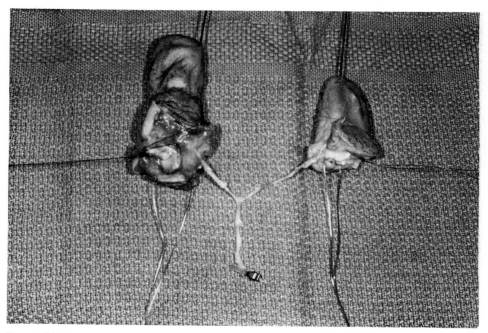

Figure 10.12 Vein grafts in the shape of a 'Y' aid in revascularizing adjacent digits. The distal limbs can be anastomosed to the larger digital arteries and the proximal limb anastomosed to a common digital artery outside the zone of trauma

Nerve repair

The same careful attention must be afforded to the nerve repair as with the vascular reconstruction. In more proximal amputations careful orientation of the group fascicular patterns is particularly important. Hemostasis with the bipolar coagulation is also necessary to offset the development of a hematoma at the neurorrhaphy site. In the forearm, the repair of the dorsal ulnar and radial sensory nerves will not only add to the sensibility of the replanted part but also help offset a potentially disabling painful neuroma.

At the digital level, skeletal shortening generally permits tension-free neurorrhaphies. On occasion, nerve grafting can be considered from amputated parts which are not suitable for replantation. In general, nerve grafting from uninjured sites is not advisable as the replanted part may not survive, leaving a lost digit as well as a nerve graft donor defect. Although return of sensibility can be variable in all replantations, we have noted a general correlation between the overall vascularity in the replanted digit and the sensibility achieved (Gelberman *et al.*, 1978).

Wound closure

Meticulous hemostasis and a tension-free skin closure are critical to protect the deep repairs and prevent sepsis. Often redundant skin is available secondary to the skeletal shortening; however, one should avoid the temptation to tailor the skin

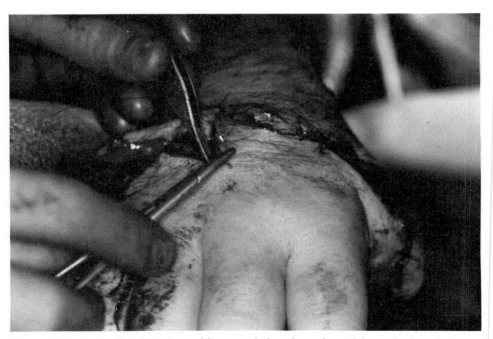

Figure 10.13 Z-plasties will help avoid a constricting circumferential scan in some instances; in this case, a Z-plasty is designed in the skin closure of a transmetacarpal replantation in a 69-year-old male

flaps as this will only lead to local compression as the digit swells in the early revascularization period. When the wound juncture is circumferential, small Z-plasties will offset a circular constricting scar (*Figure 10.13*).

The liberal use of thin split thickness skin grafts will ensure tension-free closures in those cases where insufficient local skin is available. The skin grafts may be applied, if necessary, directly over the vascular reconstructions. These should be 'pie-crusted' and sutured in place but left exposed without a tie-over bolus dressing which would prohibit drainage and potentially constrict the underlying tissues.

Devascularized parts with large muscle masses should have compartment releases by fasciotomies as part of the replantation procedure. Split thickness skin grafts will readily recover these fasciotomy sites. Small suction drains are advisable to minimize potential dead spaces.

POSTOPERATIVE MANAGEMENT

Dressing

The postoperative dressing must be non-constrictive, supportive, and permit accessibility of the replanted part for both visual as well as temperature monitoring. The wounds are coated with antibiotic ointment and covered with longitudinal strips of impregnated gauze. Circumferential wrapping of dressing material must be avoided to prevent local constriction as the replanted part swells in the early postoperative period. The entire limb is then placed in a soft bulky wrap such as Dacron batting and supported by plaster splints. We generally wrap the limb in two pillows, which maintains elevation as well as protecting the part from injury.

The dressing is routinely left undisturbed for 5–7 days unless excessive drainage or bleeding develops.

Monitoring

Optimally, the patient can be monitored in a unit where the staff is experienced with replantation surgery. Yet even in this setting the surgeon must be precise with the postoperative instructions. The part is checked hourly for color, turgor, capillary refill, and cutaneous temperature during the initial 72 hours and thereafter every 3–4 hours. Any change is reported immediately. Although a pale digit and sluggish capillary refill suggest an arterial thrombosis, while a cyanotic, tense digit with a brisk capillary refill implies a venous occlusion, this differentiation may soon prove of little relevance, as one will soon lead to the other. Stabbing the tip of a digit with a no.11 blade is also of some usefulness in determining the site of vascular occlusion. Brisk, bright red bleeding will be found with an intact arterial supply, dark blood with venous occlusion, and the absence of bleeding with arterial occlusion. Regardless of the etiology, our experience has paralleled others in suggesting rapid re-exploration (Schlenker, Kleinert and Tsai, 1980).

A number of instruments and techniques have been developed and are in use in different replantation centers to provide an objective and accurate guide to the circulating status of replanted parts (Holloway and Watkins, 1977; Stirrat *et al.*, 1978; Glogovac, Blitz and Whiteside, 1982). Cutaneous temperature monitoring remains the safest and most reliable method to date. Normal digital temperature is between 32 and 35 °C. A drop of 2.5 °C in one hour or a sustained temperature below 30 °C indicates a circulatory problem which will result in the loss of the part unless corrected (Stirrat *et al.*, 1978). While the ambient temperature can affect the readings, the use of adjacent digits or the contralateral hand as a control will prevent error in interpretation of the values.

Medication

There is now an increasing trend away from systemic anticoagulants in the postoperative period as none of the available medications can predictably salvage an anastomotic failure secondary to technical error or damaged vessels. Aspirin (650 mg twice a day) remains an effective inhibitor of platelet aggregation, and is initiated in the emergency room via a rectal suppository and continued for 6–8 weeks post-replantation. Low molecular weight dextran administered at 20–30 ml/h is also part of the basic pharmacological regimen in most replantation centers. Its beneficial action stems from its effect as a plasma expander as well as an antiplatelet effect. It is usually continued for 5–7 days postoperatively.

Heparin, in our center, is reserved for the injuries with a wide zone of trauma or in situations where the anastomoses are problematic. A bolus of 5000 units is given intraoperatively and heparinization continued for 5–7 postoperative days. The coagulation parameters must be carefully monitored, as bleeding can result in local hematoma and vascular compromise.

Generally, replantation surgery is accomplished with axillary block anesthesia. This will provide a sympathetic block which can be sustained postoperatively either by a catheter placed adjacent to the axillary contents or adjacent to the median or ulnar nerves in the wrist. Bupivacaine (Marcaine)* injected every 6 hours will provide a continuous sympathetic block and increase local vasodilatation (Phelps, Rutherford and Boswick, 1979).

POSTOPERATIVE REHABILITATION

Once the survival of the replanted part seems assured, the patient, therapist, and surgeon embark on a rehabilitation program which will include occupational and physical therapy, vocational rehabilitation and frequently secondary surgical procedures. Mutual understanding and emotional support are an important aspect of this program.

When to initiate mobilization is determined, in part, by the level and type of amputation. At the digital level the surgeon is challenged by the desire to initiate rapid mobilization of these severe injuries while at the same time protecting the microvascular anastomoses until re-endothelization has occurred, generally within 10–14 days.

Toward the end of the first week, passive range of motion of the non-involved joints is started. Static orthoplast resting splints, elevation, and patient education comprise this early rehabilitation program.

---

* Marcaine Hydrochloride, Winthrop-Breon Laboratories, New York, NY 10016

During the third postoperative week, active range of motion of the replanted part is encouraged. Gentle retrograde massage and coban wrapping help diminish edema and non-resistive grasp, and release activities begin the arduous rehabilitation program.

Toward the end of the first postoperative month, gentle passive range of motion of the replanted part is added. Dynamic splintage can be safely tolerated and is individually tailored to the needs of each replanted part (*see Figure 10.6(e)*). The patient is encouraged in non-resistive functional tasks. It is often at this juncture that the patient begins to comprehend the magnitude of the injury and often reactive depression and anger is seen. This is a most important period of the rehabilitation, and support and encouragement are needed to help carry both the patient and family through this difficult time.

FUNCTIONAL EVALUATION

Replantation surgery is, in reality, one of many methods of reconstructing a severely traumatized upper extremity. The functional evaluation of the replanted part is, therefore, better judged when placed in contrast to the expected outcome of alternative reconstructive procedures (Burton, 1981). In addition, subjective factors such as patient acceptability and the aesthetic restoration must be included in every evaluation. Socioeconomic factors including time out of work and the overall expenses should also be considered, but once again in the same manner as with any severe trauma and subsequent reconstructive surgery.

The functional outcome is seen to correlate well with the level of the amputation, the duration of anoxia, and with the extent of trauma to both the amputated part and remaining stump. The sharp 'guillotine' amputations will generally have a more favorable outcome than those associated with avulsing or crushing injuries (Wang, Young and Wei, 1981; Tamai, 1982; Russell *et al.*, 1984).

Replantations proximal to the elbow, while tending to attract the most notoriety, remain controversial. The risks are substantial, considering the blood loss and extent of the ischemic skeletal muscle mass.

Most replantations at the forearm or higher will result, for the most part, in an assistive limb. Reconstructive procedures are commonplace and include nerve grafting or neurolysis, tendon transfers or tenodeses, and joint capsulotomies or arthrodeses. Despite incomplete function, when questioned the patient will almost always favor the replanted limb to any prosthetic alternative (Russell *et al.*, 1984). In addition, in some societies, the restoraton of even a marginally functional limb is viewed as important for social acceptability. It may be, however, that the replantation of an above elbow amputation should be reserved for the pediatric patient, the bilateral traumatic amputation, or with an unusually sharp amputation.

At the forearm level, the distal third replant offers, by far, the best chance of achieving an excellent function as well as aesthetic outcome. Protective sensibility is almost always regained and in the sharper amputations, gross two-point discrimination has been noted. Intrinsic muscle function recovery is uncommon and, therefore, grip and pinch strength will be diminished (Tamai, 1982). Cold intolerance is also commonplace. At this level the recovery of tendon glide and joint mobility is favorable. Secondary reconstructive procedures include tendon transfers aimed to provide intrinsic function, tenolyses and, less commonly, neurolyses or nerve grafting.

By contrast, in proximal forearm replantations, the severed muscle mass is bypassed by the vascular reconstructions leading to ischemic necrosis and contractures. While the capacity for sensory return makes replantation at this level superior to prosthetic function, the overall outcome is less favorable than at the distal forearm.

Replantations through the carpus or metacarpals, like the distal forearm, are excellent functional restorations and are indicated unless other injuries or illnesses are medical contraindications. Sensibility is frequently discriminatory, mobility generally good, and the shorter distance for nerve regeneration leads to a much shorter recovery time than with more proximal replantations.

Perhaps the most predictable functional outcome can be seen with thumb replantations. As the thumb functions independently, the recovery time for the patient is limited and the ultimate disability is also low. Even those amputations beyond the interphalangeal joint, if technically feasible, should be replanted as the expected aesthetic and functional result will be excellent.

At the digital level, once again overall function must be viewed against other reconstructive alternatives. The multiple digital replantation at the proximal phalangeal level will offer good sensibility, adequate pinch and grasp, and usually an acceptable aesthetic result. By the same token, the single digital replantation at this level will often have an adverse effect on the overall hand function, require prolonged rehabilitation, and will generally be bypassed for most functional requirements.

Replantations of digits amputated distal to the insertion of the superficialis tendon will provide excellent sensory return, retain proximal interphalangeal motion, and look quite normal. While cold intolerance is commonplace and permanent for some patients, these replanted digits are otherwise rarely painful.

References

BERGER, A., MILLESI, H., MANDL, H. and FREILINGER, G. (1978) Replantation and revascularization of amputated parts of extremities: a three year report from the Viennese replantations team. *Clinical Orthopaedics and Related Research*, **133**, 212–214

BIEMER, E. (1980) Definition and classifications in replantation surgery. *British Journal of Plastic Surgery*, **33**, 164–168

BUNCKE, H. J., BUNCKE, C. M. and SHULZ, W. B. (1965) Experimental digital amputation and reimplantation. *Plastic and Reconstructive Surgery*, **36**, 62–70

BURTON, R. (1981) Problems in the evaluation of results from replantation surgery. *Orthopaedic Clinics of North America*, **12**, 909–913

CARREL, A. and GUTHRIE, C. C. (1906) Results of replantation of thigh. *Science*, **23**, 393–394

CHIEN, C. W., CHIEN, Y. C. and PAO, Y. S. (1965) Further experiences in the restoration of amputated limbs. *China Medical Journal*, **84**, 225–231

CHRISTEAS, N., BALAS, P. and GIANNIKAS, A. (1969) Replantation of amputated extremities: report of two successful cases. *American Journal of Surgery*, **118**, 68

DANIEL, R. K. and TERZIS, J. K. (1977) In *Reconstructive Microsurgery*, edited by R. K. Daniel and J. K. Terzis, pp. 125–167 Boston: Little Brown

EIKEN, O., NABSETH, D. C., MAYER, R. F. and DETERLING, R. A. (1964) Limb replantation. I: The technique and immediate results. II: The pathophysiological effects. III: Long-term evaluation. *Archives of Surgery*, **88**, 48, 54, 66

GELBERMAN, R. H., URBANIAK, J. R., BRIGHT, D. S. and LEVIN, L. S. (1978) Digital sensibility following replantation. *Journal of Hand Surgery*, **3**, 313–319

GIBSON, T. (1965) Early free grafting: the restitution of parts completely separated from the body. *British Journal of Plastic Surgery*, **18**, 10–11

GLOGOVAC, S. V., BLITZ, M. and WHITESIDE, L. A. (1982) Hydrogen washout technique in monitoring vascular status after replantation surgery. *Journal of Hand Surgery,* **7,** 601–605

HALL, R. H. (1944) Whole upper extremity transplant for human beings: general plans of procedure and operative technique. *Annals of Surgery,* **120,** 12–23

HALSTEAD, W. S., REICHERT, F. C. and REID, M. R. (1922) Replantation of entire limbs without suture of vessels. *Transactions of American Surgical Association,* **40,** 160–167

HAYHURST, J. W., O'BRIEN, B. M., ISHIDA, H. and BAXTER, T. J. (1974) Experimental digital replantation after prolonged cooling. *The Hand,* **6,** 134–141

HOLLOWAY, G. A. and WATKINS, D. W. (1977) Laser doppler measurements of cutaneous blood flow. *Journal of Investigative Dermatology,* **69,** 306

HÖPFNER, E. (1903) Uber Gefassnaht, Gefasstransplantation und Reimplantation von Amputierten extremitaten. *Archiv Klinik Chirurgerie,* **70,** 417–471

INOUE, T., TOYOSHIMA, Y., FUKUSUMI, H. *et al.* (1967) Replantation of severed limbs. *Journal of Cardiovascular Surgery (Torino),* **8,** 31–39

JACOBSEN, J. H. (1963) Microsurgical technique in repair of the traumatized extremity. *Clinical Orthopaedics and Related Research,* **19,** 132–136

JACOBSEN, J. H. and SUAREZ, E. L. (1960) Microsurgery in the anastomosis of small vessels. *Surgical Forum,* **9,** 243

JAEGER, S. H., TSAI, T-M. and KLEINERT, H. E. (1981) Upper extremity replantations in children. *Orthopedic Clinics of North America,* **12,** 897–907

JOBSIS, F. F., BOYD, J. B. and BARWICK, W. J. (1979) Metabolic consequences of ischemia and hypoxia. In *Microsurgical Composite Tissue Transplantation,* edited by D. Serafin and H. J. Buncke, Jr, pp. 47–65. St Louis: C. V. Mosby

JONES, J. M., SHENCK, R. R. and CHESNEY, R. B. (1982) Digital replantation and amputation – comparison of function. *Journal of Hand Surgery,* **3,** 183–189

JONES, N. F. and JUPITER, J. B. (1985) The use of Y-shaped interposition vein grafts in multiple digit replantations. *Journal of Hand Surgery,* **10A,** 675–678

JUPITER, J. B. and KLEINERT, H. E. (1982) Traumatic amputations and replantation of amputated parts in the extremities. In *Committee on Trauma of American College of Surgeons: Early Care of the Injured Patient,* pp. 265–276. Philadelphia: W. B. Saunders

KIIL, J. (1982) The epidemiology of replantation cases. *Scandinavian Journal of Plastic and Reconstructive Surgery,* Supplement 19, 78–80

KLEINERT, H. E., JUHALA, C. A., TSAI, T. M. and VAN BEEK, A. (1977) Digital replantation – selection, techniques, and results. *Orthopaedic Clinics of North America,* **8,** 309–318

KLEINERT, H. E. and KASDAN, M. L. (1963a) Restoration of blood flow in upper extremity injuries. *Journal of Trauma,* **3,** 461–474

KLEINERT, H. E. and KASDAN, M. L. (1963b) Salvage of devascularized upper extremities including studies on small vessel anastomosis. *Clinical Orthopaedics and Related Research,* **29,** 29–37

KLEINERT, H. E., TSAI, T.-M. and JUPITER, J. B. (1981) Replantation: an overview. In *The Twenty-Fifth Anniversary Symposium of the Hospital for Special Surgery,* edited by P. D. Wilson, Jr and L. R. Straub. *Clinical Trends in Orthopaedics,* pp. 32–37. New York: Georg Thieme

KOMATSU, S. and TAMAI, S. (1968) Successful replantation of a completely cut-off thumb: case report. *Plastic and Reconstructive Surgery,* **42,** 374–377

LAPCHINSKY, A. G. (1960) Recent results of experimental transplantation of preserved limbs and kidneys and possible use of this technique in clinical practice. *Annals of the New York Academy of Science,* **64,** 539–569

LENDVAY, P. G. (1973) Replacement of the amputated digit. *British Journal of Plastic Surgery,* **26,** 398

LEVY, M. N. (1959) Oxygen consumption and blood flow in hypothermic perfused kidney. *American Journal of Physiology,* **197,** 1111

MacDONALD, G. L. JR, TOSE, L. and DETERLING, R. A. JR (1962) A technique for reimplantation of the dog limb involving the use of a mechanical stapling device and a rapid polymerizing adhesive. *Surgical Forum,* **13,** 88

MALT, R. A. and McKHANN, C. F. (1964) Replantation of severed arms. *Journal of the American Medical Association,* **189,** 716–722

MALT, R. A., REMENSNYDER, J. P. and HARRIS, W. H. (1972) Long-term utility of replanted arms. *Annals of Surgery,* **176,** 334–342

MALT, R. A. and SMITH, R. J. (1977) Limb replantation: selection of patients and technical considerations. In *Vascular Surgery,* edited by R. B. Rutherford, pp. 471–475. Philadelphia: W. B. Saunders

MAY, J. W. JR and GALLICO, G. G. (1980) Upper extremity replantation. In *Current Problems in Surgery,* edited by M. M. Ravitch, pp. 635–717. Chicago: Year Book Publishers

MAY, J. W. JR., TOTH, B. A. and GARDNER, M. (1982) Digital replantation distal to proximal interphalangeal joint. *Journal of Hand Surgery,* **3,** 161–166

MEHL, R. L., PAUL, H. A., SCHNEEWIND, J. and BEATTIE, E. J. (1964) Treatment of 'toxemia' after extremity replantation. *Archives of Surgery,* **89,** 871–879

MEYER, V. E., ZHONG-WEI, C. and BEASLEY, R. W. (1981) Basic technical considerations in reattachment surgery. *Orthopaedic Clinics of North America,* **12,** 871–895

MORRISON, W. A., O'BRIEN, B. M. and MacLEOD, A. M. (1978) Digital replantation and revascularization. A longterm review of one hundred cases. *The Hand,* **10,** 125–134

NAKAMURA, J. (1977) Late results of successful replantations of the amputated digits and hands. *Japanese Journal of Plastic and Reconstructive Surgery,* **20,** 89

NYLANDER, G., VILKKI, S. and OSTRUP, L. (1984) The need for replantation surgery after traumatic amputations of the upper extremity – an estimate based upon the epidemiology of Sweden. *British Journal of Hand Surgery,* **9B,** 257–260

O'BRIEN, B. M. (1974) Replantation surgery. *Clinics of Plastic Surgery,* **1,** 405–415

O'BRIEN, B. M., MacLEOD, A. M. and MILLER, G. D. H. (1973) Clinical replantation of digits. *Plastic and Reconstructive Surgery,* **52,** 490–503

PHELPS, D. B., RUTHERFORD, R. B. and BOSWICK, J. A. (1979) Control of vasospasm following trauma and microvascular surgery. *Journal of Hand Surgery,* **4,** 109–112

RAMIREZ, M. A., DUQUE, M., HERNANDEZ, L., LONDONO, A. and CADAVID, G. (1967) Reimplantation of limbs. *Plastic and Reconstructive Surgery,* **40,** 315–324

ROSENKRANTZ, J. G., SULLIVAN, R. C., WELCH, K., MILES, J. S., SADLER, K. M. and PATON, B. C. (1967) Replantation of an infant's arm. *New England Journal of Medicine,* **276,** 609–612

RUSSELL, R. C., O'BRIEN, B. M., MORRISON, W. A., PAMAMULL, G. and MacLEOD, A. (1984) The late functional results of upper limb revascularization and replantation. *Journal of Hand Surgery,* **9,** 623–633

SCHLENKER, J. D., KLEINERT, H. E. and TSAI, T-M. (1980) Methods and results of replantation following traumatic amputation of the thumb in 64 patients. *Journal of Hand Surgery,* **5,** 63–70

SCULLY, R. E., SHANNON, J. M. and DICKERSON, G. R. (1961) Factors involved in recovery from experimental skeletal muscle ischemia produced in dogs. *American Journal of Pathology,* **39,** 721–737

SIXTH PEOPLE'S HOSPITAL, SHANGHAI (1967) Reattachment of traumatic amputations: a summing up of experience. *China Medical Journal,* **1,** 392–401

SNYDER, C. C., KNOWLES, R. P., MAYER, P. W. and HOBBS, J. C. (1960) Extremity replantation. *Plastic and Reconstructive Surgery,* **26,** 251–263

SOLONEN, K. A. and HJELT, L. (1968) Morphological changes in striated muscle during ischemia. *Acta Orthopaedica Scandinavica,* **39,** 13–19

STIRRAT, C. R., SEABER, A. V., URBANIAK, J. R. and BRIGHT, D. S. (1978) Temperature monitoring in digital replantation. *Journal of Hand Surgery,* **3,** 342–347

TAMAI, S. (1978) Digit replantation: analysis of 163 replantations in an 11 year period. *Clinics of Plastic Surgery,* **5,** 195–209

TAMAI, S. (1982) Twenty years experience of limb replantation. Review of 293 upper extremity replants. *Journal of Hand Surgery,* **7,** 549–556

TSAI, T. M. (1975) Experimental and clinical application of microvascular surgery. *Annals of Surgery,* **181,** 169–177

VAN BEEK, A. L., WARAK, P. W. and ZOOK, E. G. (1979) Microvascular surgery in young children. *Plastic and Reconstructive Surgery,* **63,** 457–462

VILKKI, S. K. and GORANSSON, H. (1982) Traumatic amputations and the need for a replantation service in Finland. *Annales Chirurgiae et Gynaecologiae,* **71,** 2–7

WANG, S. H., YOUNG, K. F. and WEI, J. N. (1981) Replantation of severed limbs – clinical analysis of 91 cases. *Journal of Hand Surgery,* **6,** 31–38

WEILAND, A. J., VILLARREAL-RIOS, A., KLEINERT, H. E., KUTZ, J., ATASOY, E. and LISTER, G. (1977) Replantation of digits and hands: analysis of surgical techniques and functional results in 71 patients with 86 replantations. *Journal of Hand Surgery,* **2,** 1–12

WILLIAMS, G. R., CARTER, O. R., FRANK, G. R. and PRICE, W. E. (1966) Replantation of amputated extremities. *American Surgery,* **163,** 788–794

WILMS-KRETSCHMER, K. and MAJNO, G. (1969) Ischemia of the skin: electron microscopic study of vascular injury. *American Journal of Pathology,* **54,** 327–353

ZHONG-WEI, C., MEYER, V. E., KLEINERT, H. E. and BEASLEY, R. W. (1981) Present indications and contraindications for replantation as reflected by long-term functional results. *Orthopaedic Clinics of North America,* **12,** 849–870

11
The painful hand

C. B. Wynn Parry and R. H. C. Robins

INTRODUCTION

The central theme of all the preceding chapters in this book is the restoration of function in the hand after injury or disease. Although trauma is an obvious cause of pain, treatment is directed to the associated functional loss and the assumption is made that the painful aspects of the patient's disability will be alleviated by the natural processes of healing. Failure in this respect is rightly regarded as a failure of treatment or the onset of a complication. Leaving aside injuries and acute infections, the majority of disorders which the hand surgeon is called upon to treat are not painful. However, when pain does affect the hand it can do so to a devastating degree, providing problems in management which tax the fortitude of the patient and the skill and persistence of the doctor. These difficult and resistant cases have not until recently featured large in the literature because the poor results of treatment have only been matched by lack of understanding of the cause. Advances in neurology and a better appreciation of the physiology of pain have brought some insight into the mechanisms involved and so to a rational approach to treatment.

Painful conditions of the hand may be classified as local in origin, or referred from a disorder proximally in the arm, or from within the central nervous system. The local causes of pain are discussed from the point of view of diagnosis and the bearing this symptom has on the management of the patient, and the timing of surgery. Neurological causes are discussed as problems in differential diagnosis and the treatment of peripheral lesions is described whether such treatment be confined to the hand or to involve the rest of the upper limb, or indeed the patient as a whole. The common compression lesions of nerves are not difficult to understand, and hence to treat, but the severe pain associated with damaged or severed nerves, or those conditions with vascular as well as neurological features, have often defied therapy in the past. In such instances psychiatric causes were held responsible but this grey area of diagnosis is diminishing with increasing knowledge of the disordered physiology of nerve conduction. In order to appreciate what has gone wrong and, so to apply the appropriate treatment, a basic knowledge of these mechanisms is required.

NEUROLOGICAL CAUSES OF PAIN IN THE HAND

The perception of pain after nerve injury

There has been an explosion of interest in peripheral nerve disorders in neurophysiological laboratories in the last ten years and we owe a great deal to the pioneer work of Wall and his associates in the unravelling of the mysteries of painful nerve disorders.

In 1974 Wall and Gutnik showed that the fibre sprouts in an experimental neuroma, after cutting the sciatic nerve in the rat, were the source of continuous ongoing electrical discharges. Furthermore, these discharges could be arrested by antidromic electrical stimulation and could be excited by mechanical irritation. Subsequently they, and other workers, showed that when nociceptive impulses were excited in small diameter nerves and recordings made by microelectrodes in the dorsal horn in cats, these discharges could be reduced or abolished by electrical stimulation of the large diameter fibres that carry touch, pressure, and vibration. This was the origin of the 'gate' theory of Melzack and Wall (1983), in which the hypothesis is stated that the transmission of nociceptive traffic centrally is determined by the ratio of large diameter to small diameter nerve activity. This is the basis of the widespread use of transcutaneous electrical stimulation for the relief of pain clinically. Not only were fibre sprouts highly sensitive to pressure but they were also found to be very sensitive to circulating noradrenaline, and that a very tiny dose of noradrenaline could stimulate a huge discharge of electrical activity in a neuroma. It has also been shown that sympathetic blocking could arrest such discharges. Subsequently it has been shown that where poorly myelinated nerve fibres are in apposition, crosstalk may develop so that short circuits arise with a constant barrage of electrical activity conducted both peripherally and centrally. Poorly myelinated nerve fibres may become the source of ectopic foci throughout the length of the nerve. Nerve sprouts from a neuroma may not only course distally, but also centrally, back along the proximal nerve fibre for long distances, and even up to the nerve root, and these are a potent source of spontaneous discharges.

Finally, Wall and Devor (1981) have shown that there are profound central effects of peripheral nerve damage. Even one week after nerve damage dorsal root ganglia start discharging spontaneously and there are profound chemical alterations in the central nervous system at that level. Partial or complete deafferentation results in spontaneous firing of nerve cells in the spinal cord, and this spontaneous firing can spread throughout the whole of the ascending tracts of the nervous system. We thus have a situation where slight damage to a peripheral nerve may result in spontaneous electrical discharges at that site, hypersensitivity to circulating noradrenaline and profound central effects which may persist and indeed worsen over the years. It is small wonder that the clinical condition can be so devastating and that the pain can spread well outside the autonomous zone of the damaged nerve. Clearly there must be some profound central change, possibly abnormal firing and abnormal internuncial neuronal circuits to explain these phenomena. Thus damage to peripheral nerves may cause profound peripheral and central effects and these effects may continue for many years and indeed indefinitely, with gradual worsening of the condition and devastating effects on the patient and his life. Similar burning pain and hyperpathia can develop in amputation stumps, particularly after amputation of the fingers and thumb.

Advances in amputation surgery have markedly reduced these complications, for the likeliest cause of stump pain is tethering of the nerves to bone or soft tissues and careful elective surgery by experienced amputee surgeons, allowing the nerve to retract fully, very markedly reduces their incidence. However, pain of this nature may follow along incision lines where very small nerves are affected. What is the nature of this curious condition? Why should nerves when partially damaged produce such devastating symptoms? Until very recently this was a mystery and it was believed that there was some disorder of the sympathetic nervous system. It was noted by Barnes in 1954 that sympathectomy would almost always relieve the pain of causalgia. Early workers including Weir Mitchell (1872) had recommended resection of the nerve, thus hopefully cutting out the source of the pain, but in many such cases the pain returned and patients were subjected to multiple procedures, often with serial amputations, and yet the pain persisted. Clearly, removing the peripheral source of pain was not successful and now we realize that this is because the pain by then had become settled in the central nervous system.

Differential diagnosis

Pain of neurological origin, felt in the hand, can arise from two sources, either from local lesions or referred from a distant source. Local causes include amputation stumps, nerve irritation from scarring, compression of the median nerve in the carpal tunnel and direct involvement of nerve with nerve tumours. The palmar cutaneous branch of the median, and the superficial radial nerve, may be divided accidentally by surgery. Remote causes include cervical rib, cervical spondylosis and post-irradiation neuritis. It is usually not difficult to differentiate between local and remote causes, but there are certain circumstances where difficulty may be experienced and special investigations such as electromyography and evoked responses are required.

In carpal tunnel syndrome and cervical spondylosis the pain is associated with paraesthesiae and numbness involving the median innervated fingers. However, patients can be adamant that the little finger is also involved and this can confuse the examiner into believing that there is also an associated ulnar nerve entrapment in Guyon's canal, or that these are symptoms of a generalized neuropathy. It is worth asking the patient when he or she awakes at night to outline the area of paraesthesiae with an indelible pencil and both the patient and the examiner may be surprised to see how the exact territory of the median nerve may be delineated, despite there being a belief that the little finger is also involved. Wynn Parry (1981) has shown that functional testing using objects and textures with the patient blindfolded shows little or no abnormality, even in quite late stages of this condition. In some cases it may be difficult to establish whether the symptoms are due to pressure on the median nerve at the wrist or elbow, or whether the symptoms are arising from pressure on cervical roots in the neck, associated with cervical spondylosis or disc prolapse. It is well recognized that rotator cuff lesions can give paraesthesiae and pain referred to the hand. It may be that such patients have a mild median nerve compression, and an increase in nociceptive input from a lesion elsewhere in the upper limb may make manifest this subclinical condition. It is often found that relief of one parameter of this multiple pathology may relieve pain in the others. If a painful rotator cuff lesion is successfully treated by steroid injection or physiotherapy, or neck pain is treated by physiotherapy in the form of traction, manipulation or a collar, the symptoms of paraesthesiae in the hand may be completely relieved. The use of electrodiagnosis has made it possible to provide a definitive diagnosis of median nerve compression in nearly all patients. The most sensitive test is disturbance of the sensory action potential as measured by stimulating the index or middle fingers and thumb with ring electrodes and recording the response over the wrist; the so-called orthodromic technique. The antidromic technique in which the nerve is stimulated at the wrist, and the sensory potential recorded with electrodes on the fingers, is perfectly acceptable. Compression of the median nerve is shown by diminution of amplitude of the sensory action potential and delay in its latency. Sometimes the action potential may be within the normal range and yet can be shown to be smaller in amplitude than that of the ulnar nerve, stimulating the little finger and recording over the ulnar nerve at the wrist. The ulnar sensory action potential should be smaller than that of the median and when there is such a discrepancy it is clear that there is compromise of the median sensory branch. A most recent refinement described by Mills (1985) involves stimulating the median and ulnar nerves in the palm and recording equidistantly at the wrist over the two nerves, a difference of more than 0.5 ms latency indicating an involvement of the median nerve. EMGs should also be carried out on the abductor pollicis brevis (ABP), the muscle most likely to be median supplied and not the seat of an anomalous nerve supply involving branches from the ulnar nerve. A delay in latency between the wrist and abductor pollicis brevis of more than 5 ms is abnormal and there is evidence to show that the degree of slowing is related to the response to treatment. If the patient has more than 7 ms delay he is extremely unlikely to respond to other than surgical measures. Denervation in the form of spontaneous fibrillation and large motor units on effort are also indications of nerve damage, but these are late signs and hopefully the diagnosis will be made before their appearance. It is always important to measure the ulnar sensory action potential, not only to gain a comparison in amplitude in very mild cases, but also to make sure that there is not a generalized neuropathy, of which the median nerve compression is the first sign. If the ulnar action potential is also diminished then investigation should be carried further by measuring the sural action potential and motor conduction in the arms and legs. Although it is possible for the median nerve to be compressed at the wrist in the presence of totally normal motor and sensory conduction using the most refined techniques, it is rare, and surgery to decompress the nerve should seldom be advised in the absence persistently of any abnormal electrophysiological signs. Compression of the median nerve at the elbow in the so-called pronator teres syndrome will be shown by the detection of denervation in the forearm muscles such as flexor pollicis longus, or flexor digitorum superficialis. Unless there has been a severe degree of root damage, sensory and motor conduction are entirely normal in cervical spondylosis, or other conditions causing irritation of nerve roots.

Paraesthesiae in the hand from cervical spondylosis is usually due to C6 or C7 root involvement and denervation will not be seen in the small muscles of the hand. It is unfortunately rare to find denervation in the nerve root territories involved, for example, in biceps, deltoid, triceps or extensors of the fingers, and if it is so found the diagnosis will be obvious. Occasionally measuring the reflex responses may show a significant slowing on the affected side. Sensory evoked potentials stimulating the median and ulnar nerves at the wrist, whilst recording over the brachial plexus and over the cervical spine, can sometimes show a slowing on the affected side but, again, these sophisticated tests are rather disappointing and rarely give a clear-cut answer. One has to depend on a very careful history and clinical examination. If rotating the neck towards the side of symptoms increases symptoms, and if gentle manual traction relieves the symptoms, this is clear evidence of nerve root compression in the cervical region. As over half the population over the age of 45 have radiographic changes of spondylosis, such appearances do not necessarily indicate the cause of symptoms. The demonstration of marked narrowing of an intervertebral foramen with encroachment of osteophytes is a very helpful sign but usually radiographs are taken to exclude sinister causes such as vertebral collapse from primary or secondary tumours, or chronic infection.

The question arises as to whether all patients suspected of having median nerve compression at the wrist should be subjected to electrophysiological investigation. In an ideal world this should be so. Too many patients are seen, in whom operations have been carried out, who have subsequently been shown to have either nerve compression at the elbow or at the root of the neck. This, however, is a very common condition and electrophysiologists are in relatively short supply. If there is the slightest doubt about the diagnosis then we believe that patients should be referred for electrophysiological studies and certainly the operation should be conducted by a skilled surgeon and not left to junior staff. There are a whole range of possible complications following this operation including pain from scarring, causalgia from division of the palmar cutaneous branch, infection and tethering of the scar to underlying tissues. Obviously the surgeon will suspect and exclude hypothyroidism, acromegaly, amyloid disease and, commonest of all, rheumatoid arthritis. The symptoms of median nerve compression at the wrist can precede the appearance of joint swellings by up to two years, and all patients in whom there is any swelling of the flexor tendons or puffiness in the palm should be suspected of having rheumatoid arthritis and should be followed up carefully. It is difficult to know how many patients benefit permanently from local steroid injections. If the EMG findings indicate only very mild compression, there is no denervation, and the patient is not keen on operation, it would seem reasonable to try one or possibly two steroid injections. We favour the use of soluble preparations such as Codelsol, for Brooks has noted that when hydrocortisone is used the crystals can remain around the nerve for years. Carpal tunnel symptoms arising during pregnancy usually subside spontaneously after delivery.

Cervical rib and thoracic outlet

There was a vogue not long ago to attribute paraesthesiae and pain down the inner side of the arm into the hand to compromise of the brachial plexus and subclavian artery at the root of the neck by cervical ribs or bands, or by a tight scalenus anterior. The condition was certainly overdiagnosed and many people were unnecessarily subjected to surgery which at the best of times is difficult and can be dangerous. The classical neurological picture is of a wasted abductor pollicis brevis with paraesthesiae on the inner side of the arm and hand, and some blunting of sensation over the little finger. Electrophysiologically the median sensory action potential is normal and the ulnar sensory action potential is reduced, with denervation present in either or both C8 and T1 muscles. This picture, however, is the late stage of nerve compression and one would certainly want to make the diagnosis long before it had been reached. Unfortunately, electrophysiology is not very helpful in this respect, for sensory and motor conduction is usually normal, and denervation absent. However, some patients have been seen with normal motor and sensory conduction but with denervation in one or other of C8 and T1 supplied muscles of the hand, and this has proved a valuable indication of nerve compromise. Unfortunately sensory evoked responses are not contributing as much as was hoped, but if they are positive, and if there is clear evidence of delay compared with the unaffected side, this will be helpful. Patients classically complain of a deep-seated ache at the root of the neck with pain travelling down the arm, usually on the inner side of the forearm and hand, with paraesthesiae and painful 'shoots' in the ulnar distribution of the hand. In the early stages there is no objective sensory loss, no wasting, no reflex changes and a lack of power, only in relation to the pain. Patients complain of an exacerbation of pain when lifting and carrying and raising their arms above their head. They feel a sense of heaviness in the whole upper limb. Sometimes pressure over the plexus at the root of the neck can reproduce the pain and if it does so on one side and not on the other this may well be significant. Radiographs can be problematic. The demonstration of a cervical rib or a large transverse process does not necessarily mean that this is the cause of symptoms as it is well known that such chance findings are compatible with a complete lack of symptoms. On the other hand, it is possible to have well-defined pressure by a band which is not visible on a radiograph. Digital arterial subtraction tests can be helpful and are well worth carrying out in difficult cases. It must be accepted that the diagnosis of this condition is difficult and treatment by no means always successful. This indeed is one of the areas for surgical *chasse gardée* reserved for the highly expert surgeon.

Other important causes of nerve compression at the root of the neck are Pancoast tumours and scarring of the brachial plexus following irradiation for carcinoma, usually of the breast. This latter is a particularly distressing condition. Some two years or more after excision of a carcinoma and radiotherapy the patient begins to notice painful paraesthesiae in the hand; this may well present as if it were a carpal tunnel syndrome and many patients have been subjected to nerve decompression when careful EMG studies would have shown that the lesion extended beyond the territory of the median nerve, to involve the ulnar nerve and even more proximal structures as well. The pain increases and paralysis steadily worsens until the patient's arm becomes flail and extremely painful. The pain is due to a combination of peripheral components, for example causalgia, and central deafferentation, and is extremely difficult to treat. Just occasionally some patients get relief from surgery – excision of fibrosis and application of an omental graft. Of course, the neurological conditions cannot be improved, and all too often the pain can be made worse, and as the operation is fraught with vascular danger it is rarely performed. Transcutaneous electrical stimulation is described later and should be tried, and in very severe desperate cases a Nashold procedure should be considered.

Ulnar neuritis

Here again is a condition that is overdiagnosed and frequently overtreated. Classically, the patient may damage the ulnar nerve from fractures around the elbow or suffer delayed damage from cubitus valgus, though this is probably less common than the textbooks would allow. Osborne's band (Osborne, 1957, 1970) can cause compression of the nerve and may be associated with osteoarthrosis. Severe arthritis, whether caused by osteoarthrosis or rheumatism, can also cause ulnar nerve compression at the elbow. It cannot be too strongly emphasized that if the patient is complaining of sensory symptoms in the forearm, then the condition is certainly not due to ulnar nerve entrapment at the elbow, for the ulnar nerve does not supply any sensation in the forearm. It is distressing in the extreme to see patients presenting with severe causalgia following ulnar nerve transposition at the elbow when their symptoms have quite clearly been due to more proximal damage. A well-established case will show some wasting in the intrinsics, some dullness to sensory testing in the ulnar distribution in the hand and a positive Tinsel sign at the elbow. Treatment instituted before these changes develop give results that are much superior to those when treatment is delayed until there are overt neurological signs.

Here electrophysiological techniques are of extreme value. If the sensory action potential from the little finger to the wrist is normal, and of comparable amplitude to the other side, then it is extremely unlikely for there to be any compromise of the ulnar nerve at the elbow. Confirmatory signs of ulnar nerve compression electrophysiologically are: reduction in the sensory action potential, reduction in the nerve action potential measured by stimulating the wrist and recording above the elbow, in both cases compared with the normal side, the demonstration of entirely normal sensory conduction between the elbow above the site of compression and recording in the axilla. There will also be reduction in amplitude when stimulating at the elbow and recording over the abductor digiti minimi. Finally, there may be denervation in the ulnar supplied muscles. All these tests may be normal, and the only abnormality be a delayed latency stimulating above the elbow and recording in the flexor carpi ulnaris, as described by Payan in 1969.

Operation for relief of pressure at the elbow should be as simple as possible. Division of a band is very likely to relieve symptoms of pressure. If there is a very clear-cut abnormality of the nerve bed the band should be transposed deep to the nerve. In our opinion transposition is seldom necessary. There are very real and disastrous complications of ulnar nerve transposition: in particular, the development of severe causalgia with hyperpathia in the ulnar distribution of the hand and paroxysmal shooting pains down the arm and also severe hyperpathia in an oval area all round the scar of the elbow. This can be such that the patient cannot wear any clothing around the arm and is severely hampered functionally. It is our view that transposition of the ulnar nerve is seldom indicated and should never be effected unless there is clear-cut electrophysiological evidence of nerve compromise. If there is any doubt the surgical hand should be stayed and repeated electrophysiological tests undertaken. Some of the most devastating cases of causalgia that we have to deal with follow ulnar nerve transposition and in many cases, it is sad to relate, for conditions that are subsequently shown to be not due to ulnar nerve involvement at the elbow, but to some other neurological disorder, such as pressure at the root of the neck or a generalized neuropathy.

Painful peripheral nerves – causalgia

In a small proportion of patients, probably between 5 and 10 per cent, partial damage to peripheral nerves can lead to extremely distressing chronic pain, known as causalgia. It is almost always burning in character and there is classically hyperpathia in the distribution of the nerve such that light touch causes severe pain to a degree that patients will not allow the part to be touched. In time the pain may spread well outside the autonomous zone of the affected nerve. Common conditions producing this in practice are: neuromata of the median nerve at the wrist, ulnar neuritis at the elbow, amputation stumps, entrapment of digital nerves, scarring in the palm and Sudeck's atrophy. In a few cases the burning pain will subside with time, either spontaneously or after treatment, but the interval may be so long that irreparable changes in the skin, muscles, bone and psyche may develop. Some patients even commit suicide (White, Heroy and Goodman, 1948).

Weir Mitchell (1872) quotes Paget's description of the colour changes in the skin and these again have never been bettered. 'The fingers become glossy, tapering smooth hairless, almost void of wrinkles. Pink or ruddy or blotched as if with permanent chilblains and commonly also very painful.' Weir Mitchell describes the skin changes as 'cracks in the skin with yellow and brown scales being a very constant feature, sometimes with an eczematous eruption.' Occasionally this eruption would ease the pain and very occasionally these eruptions would appear on the other, unaffected hand. In the foot there was a curving of the nail, less marked than in the fingers but with distressing ulceration which might break out again and again despite every care and attention. Painful swelling of joints might develop after a few days, becoming stiff and sore and even proceeding to ankylosis. 'One may be at some loss', Weir Mitchell goes on, 'to discern a difference from subacute rheumatism of the same parts.' When the deprived nutritive state has lasted for some months the hair commonly disappears from the fingers affected and the nails undergo remarkable alterations. They suffer only in those fingers the neural supply of which has been interfered with, so that the nails in the median distribution may be contorted and that in the little finger be unaffected. Alteration in the nail consists of a curve in its long axis and extreme lateral arching and sometimes a thickening of the cutis beneath its extremity. Protuberant and oddly curved nails develop. 'The whole surface of the skin supplied by the affected nerve becomes hyperaesthetic and the senses grew to be only avenues for fresh and increasing tortures until every vibration, every change of light and even the effort to read brought on new agony.' The onset of this curious condition was often immediate and Weir Mitchell's book is full of the most extraordinary descriptions of the reaction of the patients to injury. A private shot through the brachial plexus became wildly excited crying 'murder' repeatedly and accusing those near him in the ranks of having shot him. 'He did not fall.' An officer shot through the right median nerve was helped away to the rear 'talking somewhat incoherently about matters foreign to the time and scene.' Another patient felt that he had been struck by a stick and angrily accused a comrade of the trick. Many of the cases of causalgia seen in civilian life may follow some time after nerve damage, in particular after median nerve repair at the wrist when the nerve begins to reinnervate the skin and muscle; some three months after nerve repair the severe burning pain may commence. The immediacy of onset, however, in gunshot wounds indicates that the cause of the pain must have a central component, for there is not time for changes to develop peripherally to explain the symptoms. The characteristics of the pain are remarkable. Again, we turn to Weir Mitchell (1872) for the characteristic clinical picture:

'Joss H. Corliss, late Private of B Company, 14th New York State Militia, aged 27, a shingle dresser enlisted April 1861. At the second battle of Bull Run, 28th August, 1862, he was shot in the left arm 3 inches above the internal condyle and the bullet emerged one and a quarter inches higher. He was ramming a cartridge when hit and thought he was struck on the crazy bone by some of the boys for a joke. Resection of the median nerve was no good. A week after he was shot in the right arm, he was weak and could not feed himself. By April 1864 he was better, he had pain in the median distribution but excessive pain in the ulnar. He kept his hand wrapped in a rag, wetted with cold water and covered in oil silk. Moisture was more essential to him than cold, he keeps a bottle of water about him, with a wet sponge in his right hand and keeps water in his boots. It is as if a rough bar of iron was thrust to and fro through the knuckles and a red hot iron placed at the junction of the palm and thenar eminence with a heavy weight on it and the skin rasped off his finger ends. The rattling of a newspaper, a breath of air, the step of another across the ward, the vibrations caused by a military band or the shock of the feet in walking gives rise to increase of pain. He insisted that the observer wet his hand before touching him. Cold weather eased his pain, heat made it worse.'

The effect of noise and vibration, so graphically described in Private Corliss's case, is reflected also in the experience, in the Second World War in the United States Air Force. In Texas a large military hospital was situated a mile from an airfield. The Commanding Officer of the hospital was able to persuade the officer commanding the air force base to reroute his aircraft so that they did not fly directly overhead, for every time they did so all his patients (and there were many) with partial nerve lesions and causalgia would get an extreme exacerbation of their pain.

The term 'causalgia' which means 'burning pain' was invented by Weir Mitchell and his description of the characteristic features of the condition have never been bettered.

The natural history of this condition is distressingly chronic. Weir Mitchell's son was a neurologist, and he followed up a number of his father's patients 27 years after their original injury. *Table 11.1* presents this follow-up, which has been compiled from both the Weir Mitchell's books (1872, 1895).

It is certainly the experience of patients attending the peripheral nerve injuries clinic at the Royal National Orthopaedic Hospital (RNOH) that the untreated course of this condition is disappointing. Indeed, the average time that patients had suffered pain before referral to this specialist unit was 3½ years, and for many six years or more.

Table 11.1 Causalgia: 27 year follow-up by J. K. Weir Mitchell (1895), patients of S. Weir Mitchell (1863)

Nerve	Numbers	Severe pain	Relief
Ulnar and median	6	3	3
Brachial plexus	5	5	0
Sciatic	4	2	2
Median	3	2	1
Ulnar	2	2	0
Facial	1	1	0
Cutaneous of thigh	1	1	0

$n = 22$.

In Weir Mitchell's series only 12 had complete relief out of the 23 patients, and in one case six operations for excision of a damaged nerve had been carried out before relief was obtained, and even in this patient pain returned after 18 months. This again is a very distressing feature of the condition and repeated attempts to treat these patients surgically are doomed to failure.

Reflex sympathetic dystrophy: Sudeck's atrophy

In 1900 Sudeck described an acute atrophy of bone associated with swelling, pain and loss of function. Classically Sudeck's atrophy has two stages: first, in the days and weeks immediately after injury, swelling, redness, hotness and burning pain in the affected hand or foot; later this progresses to a cold, clammy, pale, stiff hand with, in severe cases, virtually a frozen hand or foot, such that no movement, active or passive, is possible. The original description was of a disorder of the foot but it is now clear that the condition is much more common in the hand. Of the number of terms which have been applied to this condition the most commonly accepted now are reflex sympathetic dystrophy or Sudeck's atrophy. There is a remarkable similarity clinically between the painful sequelae of peripheral nerve damage or causalgia and Sudeck's atrophy, for both are associated with severe spontaneous pain, hyperpathia, swelling of the affected hand, colour changes, muscle wasting and atrophy of bone. Most authorities now agree that these conditions are at either end of the same neurological spectrum, pain following partial nerve lesions or major causalgia, and minor causalgia where the damage is to the very fine terminal axons. Sudeck's atrophy often follows relatively trivial trauma such as a minor fracture of the wrist and it is more common after closed injuries than open ones. It can follow such conditions as frozen shoulder, coronary thrombosis, and even intracranial neoplasms.

The brachial plexus

Reference must be made to complete brachial plexus lesions in which the patient with the flail limb is at risk for developing intractable pain.

The traditional treatment of amputation of the flail arm, followed by arthrodesis of the shoulder and fitting of a prosthesis, is, in our view, no longer acceptable. The vast majority of patients with brachial plexus lesions have total lesions, which means that they have no proximal shoulder control. Without this it is impossible to activate an artificial limb appliance, for the elbow locking and unlocking depends on shoulder protraction by serratus anterior. It is now generally accepted that such patients will rarely use an artificial limb, but will accept a functional splint which is virtually a prosthesis over the patient's own paralyzed arm (Wynn Parry, 1981). It consists of a shoulder support, which prevents subluxation, an elbow locking device so the patient can put his elbow in one of four or five positions, and a forearm support which carries a platform, into which slot the standard artificial limb appliances such as a split hook, manipulated by a harness on the contralateral shoulder. These splints allow the patient to support objects in the paralyzed arm whilst using the normal arm. The flail arm splint allows the patient the best of both worlds. He retains his arm, but he has function. Most patients abhor the idea of an amputation and do not feel that they would be able to go to swimming pools or on the beach with a stump. It cannot be overemphasized how important it is for the patient to understand that amputating a flail arm will have no effect on the pain he suffers. The pain is central and does not arise from the deafferented limb. The nature of the pain must also be explained to the patient, and it is feared that there are still physicians and surgeons who do not realize this fact and are advocating amputation as a pain-relieving procedure. This can only lead to total disillusionment and disaster. Of 200 patients with total arm paralysis after brachial plexus lesions splinted this way at RNOH, 70 per cent were using them regularly for work, hobbies or do-it-yourself activities one year later. The single most important way of coping with intractable deafferentation pain, which is particularly severe in avulsion lesions of the brachial plexus, and felt almost invariably in the anaesthetic hand, is by distraction. When patients are fully absorbed in work or demanding hobbies, their pain can become reduced to manageable proportions. It is the central inhibitory pathways that are brought in, originating from the periventricular grey matter in the thalamus and relaying directly via the raphe nucleus to laminas 1 and 5, where all the spontaneous nociceptive activity arises. Drugs are of little of no use in this severe deafferentation pain. A few patients find large doses of dihydrocodeine helpful, but most have abandoned analgesics. The side-effects are too great and the effects too transitory.

Treatment

In their 1974 paper in *Nature*, Wall and Gutnik showed that electrical stimulation could reduce or abolish spontaneous firing of a neuroma. Wall and Sweet (1967) were the first to use transcutaneous stimulation in patients with severe pain and showed that it could be highly successful. Transcutaneous nerve stimulation is now an accepted form of treatment for pain. It appears to have both peripheral and central effects. It reduces, or abolishes, the spontaneous firing from the seat of damage, and by stimulating 1A afferents causes the secretion of chemical substances in the spinal cord which may damp down the spontaneous firing induced by partial deafferentation, or prevent their transmission by interfering with the secretion of substance P. The exact mechanism has yet to be worked out, but there is no doubt at all about the efficacy of this treatment, provided it is properly given.

The hypersensitivity to noradrenaline is an important feature of these conditions. The first really effective treatment for causalgia was introduced by Barnes in 1954, when he pointed out that almost all cases of causalgia from gunshot wounds could be relieved by sympathetic block, or sympathectomy. In fact, some workers have defined causalgia as that pain that responds to sympathetic block. This is now known to be going too far but there is a germ of truth in the statement. In Barnes' series there were some dramatic results. Patients who had severe burning pain, only relieved by immersing the arm or leg in cold water for hours on end, could, immediately after sympathetic block, use their limb normally. Barnes reported 22 patients who had sympathectomy carried out for causalgia, and in 15 there was dramatic long-lasting success.

Guanethidine blocks

The introduction of guanethidine blocks by Hannington-Kiff (1974) has revolutionized the clinical management of these conditions. Guanethidine blocks are more long-lasting and much easier to carry out than sympathetic block, obviating the need for sympathectomy in most cases. Modifying his technique by not using any sedation encourages the patient to try and desensitize the hypersensitive and hyperpathic skin by as normal use as possible in the occupational therapy and workshops, whilst the guanethidine effect is still present.

Several reports have appeared indicating the prolonged effect of guanethidine blocks and their profound effect on temperature. A guanethidine block can be carried out by the house officer, whereas the stellate block requires an experienced anaesthetist. Sympathectomy can be dramatic, but is often disappointing. It is well known that the sympathetic nervous system has a distressing propensity to regenerate and many patients are seen with dramatic results shortly after operation, only for the pain to return some months later.

Transcutaneous nerve stimulation (TNS)

Loh and Nathan (1978) pointed out that patients with hyperpathia are much more likely to respond to sympathetic block than those without. Consequently the first choice of treatment in somebody with severe hyperpathia would be guanethidine blocks. However, patients in whom hyperpathia is either absent or only slight, may respond to sympathetic block, and this is therefore a treatment to try. If it fails, transcutaneous nerve stimulation (TNS) is the next choice. This will be the logical first choice if the patient is suffering from active nerve pain, such as paraesthesiae, tingling, shooting pains, and with marked mechanosensitivity of the peripheral nerves. Far too often transcutaneous nerve stimulation has been misused. The patient is handed a stimulator at a pain clinic, with only the briefest instructions as to its use, and often returns it, having tried it for only half an hour or an hour at a time, claiming it has failed.

The proper use of transcutaneous nerve stimulation is as an inpatient procedure. All patients admitted to the Rehabilitation Centre of the RNOH are treated by a skilled physiotherapist who will experiment with different electrode placings, with different settings of transcutaneous nerve stimulation and different timing of use. Almost all patients wear the stimulator for many hours on end, sometimes all day and sometimes all night. The electrodes must always be placed proximal to the pain, not over its site, where it would be ineffective. The idea is to get as much afferent input as possible along the affected nerve, proximal to where it is damaged, or where there is no afferent input; for example, in total deafferentation in phantom pain or brachial plexus lesions, as near to the input as possible. For example, in a total brachial plexus lesion, the electrodes will be placed over the neck, the root of the neck, the anterior part of the chest wall, stimulating C3 and 4, or over the inner side of the upper arm over T2. The object is to stimulate as much electrical activity around the cells which are spontaneously firing, in the hope of suppressing their activity.

Patients are encouraged to wear their stimulator during work or hobbies. The new models which are light, portable and comfortable to wear, make this a distinct possibility. Many patients go about their daily affairs wearing their stimulator all day. Others find the distraction of work is enough to keep the pain at bay, but when they relax in the evening the pain reasserts itself and it is then that the application of transcutaneous nerve stimulation for some hours in the evening or during the night can be most helpful. One must beware of letting the patient give up the treatment too soon. Patients are encouraged to go through all four seasons of the year without significant pain before returning the stimulator. They may be substantially relieved of pain by transcutaneous nerve stimulation or guanethidine blocks, but, with the onset of a severe winter find that cold exacerbates the pain and it is then that the stimulator can be most useful.

Physiotherapy and occupational therapy

It has already been emphasized that there is a profound central disturbance after peripheral damage and this means that there are abnormal circuits firing centrally. The only way to re-establish normal neural patterns is by encouraging the patient to use the limb normally in functional activities. In physiotherapy, occupational therapy and remedial workshops, patients are encouraged to use their limb in various activities that are interesting and absorbing in order to restore normal neural patterns centrally. This, of course, can only be done when pain is sufficiently reduced to allow them to use the limb.

Thus, the recommended regime for a patient with severe causalgia affecting the median nerve would be guanethidine blocks until the pain was controlled, then attendance at a physiotherapy department for desensitization techniques, stroking, rubbing, using the hand in exercises, followed by activity in occupational therapy – carpentry, metalwork, needlework, art of various kinds. If necessary, a stimulator can be worn as well.

Drug treatment

Drug treatment of causalgic pain is particularly disappointing, for the standard analgesic and anti-inflammatory drugs are of no value. The effect of carbemazine (Tegretol), or one of its analogues, such as sodium valproate, should be tried if the patient has severe shooting pains indicating that there are paroxysmal central discharges, as in trigeminal neuralgia. But they have no effect on the constant burning pain or hyperpathia. Steroid therapy is ineffective in Sudeck's atrophy.

Results of treatment

In 1979 the first 103 cases of severely painful peripheral nerve injuries treated at the RNOH by an intensive rehabilitation regime, using sympathetic block and transcutaneous nerve stimulation were reviewed and gave some 55 per cent of good results. The lesson learned was not be too timid towards sympathetic blocks. Originally, after one or two guanethidine blocks, if only marginally effective, the treatment was abandoned. Now at least six blocks are given before abandoning the method. Very often one obtains a slight improvement for an hour or two after the block, only for the pain to recur. But the fact that pain may be reduced or abolished, even for a short period, is highly significant and encouraging. Many patients have had as many as 12 blocks, and in two cases 28 and 31 blocks respectively.

Five years later the experience of a further 69 patients with severe intractable peripheral nerve pain was reported (Withrington and Wynn Parry, 1984). *Table 11.2* shows the results in these patients and *Table 11.3* shows the operations carried out specifically to relieve pain. It will be seen that just over two-thirds of patients achieved substantial or complete relief of pain, and this in patients who had had a long history of pain and often many procedures to attempt to relieve it. The most disconcerting result from these experiments was the very high proportion of failures when attempting to relieve the pain by surgery.

Table 11.2 Painful peripheral nerve lesions at the Royal National Orthopaedic Hospital (RNOH) 1979–1983

		Helped	*Not helped*
Median nerve	(18)	12	6
Ulnar nerve at elbow	(12)	7	5
Ulnar nerve at wrist	(2)	2	0
Digital nerve	(22)	16	6
Superficial radial nerve	(3)	3	0
Scar	(6)	4	2
Others	(6)	5	1
		49	20

Transcutaneous nerve stimulation helped 30 out of 59 patients treated. Guanethidine helped 29 out of 58 patients treated. Eleven patients were helped by both.
Of 50 patients who had 71 operations for pain, one was successful.

Table 11.3 Painful peripheral nerve disorders at the Royal National Orthopaedic Hospital 1979–1983

	Operations for pain (71)	
Median	excision of neuroma	4 (two grafts)
	neurolysis	12
Ulnar	transposition	16
	excision of neuroma	3
	neurolysis	3
Digital	excision of neuroma	16
	crushing	1
	trimming of stump	2
	neurolysis	1
Superficial radial	excision of neuroma	1
	neurolysis	3
Excision of scar		7
Others	neurolysis	2

Indications for surgery

Warnings against the use of surgery to relieve peripheral nerve pain have been issued over the years by many authors. Livingston (1943) remarked that the pain has a remarkable ability to find a new route when the customary channels have been blocked. This, of course, is very true for central pain as well as peripheral pain, and most neurosurgeons have abandoned cordotomies, rhizotomies and tractotomies for patients with benign, intractable pain – that is, pain that does not threaten life and which the patient may well have been suffering for decades. Such procedures are acceptable in terminal cancer pain but not in benign pain.

Leriche in 1939 stated 'nerves are not made to be divided'. It is, after all, the function of the nerve cells to discharge and if they are prevented from so doing by division of their input, they will tend to respond by increased activity in order, as it were, to draw attention to themselves. Snyder (1961) who reported over 150 surgical methods of trying to alleviate peripheral pain by surgery, pointed out that treatment often causes temporary relief, to return 4–10 weeks later as a second neuroma forms.

The following recommendations are made regarding surgery. First, only one local procedure is generally allowed. In the case of amputations, an unsatisfactory stump should be revised, in order to cover the end with a suitable cushion of soft tissue and to place the scar where it will not be subjected to repeated pressure. Adherent neuromata are resected and allowed to retract into muscle or fatty subcutaneous tissue. Burying the ends in bone is inadvisable, because it only serves to tether them, and to encourage further spontaneous firing. Second, in peripheral nerve division, continuity should always be restored if possible. Peripheral nerve surgery demands the highest quality in technique and should be left to skilled hand surgeons. Internal neurolysis is always to be condemned; more damage is done as a result. Sympathectomy, if it is to be carried out, also demands the highest technique, as damage to the lower trunk is likely to occur in inexperienced hands. Anatomy must be very carefully respected, particularly in operations for carpal tunnel decompression. There is a definite morbidity after this procedure and severe causalgia can follow division and damage to the palmar cutaneous branch of the median nerve.

Long-term follow-up is extremely important, for pain may be abolished for some weeks, only to return some months later.

Intensive full-time and comprehensive rehabilitation is essential for these patients. Return to work or to meaningful and absorbing activities in the house is the single most valuable way the patient can come to terms with his pain. Thus, a rehabilitation programme must include assessment and, where necessary, retraining for work and a determined effort to place patients back in the community. For patients, with avulsion of the brachial plexus, suffering phantom pain after amputation, where the pain is destroying their life and that of their family, and in whom all other measures have failed, then the Nashold procedure or dorsal root entry zone rhizotomy can be considered. The rationale here is to destroy those cells of the spinal cord where the spontaneous firing occurs, thus getting, as it were, to the root of the the problem.

Nashold has published a series of over 100 patients with a 70 per cent success rate (Nashold and Ostdahl, 1979) confirmed by the experience of Thomas of London (unpublished reference). There are, however, side-effects from this procedure in the ipsilateral proprioceptive loss in the leg and possible locomotor dysfunction.

However, if the possibilities and complications are carefully explained to the patient, and he agrees that life is not worth living without some attempt to relieve the pain, then this procedure is justified. It is, to some extent, still experimental and must be confined to centres of expertise and to those where patients can be very thoroughly evaluated before surgery over a prolonged period, assessing them as people both at work and at home, and with a prolonged rehabilitation postoperatively. It is well known that patients are less likely to feel phantom pain and more likely to come to terms with the pain if they are regular prosthetic users. This again implies an intensive continuing rehabilitation programme.

The future

Recent progress has come about through the close liaision between basic scientists and clinicians. Much remains to be done in this difficult field, for, despite success in a significant number of patients with these appalling pains, there is still 30 per cent of patients who cannot be helped. Exciting research continues in the experimental field. The demonstration that axoplasmic blocking techniques can arrest spontaneous activity in damaged peripheral nerves encourages the hope that some substance will emerge that will not be damaging to nerve, but can rest it for prolonged periods without producing degeneration and allow more normal patterns of central activity to be reasserted. Doubtless there will be new encephalin and endorphin analogues available to help relief of central pain. Possibly there will be new developments in precursors, such as tryptophan, which help replace the patient's depleted stores as a result of chronic pain. Possible refinements of electrophysiological techniques will allow the routine study with microelectrodes and firing in human damaged nerve with clinical assessment of the effects of pain-relieving modalities.

From the clinician's point of view there is still, as there always has been in clinical medicine, enormous scope for careful and detailed clinical descriptions of these disorders and recording of the various factors that alleviate or aggravate the pain. As we have seen, very little has been added to our description of the clinical nature of these conditions since Weir Mitchell's beautiful publication of 1872, but he was denied the access to laboratory experiments and the demonstration of the nerve cell in action which we are now privileged to be able to study. Let us hope that in the foreseeable future there will be further striking advances in this difficult, challenging but fascinating field.

LOCAL CAUSES OF PAIN IN THE HAND

While the bulk of this chapter is directed to those conditions where pain in the hand is the presenting and dominant complaint, it is pertinent to refer also to certain principles in diagnosis and management, and to the relevance of careful history-taking and precise examination. Detailed discussion of most of these topics will be found elsewhere in this book.

Trauma

Open wounds of the hand, with or without fractures or damage to deep structures, are obvious and pain is an accompanying feature. Occasionally pain seems to be disproportionate to the severity of the injury. A possible cause to be considered is the direct penetration of a nerve, the median for instance, by a foreign body or spicule of bone.

Closed injuries of the wrist and hand are notorious for misdiagnosis by inexperienced doctors. The occasional delayed radiological appearances of a fracture of the scaphoid bone is well-known, but overcaution is often exhibited, a situation which will be referred to later. Dislocations in the carpus and hand are more commonly missed than fractures, despite the fact that they are the most painful and that, whereas the pain from a fracture is eased by traction or immobilization, the pain of a dislocation is only relieved by its reduction. The bone at greatest risk is the lunate. While it is excusable in the emergency room to overlook a dissociation between the lunate and scaphoid, it is hard to condone failure to diagnose a semilunar dislocation because the severity of the pain, the degree of swelling and the restriction of motion in the wrist should lead the least experienced doctor to re-examine the radiographs, and X-ray the other side for comparison.

Many patients referred to hand clinics, rather than to the emergency room, suffer from the effects of trauma, real or implied, and a careful history is required to determine its relevance. The only complaint may be of pain in relation to a joint, where the most important physical sign is the localization of tenderness in response to active or passive motion. On this basis a diagnosis can usually be made between specific lesions of tendon or ligament and those affecting the whole joint complex. Radiographs may show flakes of bone indicative of avulsion of important soft tissue attachments. Pain and swelling disproportionate to the radiological appearances may be explained by a dislocation reduced spontaneously or by the patient. A careful history should determine whether this was so.

The principle to be emphasized is that complaints of pain persisting after injury are not to be dismissed as exaggerated until several possibilities have been excluded: one is that the injury was more severe than at first suspected, as mentioned above; another is partial injury to a nerve, a potentially serious problem already discussed; third is a retained foreign body, a situation of which the patient may be unaware and complain only of local soreness or a tender lump. A pricking feeling can be caused by an unsuspected spicule of glass. In rural areas blackthorns often penetrate the hand, usually a flexor sheath in the distal palm or a metacarpophalangeal joint on the dorsum. If a patient 'thinks it is all out', and there is still persisting tenderness, it may reliably be assumed that the tip of the thorn has been left behind, providing a focus for chronic infection.

Infection

Acute infection in the hand is seldom difficult to recognize. Pain occurs early and is particularly severe in two situations, the distal pulp and the flexor sheath. In each case the reason is the same: tension in a closed compartment, one bounded by the fibrous septa dividing up the fibrofatty tissue, the other by the synovial sheath of the tendon. In septic tenosynovitis the pain is greatly increased by passive extension of the digit. Most hand infections arise in normal tissue but pain occurring in a previous inclusion dermoid cyst is an indication of secondary infection. Chronic infections such as tuberculosis are remarkably painfree, even when gross synovial disease causes compression of the median nerve.

Postoperative pain

Operations on the hand should not be unduly painful. If a patient complains of pain to a degree necessitating powerful analgesic drugs a cause must be sought – infection, haematoma or ischaemia. The dressing should be taken down under sterile conditions. A haematoma, if present, is released and, if necessary, the wound is opened and resutured. The most common cause of pain is a tight bandage or constricting dressing which demand urgent attention in order to prevent the potential risk of actual ischaemic changes. The usual mistake is to apply too much pressure to a bandage passing through the web between the index finger and thumb.

Ischaemia

Excluding open vascular injuries, the causes of ischaemia in the hand are blunt trauma causing arterial thrombosis or iatrogenic factors such as intra-arterial injection or external pressure from tight postoperative bandaging mentioned above. In Volkmann's contracture the functional loss is in the hand, but the site of pain is the forearm.

The vascularity of the hand is very variable and on it depends the degree of ischaemia which may result from thrombosis of one of its arterial components. The ulnar artery is the one most likely to be affected because of the tendency for the ulnar side of the hand to be used as a hammer. The dominant complaint is of severe pain, usually unaccompanied by signs of vascular insufficiency. Costigan, Riley and Coy (1959) reported that in one of their two cases the accompanying paraesthesiae were relieved by resection of the affected length of vessel and attribute the ulnar neuritis to pressure on the nerve by the thrombosed vessel.

Recently Richards and Urbaniak (1984) have described two patients with spontaneous retrocarpal thrombosis of the radial artery, causing pain with cold sensitivity and treated by resection of the affected length of vessel and vein grafting. Thrombosis of a persistent median artery has been shown to cause acute pain in the palm with colour changes in the long finger (Aulicino, Klavans and DuPuy, 1984). After resection of the thrombosed artery the backflow through the arch was greater than the flow from the proximal cut end, so no grafting was carried out. Most cases of radial artery thrombosis follow percutaneous indwelling catheters for monitoring cardiovascular function. Crossland and Neviaser (1977) report 60 cases of ischaemia in a series of 600 patients with radial artery catheterization over a period of five years. They emphasize the importance of performing Allen's test to ensure the adequacy of the circulation before the procedure is implemented, and the careful watch for signs of impending circulatory embarrassment. Allen (1929) described a method of determining the blood flow through the arteries at the wrist by compressing both radial and ulnar vessels while the fingers are flexed and extended to empty the hand of blood. The pressure on the radial artery is then released and the circulatory return is observed. The procedure is then repeated and the pressure on the ulnar artery is released. The opposite hand can be tested for comparison. If the hand becomes incompletely revascularized until both vessels are released it indicates that one artery is occluded or the palmar arch incomplete. The normal filling time is about 5 seconds. McCready *et al.* (1984) have described a similar problem after brachial artery puncture in the cubital fossa.

The options with regard to treatment of arterial thrombosis in the hand have been summarized by Urbaniak and Koman (1982): intra-arterial reserpine or tolazoline hydrochloride; serial stellate ganglion blocks; surgical sympathectomy; or resection and ligation of the thrombosed segment with or without vein grafting. In practice, surgery on the artery is usually required and should not be delayed.

Digital arthritis and tenosynovial disease

Osteoarthrosis commonly affects the terminal joints of the fingers and, although unsightly in women, is seldom painful enough to demand surgery unless accompanied by severe instability or the presence of a synovial cyst. The latter are a nuisance, awkward to excise because of thin overlying skin and the close relationship to the extensor tendon. Moreover they will recur if incompletely removed. Although tender if knocked, they are not spontaneously painful and such symptoms may be related to underlying arthritis. Osteoarthrosis of the proximal interphalangeal joints is likely to be attributable to previous trauma, usually an intra-articular fracture.

An osteophyte on the metacarpal head is an uncommon cause of painful locking of the finger, which must be suspected if the interphalangeal joints are not flexed. The common cause is the impaction of a swelling on the flexor tendon at the entrance to the fibrous flexor sheath. In rheumatoid patients the lesion may be found at the decussation of the superficialis tendon with large synovial nodules on either tendon or both. Tenosynovial disease, rheumatoid or otherwise, may be treated either by injection of hydrocortisone into the sheath or by surgical decompression. The small tense ganglion found in the distal palm and causing pain on gripping should be treated by excision together with the segment of fibrous sheath from which it arises.

The biggest problem of osteoarthrosis in the hand is the carpometacarpal joint of the thumb. Similar symptoms are produced by involvement of the joint between the scaphoid and trapexium, or by pantrapezial arthritis, where degenerative disease affects all the bones articulating with the trapezium, leaving the rest of the carpus free. Osteoarthrosis at the base of the thumb is extremely common and by no means always painful. It is surprising that it so seldom is a sequel to Bennett's fracture dislocation. A joint which becomes stiff is less painful than one which is unstable. Pressure along the length of the thumb accompanied by a rotational movement will make the diagnosis. Instability may be judged by pressure of the examiner's thumb over the base of the metacarpal while its head is alternately adducted and abducted. Conservative treatment is by injection of intra-articular hydrocortisone or the provision of a light removable splint. If pain has been provoked by a single episode of trauma or by recent recurring strains, a three-week period in a plaster cast is advisable. The choice of surgery is between excision or implant arthroplasty or arthrodesis.

Neoplasia

Neoplasms in the hand are rarely malignant, and those which are benign seldom cause pain except by pressure on a nerve if of soft tissue origin or by pathological fracture if they arise in bone. The latter is particularly true of the common enchondroma.

A notable exception is the glomus tumour which, though uncommon, is not rare and often situated near the finger-tip and particularly under the nail. Carlstedt and Lugnegard (1983) reviewed 18 patients with glomus tumour in the hand. They emphasized the intense pain with mechanical stimulation of the tumour and temperature sensitivity. In five cases the tumour was subjected to light and electron microscopical analysis. Niechajer (1982) distinguishes the solitary painful lesion from multiple glomus tumours, a rare clinical and genetic entity, with an autosomal dominant mode of inheritance. Corrado *et al.* (1982) describe the use of thermography in the diagnosis. It is the author's experience that the condition is liable to go unrecognized for a long time because the diagnosis is not considered and the patient may well be labelled as hysterical. The site of the lesion, the exquisiteness of the pain in response to touch and temperature should raise a high level of suspicion. The tumour is recognizable at operation as a small nodule with a bluish tinge. Its removal gives instant relief from pain.

Of bony tumours, osteoid osteoma is a rare cause of pain, which characteristic-ally is most prominent at night, and relieved by aspirin. Radiographs show a nidus surrounded by a zone of sclerosis. Operative resection relieves the pain. Generally the subject of individual case reports, a recent review of osteoblastoma (Chaise and Witvoet, 1984) refers to only six cases in the English literature. Since the signs are non-specific, and the radiological appearance of cystic changes in bone not diagnostic, the symptom of pain is important. The lesion is benign and the surgery therefore conservative.

THE PAINFUL WRIST

The obvious causes of pain in the wrist are recent fracture, osteoarthrosis and rheumatoid arthritis. These will not be considered further except to emphasize that physical signs on both sides of the wrist will distinguish arthritis from tenosynovitis.

Not infrequently complaints of pain in the wrist are accompanied by an inconclusive history and a paucity of physical signs. Radiological investigation, in addition to routine anteroposterior, lateral and oblique views may include magnified views, tomography, radiographs taken at extreme ranges of motion or cineradiography, films taken with gripping and loading, arthrography, or bone scans. The opposite wrist is often used for comparative views. To these techniques may now be added arthroscopy (Bora, 1985). At present this is mainly for diagnostic purposes, allowing inspection of the articular surfaces of the wrist joint with its ligamentous connections and triangular fibrocartilage. It has a particular place in assessing the integrity of a non-union of the scaphoid under direct vision and observing whether any radiocarpal arthritis is present. The arthroscope can be controlled with one hand, and the wrist viewed either by direct vision or on a television screen.

While most causes of wrist pain can be diagnosed on clinical examination, it must be admitted that some remain in doubt after all investigations have been exhausted. Most patients in this category are young women and the symptoms most often on the ulnar side. The authors agree with Urbaniak and Roth (1982): 'Rest, splintage, non-steroidal anti-inflammatory agents, and the passage of time will, fortunately, resolve many painful wrists with no specific diagnosis. The knowledgeable surgeon should not be too quick to explore the wrist.'

Pain on the radial side of the wrist

A history of injury and complaint of pain on the radial side of the wrist immediately, and quite properly, raises the suspicion of a fracture of the scaphoid. Sometimes this anxiety is carried to extremes and the patient subjected to repeated radiographic examination long after the possibility of fracture has passed. Alternative diagnoses, recognizable on radiographs, are rotary subluxation of the scaphoid due to disruption of the ligamentous attachment to the lunate, osteoarthrosis around the trapezium or between the scaphoid and radial styloid or a deposit of calcification in the same area. Episodes of acute calcification when they occur, and they are uncommon at the wrist, pursue a similar course to the well-known condition of a ruptured deposit at the shoulder: sudden onset of severe pain with spontaneous resolution in a period of weeks. Rest and support are usually sufficient, and a steroid injection may help. In practice, the commonest cause of pain on the radial side of the wrist, excluding fracture, is the de Quervain lesion, stenosing tendovaginitis of the abductor pollicis longus and particularly extensor pollicis brevis tendons. The diagnosis is made by the localization of tenderness and the application of Finkelstein's test. The patient flexes the thumb into the palm and curls the fingers over it. With the tendons thus put on the stretch the examiner deviates the wrist ulnarwards, a manoeuvre which provokes the pain. Treatment is either immobilization or injection of hydrocortisone into the sheath, usually successful if an effusion is present. If the fibrous tendon sheath is visibly thickened surgical decompression is preferable and gives instant relief. Care must be taken not to damage the terminal sensory branches of the radial nerve, and also to ensure that all the tendons are decompressed, anatomical anomalies being very common.

Central wrist pain

Pain localized centrally on the back of the wrist may have four specific causes. After recent injury a dorsal capsular sprain or flake avulsion fracture is common. Local tenderness and a detached bone fragment seen on the lateral view often make the diagnosis easy, but a negative radiograph merits a repeat a few weeks later when a shadow may appear in the detached soft tissue. Tenosynovitis of the extensor tendons is readily diagnosed from the presence of soft synovial swelling along the line of the tendons and the presence of crepitus felt on movement of the wrist or fingers. Dorsal ganglia are common and when large are usually painless as well as obvious. They all arise from the carpal joints and usually appear in the interval between the radial extensor tendons of the wrist and the extensors of the fingers. When still small they may cause pain by being pinched between the carpal joints on movements of the wrist. At this stage they may not be readily felt clinically, although they may be a perfectly reasonable cause of central wrist pain. Kienböck's disease, osteomalacia of the lunate, is the condition to which the surgeon must always be alert. The symptom of pain and the signs of local tenderness and restricted motion of the wrist joint precede the radiographic appearance of increased bone density and loss of height in the lunate. If the diagnosis is suspected but not confirmed by radiographs, the films should be repeated after two months. Meanwhile the wrist should be rested in a cast because, contrary to frequently expressed opinions, the condition may resolve spontaneously if treated early. Once the lunate has collapsed, surgery is likely to be required.

The many operations which have been devised indicate that no one of them is curative. Removal of the lunate causes a carpal shift, and the eventual outcome is often the need for arthrodesis or excision of the whole of the proximal row of the carpus. Lengthening of the ulna or shortening of the radius have been recommended as a means of unloading the lunate by increasing the load down the ulnocarpal column. Such procedures do not affect the rotary subluxation of the scaphoid which accompanies lunate collapse and are therefore only applicable in the early case.

In order to fill the space left by the excised lunate, flaps of soft tissue were first used, and later acrylic implants (Agerholm and Goodfellow, 1963). Swanson (1970) reported the operation of replacement with an implant of silicone rubber. This works well as a spacer, but under relatively small loading, as in gripping, the implant may collapse and the scaphoid rotate. In an effort to counteract this problem, Watson, Ryu and Dibella (1985) have proposed a fusion of the scaphoid, trapezium and trapezoid as a primary procedure. The principle is to relieve the compressive stress on the lunate and treat the subluxation of the scaphoid. The operation may be performed with the diseased lunate *in situ*, or the bone may be replaced by a silicone implant at the same time or later if symptoms continue. Moreover, the fusion can be carried out after lunate replacement if pain persists. The long-term results of this procedure are awaited.

Pain on the ulnar side of the wrist

The causes of pain on the ulnar aspect of the wrist are tenosynovitis of the flexor carpi ulnaris, chronic strain of the ulnar collateral ligament and derangements of the inferior radio-ulnar joint. Synovial thickening and effusion affecting the tendon sheath of flexor carpi ulnaris may be a presenting sign of rheumatoid arthritis and thus a surgical decompression will give an opportunity for biopsy. Pain arising from the ulnar collateral ligament is diagnosed by the localization of tenderness and the provocation of symptoms by stretching the wrist into radial deviation. Injection of local analgesic and hydrocortisone is the treatment of choice; three weeks in a cast may be indicated after recent injury. Later cases may benefit from manipulation of the wrist under general anaesthetic.

Pain affecting the inferior radio-ulnar joint may have an obvious cause due to growth discrepancy, trauma or chronic arthritis. On the other hand, patients may complain in this area of pain which is unsupported by physical signs. The temptation to carry out exploratory operations or procedures involving the triangular fibrocartilage should be resisted, as they are seldom successful and may give a cause for symptoms where none existed before. Such conditions are usually self-limiting and treatment should be conservative by providing a wrist-strap or other light support. Similar considerations apply to habitual subluxation of the lower end of the ulna.

Diseases and disorders of the inferior radio-ulnar joint are traditionally treated, if the symptoms merit it, by excision of the lower end of the ulna. If this operation is performed only about 1 cm of bone should be removed and the stump stabilized by suturing over its end a flap of capsule from the joint. Bowers (1985) has indicated the importance of preserving the functional elements of the ulnocarpal ligament complex. For patients with rheumatoid arthritis or osteoarthritis, whether or not as a sequel to trauma, he recommends a hemiresection of the ulnar head with interposition of tendon graft and capsular flap. Care must be taken to avoid impingement between the remaining styloid process and the carpus.

SUMMARY

This brief survey of the possible causes of pain in the wrist and hand serves to emphasize certain principles:

(1) Diagnosis often depends on an understanding of biomechanics or applied neurophysiology, and how these mechanisms may be affected by a disease process or in response to trauma.
(2) In difficult cases a multidisciplinary approach is the most promising, and the surgeon should not be reluctant to consult with specialists in other fields.
(3) The confidence of the patient is all-important and surgery ought not to be delegated to inexperienced staff.
(4) When in doubt, do not operate; failed surgery complicates the problem.
(5) Record progress meticulously; the greatest encouragement to the patient is the sign that he or she is getting better.

References

AGERHOLM, J. C. and GOODFELLOW, J. W. (1963) Avascular necrosis of the lunate bone treated by excision and prosthetic replacement. *Journal of Bone and Joint Surgery*, **45B**, 110–116

ALLEN, E. V. (1929) Thromboangitis obliterans: methods of diagnosis of chronic occlusive arterial lesions distal to the wrist with illustrative cases. *American Journal of Medical Science*, **178**, 237

AULICINO, P. L., KLAVANS, S. M. and DUPUY, T. E. (1984) Digital ischemia secondary to thrombosis of a persistent median artery. *Journal of Hand Surgery*, **9A**, 820–823

BARNES, R. (1954) Causalgia. A review of 48 cases in *Peripheral Nerve Injuries*. Report of Medical Research Council, pp. 156–185

BORA, F. W. (1985) Wrist arthroscope. *Journal of Hand Surgery*, **10A**, 308–

BOWERS, W. H. (1985) Distal radioulnar joint arthroplasty: the hemiresection–interposition technique. *Journal of Hand Surgery*, **10A**, 169–178

CARLSTEDT, T. and LUGNEGARD, H. (1983) Glomus tumour in the hand. A clinical and morphological study. *Acta Orthopaedica Scandinavica*, **54(2)**, 296–302

CHAISE, F. and WITVOET, J. (1984) Benign osteoblastoma of the hand. A case report. Review of the literature. *Semaine des Hôpitaux de Paris*, **60(1)**, 49–51

CORRADO, E. M., PASSARETTI, U., MESSORE, L. and LANZA, F. (1982) Thermographic diagnosis of glomus tumour. *The Hand*, **14(1)**, 21–24

COSTIGAN, D. G., RILEY, J. M. and COY, F. E. (1959) Thrombofibrosis of the ulnar artery in the palm. *Journal of Bone and Joint Surgery*, **41A**, 702–704

CROSSLAND, S. G. and NEVIASER, R. J. (1977) Complications of radial artery catheterization. *The Hand*, **9**, 287–290

HANNINGTON-KIFF, J. (1974) Intravenous regional sympathetic block with guanethidine. *Lancet*, **1**, 1019–1020

LIVINGSTON, W. K. (1943) *Pain Mechanisms. A Physiological Interpretation of Causalgia and its Related States*. New York: Macmillan Co.

LERICHE, R. (1939) *The Surgery of Pain* (translated by A. Young), pp. 48–52. Baltimore: Williams and Wilkins Co.

LOH, L. and NATHAN, P. W. (1978) Painful peripheral states and sympathetic blocks. *Journal of Neurology, Neurosurgery and Psychiatry*, **41**, 664–671

McCREADY, R. A., HYDE, G. L., BIVINS, B. A. and HAGIHARA, P. F. (1984) Brachial artery puncture: a definite risk to the hand. *Southern Medical Journal*, **77(6)**, 786–789

MELZACK, R. and WALL, P. D. (1983) *The Challenge of Pain*. Harmondsworth: Penguin Books

MILLS, K. R. (1985) Orthodromic sensory action potentials from palmar stimulation in the diagnosis of carpal tunnel syndrome. *Journal of Neurology, Neurosurgery and Psychiatry*, **48**, 250–255

NASHOLD, B. S. and OSTDAHL, R. H. (1979) Dorsal root entry zone lesions for pain relief. *Journal of Neurosurgery*, **57**, 59–69

NIECHAJER, I. A. (1982) Multiple glomus tumours. Special reference to radiological findings. *Scandinavian Journal of Plastic and Reconstructive Surgery*, **16(2)**, 183–190

OSBOURNE, G. V. (1957) The surgical treatment of tardy ulnar neuritis. *Journal of Bone and Joint Surgery*, **39–B**, 782

OSBOURNE, G. V. (1970) Compression neuritis of the ulnar nerve at the elbow. *The Hand*, **2**, 10

PAYAN, J. (1969) Electrophysiological localisation of ulnar nerve lesions. *Journal of Neurology, Neurosurgery and Psychiatry*, **32**, 208–220

RICHARDS, R. R. and URBANIAK, J. R. (1984) Spontaneous intercarpal radial artery thrombosis: a report of two cases. *Journal of Hand Surgery*, **9A**, 823–827

SNYDER, C. (1961) The surgical handling of tissue. *Proceedings 7th Annual Convention, American Association of Equine Practice, Texas*

SUDECK, P. (1900) Uber die akute Entzundliche Knochenatropie. *Archiv für Klinische Chirurgie*, **62**, 147

SWANSON, A. B. (1970) Silicone rubber implants for the replacement of the carpal scaphoid and lunate bones. *Orthopaedic Clinics of North America*, **1**, 299–309

URBANIAK, J. R. and KOMAN, A. L. (1982) *Difficult Problems in Hand Surgery*, pp. 253–263. St Louis: The C. V. Mosby Co.

URBANIAK, J. R. and ROTH, J. H. (1982) Office diagnosis and treatment of hand pain. *Orthopaedic Clinics of North America*, **13(3)**, 477–495

WALL, P. D. and SWEET, W. H. (1967) Temporary abolition of pain in man. *Science*, **155**, 108–109

WALL, P. D. and GUTNIK, M. (1974) Properties of afferent nerve impulses originating from a neuroma. *Nature*, **248**, 740

WALL, P. D. and DEVOR, M. (1981) The effect of peripheral nerve injury on dorsal root potentials and on transmission of afferent signals into the spinal cord. *Brain Research*, **209**, 95–111

WATSON, H. K., RYU, J. and DIBELLA, A. (1985) An approach to Kienbock's disease: triscaphe arthrodesis. *Journal of Hand Surgery*, **10A**, 179–187

WEIR MITCHELL, J. K. (1895) *Remote Consequences of Injuries of Nerves and their Treatment*. Philadelphia: J. P. Lippincott

WEIR MITCHELL, S. (1872) *Injuries to Nerves and their Consequences*. Philadelphia: J. P. Lippincott

WHITE, J. C., HEROY, W. W. and GOODMAN, E. N. (1948) Causalgia following gunshot injuries of nerves. Role of emotional stimuli and surgical care through interruption of diencephatic efferent discharge by sympathectomy. *Annals of Surgery*, **121**, 161–183

WITHRINGTON, R. H. and WYNN PARRY, C. B. (1984) Painful disorders of peripheral nerves. *Postgraduate Medical Journal*, **60**, 869–875

WYNN PARRY, C. B. (1981) *Rehabilitation of the Hand*, 4th edition. London: Butterworths

12
Future developments in hand surgery: a British view

Neil Watson

INTRODUCTION

I have decided to conclude this volume with a look into the future. The purpose of a book such as this, in fact the whole object of the Butterworths International Medical Review series, is to bring together a review and assessment of current practice in a particular specialty. The volumes are therefore written by active practitioners for active practitioners, and their trainees. The very word practice invites comment, for it is the starting point for such a review. 'Current practice' is the distillation of knowledge and experience from past and present practitioners. It forms the basis of our day-to-day practical work, be it subconsciously when we are dealing with the familiar, or consciously when we seek help and advice from more experienced colleagues (or 'the literature') if confronted with the unfamiliar. 'Current practice' has also medicolegal connotations; our assessments of disability, recommendations for treatment and prognoses are based upon our understanding of what it is, and it constitutes the 'baseline' from which may be viewed alleged medical negligence. But the word practice, in common usage, implies a static state, that is 'established practice'. The practice of surgery is far from static. It is both an art and a craft, to which there is an increasing scientific foundation. Knowledge expands. Techniques and materials continue to improve. As their practical applications are tried and tested so new developments, provided they bring significant improvements, are gradually incorporated into 'standard practice'. But the practical details of 'standard practice' are often taken for granted, assumed to be gleaned from what is, in many places, a haphazard 'apprenticeship'. It is hoped that the foregoing chapters have included valuable practical points.

Worthwhile surgical research has mostly come from the response to clinical problems. As the technology increases, so does the cost. No country on this earth can afford comprehensive health care for all, free at the time of use. So what may be 'current practice' in an affluent community can be impossible or inappropriate in another. Thus new questions are posed for contemporary surgeons. These relate to cost and efficacy of treatment – not so much 'what can we do?' but, now, 'what can we afford to do?' Even more important, perhaps, the demanding question 'what is likely to be the functional benefit of this procedure for this patient' must be answered by the honest surgeon. They must also contribute to the collection of data which results in 'medical audit', a bureaucratic term sending shivers down the average surgeon's spine, but essential if scarce resources are to be allocated equably, particularly in the public sector. The private sector is not immune from such accountability either. Insurance companies are justifiably worried about spiralling costs of health care. Can we improve the current standard and efficency of practice in hand surgery and if so how? What problems in our specialty are as yet unresolved?

It is with these thoughts that a look into the future, through the loupes of critical observation of the present, can concentrate our minds so that we may help to mould the development of hand surgery constructively. In many places, of course, it is well established, particularly in North America, Australasia and some of the European countries. By contrast there are fewer than ten surgeons in Britain whose practice is entirely in hand surgery. Horne and Hueston (1985) reported, interestingly, that of 212 'hand surgeons' attending an international hand surgery congress only 14 per cent were in full-time hand surgery, and 50 per cent spent less than 50 per cent of their time engaged upon it.

Let us examine some aspects of our specialty and project ourselves forwards in time.

The best place to start is at the beginning.

TRAINING

By this I mean not only training in hand surgery, but also the background of education that precedes entry to medical school and the contents of the medical school curriculum. We live in a changing world. There is an increasing awareness and concern that preparation for, and selection of, entrants to medical schools is too rigid and unimaginative. The competition for entrance to medical schools is fierce. This is not surprising. Remuneration of doctors, their job satisfaction and their social standing will ensure, for the foreseeable future, that competition will remain keen. But modern medicine requires a spread of skills. The emphasis on the sciences has, in my view, been too great. Of course, progress in medicine requires enquiring, scientifically trained minds of the highest calibre, particularly in the fields of cellular biology, immunology, genetics and the like. I would suggest though that clinical medicine, and especially clinical surgery, in which areas the majority of doctors spend the whole of their working lives, demand attributes of personality, application and technical skills which do not spring naturally from a purely scientific training. Some of these characteristics are undoubtedly innate, but others can certainly be taught. For the surgeon's technical skills have been undervalued. Perhaps we should include tests of manual dexterity in our assessments.

In turn the teaching, particularly within medical schools, is often performed by erudite research workers, cut off from the hurly-burly of clinical medical life. Worse still, these 'academics', and many doctors, lack interest and training in the use of the written and spoken word, by which most learning takes place, especially in the early stages. It has been repeatedly pointed out by Asher and others that the 'gifted', or 'natural' writer or speaker is an exceptionally rare species. Those that achieve eminence in either, or both, do so as a result of their own industry. The cynic reaches for the saying 'those that can, do, and those that can't, teach'. Others add that 'those that can't do either, write'.

More truthful is another chestnut that goes; 'it takes a month to prepare a five-minute talk, a week to prepare a ten-minute talk and you can talk for an hour about anything with no notice at all'. For therein lies the uncomfortable reality; good writing and good speaking require a lot of work. Most busy doctors do not wish to devote time to either; but when their professional expertise demands the attention of their peers the pressure to do both increases. Industrious research workers often take ill-prepared time out from their work to lecture medical students.

New teaching methods are with us. There will be a rapid expansion of these. The use of videotapes and computer disc configured material is at a pubertal stage. An imminent growth spurt is inevitable, and this will enable more people to have access to the better teachers.

Undergraduate education

Preclinical studies

Numeracy and literacy are essential prerequisites for a modern education. The ability to type, and thus use a computer terminal, is fundamental in the information age in which we live. As more and more medical and scientific information is stored electronically so we can expect books and scientific journals to head the same way. So familiarity with these formats is required in order to learn from, and contribute to, these sources. Our collective resistance, if not fear, of computers is irrational. As hardware and software becomes increasingly 'user friendly', and the systems become more standardized, the remaining obstacles will crumble. Recruitment of some proficient programmers and systems analysts into medicine will hasten the integration of applications to clinical practice. The entry of more arts graduates to the profession will disseminate an improved standard of literacy, and the presence of more statisticians will help to crunch the ever-increasing numbers in ways which make them more understandable and helpful. Some mechanical and electrical engineers, materials scientists and chemists will in turn take part in integrated courses so that their subsequent medical involvement will be closer and the present 'language barriers' broken down. The presence of a wider spectrum of colleagues at medical school will broaden the minds of future doctors. The curriculum of the medical school will need modification, both in content and in duration, to cater for the differing requirements of a less uniform group of medical students. 'Pure' medical students, in turn, will have access to, and take part in, a wider number of disciplines than at present. Nor should medical students of the future be party to the steady decline in sporting and other extracurricular activities that has occurred in recent times: 'All work and no play makes Jack a dull boy.'

Within the medical schools an urgent reappraisal of what is taught, and not taught, is necessary. Overall students appear to be saturated with information, much of it 'small print' and inappropriate for undergraduates. At the same time enormous gaps of important practical knowledge are obvious. Whatever is the purpose of a medical student knowing the course and relations of the greater superficial petrosal nerve if the segmental value of the biceps jerk is unknown? The integration of clinical problems to the preclinical course, already a fact in a number of medical schools, will become normal.

Clinical studies

The demise of the intensely practical old-fashioned 'clerkships' and 'dresserships' is to be lamented. It seems possible for students to qualify with remarkably little in the way of experience in talking to, and examining patients, let alone any familiarity with simple procedures. The majority have never been instructed in how to insert a simple skin suture, sometimes not even a lumbar puncture needle, and hardly ever an intercostal drain. Part of the problem is said to be the enormous demands on the students' time which has resulted from the necessary fragmentation of medicine into so many specialties, each one of which believes its importance to be greater than the others and insist, via their powerful professorial heads, that all students should be introduced to their sometimes obscure little worlds. The teaching hospitals of course are now constituted of many such mini-empires, now that there has taken place such a dissemination of expertise into the periphery. This trend will continue, making it more and more important for medical students to undertake much of their clinical time outside traditional teaching hospitals. Paradoxically it is still the case that a large number of medical students find themselves attached for long periods of time to 'general surgical' units which have long since ceased to practise surgery in general. Many, too, spend fleeting moments in areas of clinical practice likely to occupy much of their working life as general practitioners, which a lot of them will become.

A truncation of the clinical programme is needed so that it is of a general practical nature. Another paradox in an era of specialization. To this more watertight, somewhat narrower, base of clinical examination and assessment may then be securely fastened the initial building blocks of, perhaps, a more specialized career. 'My doctor is not an examining doctor', a comment made by so many patients, should then become an epitaph and not remain a criticism.

Early graduate experience or general professional training

The prestige still attached to obtaining 'teaching hospital' positions has not disappeared, but it will for the 'just graduated'; most of the reasons have been alluded to already. They are those of ultraspecialization whereby a newly qualified doctor may find himself looking after a handful of rarities under investigation; what he needs, of course, is a ward full of patients with more common conditions under treatment. This is likely to be away from the teaching centre, so the first year of housejobs or internships will be spent in the 'periphery'. As the interests and inclinations of the doctor become clarified during this year, if they were not already, the broad choice of 'specialty' can more intelligently be made; then perhaps should be the time to return to the teaching centre.

Specialist training for hand surgery

Horne and Hueston (1985) found that 90 per cent of a group of hand surgeons emanated from an orthopaedic or plastic surgery base. The situation seems likely to remain like this. But neither specialty can consider itself a complete provider of the various skills now incorporated into modern hand surgery practice. Any changes to methods whereby surgeons acquire or are given a formal training in hand surgery will depend on the evolution of the specialty, both in terms of the numbers of practitioners and the nature of their practice.

Since many, if not most, orthopaedic and plastic surgeons are called upon to deal with hand problems at some time in their career, if not for all of it, the basic training in these two specialties must contain enough practical instruction and experience to deal with common conditions. Sadly this is often not so. In my view, many orthopaedic surgeons are mostly woefully short, if not wholly devoid, of any experience in basic plastic surgical techniques relating to skin cover and local skin flap design. The image of the muscular bonesetter has been tempered, to some extent, by general refinement of surgical techniques and an increasing awareness of the importance of precision and delicacy in the handling of tissues, to ensure their continuing viability and to minimize the unwanted complications of haematomata and infection. But there is still room for improvement. Many have never used loupes, let alone a microscope. Plastic surgeons, from my biased viewpoint, often hold a rather conceited view that they are the only surgeons who should be allowed to operate on the hand, such is their alleged 'finesse'. However, they too tend to have significant gaps in surgical knowhow, mainly with reference to contemporary methods of skeletal fixation and joint replacement, but also to more basic objectives of early restoration of function. This criticism relates also to the overall assessment of disability, for example in rheumatoid disease, and multiple injuries, neither of which is traditionally part of the ethos of general plastic surgery.

Future changes

In some centres hand surgery fellowships are well established. More will certainly follow, since this seems the ideal way in which the finishing touches can be applied. For those whose background is orthopaedic surgery a hand fellowship with a hand surgeon whose background was plastic surgery would appear desirable, and vice versa. In practical terms the establishment of such fellowships can only be achieved to best effect when the location of the fellowship is in a place where hand surgery forms the vast majority of the workload of the unit, since the attachment will be for a relatively short period.

Furthermore the ability to teach surgery is given to few. It is not easy to delegate cases of a complex technical nature, nor is it appropriate to do so. For the learner must have passed successfully up a scale of procedures of increasing complexity under supervision before he can properly undertake the difficult case.

There is a bit of a 'Catch 22' situation here. It has already been pointed out that the number of practitioners working full time in hand surgery is relatively small. This is surprising. It is widely accepted that out of all patients attending an emergency department for reasons of injury, between 25 per cent and 30 per cent can be expected to have a hand injury. This proportion is similar to the ratio between urological and general surgical emergency admissions. (There cannot be many general hospitals now without at least one urologist.) The expansion of hand surgery is long overdue, particularly in Britain, where large numbers of hand injuries are dealt with by junior doctors with little or no supervision or experience. Better that these individuals recognize their inadequacies and close the skin than continue to lunge traumatically through keyholes in their desperate search for nerve and tendon ends. 'Senior' doctors are progressively less enthusiastic about becoming involved in emergency surgery, particularly since so much of it tends to be done outside 'office hours' though, in truth, that is frequently for logistical and not medical reasons. Earlier chapters in this book have emphasized the importance of high-quality primary management of hand injuries and infections. Practising hand surgeons around the world necessarily are involved with this vital aspect of the specialty; many more should be.

Specialist training varies significantly from country to country, and even within countries. 'Specialist' British surgeons are generally older and have spent more time in general surgery than their North American counterparts. There are some tangible advantages to this, but also disadvantages, the chief of which is the age of appointment to a 'definitive' post. It seems wholly ludicrous that a large number of fully trained surgeons are forced to queue up in a log jam until vacancies in the popular specialties, and locations, arise. As 'off duty' time increases the acquisition of a 'complete' training will either take longer or be less complete.

An expansion in the consultant grade is certainly required in Britain. It has been resisted by elements of the profession, perhaps fearing encroachment of private practice, and also by the 'administration' fearful of its cost. Neither fear is wholly rational. As waiting lists increase in the face of shortage of facilities so health insurance expands and with it private bed capacity. For the administration a greater proportion of senior doctors offers greater efficiency in the use of resources; the argument that such efficiency is more expensive in the totality of provision of a national health service has yet to be substantiated, to my satisfaction.

There is therefore, in Britain, both a need for expansion of hand surgery, and a pool of surgeons from which may be hooked future practitioners. The number of plastic surgeons is too small, and many of them are tucked away in 'regional centres' which embody many of the disadvantages of our teaching hospitals outlined above. They need to get out and about.

The nature of what surgeons are being trained to do merits some thought also. Orthopaedic surgery has expanded enormously. Following the virtual demise of poliomyelitis and the dramatic reduction in frequency both of bone and joint tuberculosis and the other forms of chronic infection in the 'developed' world, there followed a rapid growth in joint reconstruction for the treatment of arthritis. Arguably the single greatest contribution to surgery this century, aside from anaesthesia, blood transfusion and antibiotics, total hip replacement accounts for a large proportion of the elective operating time of the average orthopaedic surgeon. To it is now added replacement of the knee and other joints. Operative treatment of congenital abnormalities of the hip and foot and of scoliosis also account for a significant part of the work. Arthroscopic surgery has established itself. In many places, however, the trauma 'epidemic', particularly that part of it which follows motorcycling accidents and the treatment of fractures of the neck of the femur, is of such proportions that the very logistics of providing an elective orthopaedic service are threatened, if not obliterated, for large parts of the year. The complexity and sophistication of modern methods of fracture management demand new equipment and the skills and judgement necessary to use it effectively. So the breadth of orthopaedic surgical activity has widened greatly. So much so that no single orthopaedic surgeon could pretend to be proficient in all departments. While many of these activities were previously restricted to 'centres' the overall standards and repertoire have improved so much in the 'periphery' that referral to such centres is less often necessary. The result is likely to be an unbalanced 'case mix' at the 'centre'. Just as the newly qualified doctor may find himself looking after rarities, so the trainee surgeon can finish up ill-equipped to deal with a busy 'surburban' practice if all his training time has been spent in a rarefied atmosphere. Training must be sensitive to this situation; further specialization can be anticipated. This might appear to be in direct confrontation with the notion, put forward above, that undergraduate and early general professional training be less specialized, but I do not believe that to be so. On the contrary it was emphasized that the more simplistic basic training is likely to form a sounder foundation for subsequent, and inevitable, specialization.

I might have implied too that 'peripheral' surgeons are likely to be less specialized. To some extent this is true, but as specialization inevitably develops, specialists will not, and certainly are not now, confined to large centres. Our present (British) ideas of specialization are anyhow outdated in comparison to many other places, for, even within hand surgery itself we see already subspecialization, for example the care of the rheumatoid hand.

In Britain plastic surgery too has remained, in many places, relatively isolated. This, I would submit, continues to be detrimental to the integration of plastic surgery to the whole. Perhaps plastic surgeons prefer to stand off in this way, as, apparently, do neurosurgeons. But the separation of these skills is not desirable, particularly in the acute care of the injured, where expertise in both is often required, and required urgently, for treatment of patients not ideally suited for transfer.

The future must surely see a gradual reversal of this isolationist policy, which tends to deprive both patients and surgical trainees from these specialists. Plastic surgery is after all at the root of most surgery. It seems to me that surgeons in training for any branch of surgery can, and should, benefit from secondment into plastic surgery. Indeed it should go without saying that it is a *sine qua non* for hand surgery training.

The era of specialization has been mentioned earlier. Where does hand surgery fit in? Certainly not in an isolated unit. The very large numbers of hand injuries and infections, which have been pointed out earlier, demand that expertise in their treatment be readily available in the acute setting. In other words, any hospital that receives regularly a significant number of acutely injured individuals requires 'cover' for hand surgery. Whether this takes the form of a full-time practitioner in the specialty, or constitutes a major 'interest' for a plastic, orthopaedic or other surgeon, clearly depends on numbers. Traditionally, again mentioned elsewhere in this volume, much of this vital emergency work has been left to the untrained and the unsupervised. Surely this cannot be allowed to continue for much longer.

So to return to the opening theme of this section. Formal training in hand surgery is both desirable and essential if standards are to be further improved. Discussion of subsequent topics will pinpoint areas of anticipated development in the craft and science of the specialty, which will themselves require new levels of excellence.

THE TOOLS OF THE TRADE

Magnification

In order to bring about the accurate apposition of divided tendons, nerves and blood vessels, using fine suture materials, magnification is essential. Not only is it easier but also, and perhaps more importantly, it is safer. Indeed it is not possible to handle a 10/0 suture without it. While much of the dissection and preparatory work can properly be undertaken using loupes, there can be no question that the use of the operating microscope, with variable focus and magnification, combined with a fibreoptic light source, further enhances the situation. Furthermore, the breaking strain of a 10/0 suture is below the human threshold for touch. So knots must be tied and tightened visually. This is in marked contradistinction to conventional knotting techniques in which knots are tightened largely by feel. Microsurgical methods must be learnt, since there is a necessary 'cortical' adjustment to be made in order to do this. There is no mystique in its use and the ability to use a microscope is a prerequisite for many branches of surgery nowadays. This learning is best carried out in a laboratory in which proper instruments, and not wornout rejects, are available. The learner needs good instruments. Practice models have been devised for basic manoeuvres but access to laboratory animals is required if proficiency in microvascular anastomosis is to be acquired. The situation in 'real life' is invariably more complex. Vessels have not been electively transected, size may be disparate, length, and thus tension, are often problematical, resulting in a need for vein grafting, and alternative methods of anastomosis. There can be no place for the inexperienced in these circumstances, and a background of at least 20 or 30 successful experimental anastomoses is essential before clinical microvascular anastomosis can be realistically undertaken. Nor is high-quality microsurgical neurorrhaphy any easier for similar reasons. So hand surgeons must complete a period of microsurgical training to complement the conventional armamentarium. This is not to say that all hand operations will require the microscope. Far from it. But the surgical care of the injured hand often does, as do almost all procedures involving treatment of injured peripheral nerves. Attendance at a short course is certainly better than nothing but there is no substitute for a period of regular practice until the skills are fully assimilated. Once proficient, regular employment of them is desirable to maintain both quality and speed.

Microsurgical instruments

It has already been stated that the fine sutures now available need magnification and special instruments for their proper handling. Surprisingly many such instruments are not ideally suited to this sort of activity. The finest and most controlled movement of which man's hand is capable is a rotary movement. This takes place with instruments held in the so-called 'internal precision grip' of the hand, while the forearm is rested to eliminate or minimize tremor. The instrument rests on the skin of the first web space, and is stabilized by the combined activity of the extrinsic flexor and extensor musculature. Thus placed, the precision movement, by which a suture is inserted, is brought about by action of the intrinsic musculature. For a right-handed person looking down a microscope this movement will be from 2 o'clock to 8 o'clock on an imaginary clock face. So the structure to be repaired should, ideally, cross the field in this line. Practically this will not always be possible, but movements other than these are likely to lack the same precision. In order that this basic rotary action can easily be executed, without jerking, the needle holder, and indeed other instruments, should be circular in cross-section. Their closing pressures should be minimal and they should be constructed of materials resistant to magnetization. This troublesome problem can be kept at bay by regular demagnetization of susceptible instruments, but it is annoying and always seems to occur at crucial moments. There is room for significant further improvement in instrument design.

Conventional instruments

There is scope for development here too. In particular more ergonomics could profitably be applied, taking into account similar considerations as have been discussed with respect to microsurgical instruments. More specifically, the current techniques which are used to transect tendons and nerves are relatively traumatic and thus detrimental to healing. Diamond knives, used widely in ophthalmology, offer advantages, but the sophistication of laser technology would appear to be the obvious way forward.

Microsutures

The quality of these is now excellent. Nylon or polypropylene of 75 or $100\,\mu$ diameter swaged on to 5 mm needles of scarcely greater diameter satisfy most needs. The use of coloured background material enhances visual acuity while handling such sutures and, if kept moist, helps to reduce adherence. It is hard to see dramatic changes in this area.

Tissue adhesives

It seems more likely that improvements to 'joining methods' will follow the development of biological glues. Although some have appeared, for instance fibrin, none have really found widespread application. In hand surgery the tissues to be considered are nerve, tendon and blood vessel. Suturing by even the most refined techniques still falls well short of perfection. Glues will have to be permeable to the ingrowth of microscopical blood vessels if they are to be successful and must not, of course, obstruct the flow of axonal material or blood. At present the use of biological adhesives for skin closure would appear undesirable, since a watertight skin closure would prevent the egress of blood that inevitably occurs even when vacuum drainage is used.

PROSTHETIC MATERIALS

Joints

Further refinement can be expected. Joint replacement in the hand has not achieved the level of success that has been seen in the hip and, more recently, the knee. There are several reasons why this should be so. One of the most fundamental has been the failure to translate well-established biomechanical principles, tried and tested in relation to the lower limb, to the hand. Perhaps the need to do so has not been fully appreciated nor indeed thought necessary. That is a pity. For the forces of compression and tension per unit area in upper limb joints are not wholly different from those that pertain in the lower limb. To many that seems surprising. An eminent hand surgeon recently pronounced that 'the joints of the lower limb are in compression while those in the upper limb are in tension'. This is incorrect. Muddled thinking like this has perhaps held back progress in small joint replacement in the hand. There is no theoretical reason why surface replacement of finger joints cannot be developed using similar materials to those used in the knee joint. But this leads on to the second big difficulty. Namely that many patients with joint destruction in the hand soldier on with progressively increasing deformity and disability, reaching the hand surgeon only when joint damage has reached such a point that surface replacement, even were it to be available, would be doomed to failure, due to advanced secondary changes in the soft tissues. This is so often the problem in the rheumatoid hand, dealt with in Chapter 2 of this volume. A reinforcing plea to general practitioners and rheumatologists to refer patients earlier for consideration of surgery must here be made, if we are to make the quantum leap forward that is necessary to deal with the problems that this disease produces at an earlier stage. Only by providing and demonstrating the efficacy of newer methods of joint management will advances be made.

The remarks above in no way seek to belittle existing achievements, particularly those of Swanson, whose various prostheses continue to provide great relief for large numbers of patients. He himself, I am sure, would agree that his many designs are all spacers and not joint replacements. That does not mean that they do not work; we know they do. But it should not stop us from looking for even better solutions and capitalizing on our existing experience.

Tendons

There is a need for a tendon substitute. None so far produced has fulfilled all our requirements. A more acceptable material must soon be found. With it will be associated successful methods of attachment both to parent tendon and to bone, neither of which yet exists.

Splintage materials

The continued evolution of thermoplastic materials has enabled the practising hand surgeon and associated hand therapists to construct, quickly, custom-made splints. These materials will likely be improved further, making them more compliant and, hopefully, become cheaper.

COLLAGEN METABOLISM

Much has yet to be learnt about the general and local control mechanisms of this interesting protein. Hand surgeons naturally will wish to keep themselves informed of progress. Not only in terms of its implication in the troublesome adhesions which continue to bedevil the results of flexor tendon surgery, but also its role in Dupuytren's contracture, as well as in the formation of unwanted scar tissue in crucial areas. The future is likely to bring methods by which collagen synthesis may be controlled. It is conceivable that these could take the form of local and general chemical agents; but mechanical and electrical factors, at present under evaluation in relation to other tissues, notably bone, of which collagen is a major constituent, must not be discounted. The role of collagen in the development of arthritis has been discussed by Peimer in Chapter 3 of this book.

HOMOTRANSPLANTATION

As yet this has not featured in the field of hand surgery; however, it could in due course. Attempts to use major nerves as homografts have hitherto been unsuccessful due to two main factors: first, immunological problems have not been completely resolved; second, the nerves underwent 'core' necrosis, since they were not formally revascularized. The prospects of solving both difficulties are good. Increasing experience in the use of drugs to suppress the immune mechanism, gained from other transplant programmes, will undoubtedly be transferred to this application. The concept of a vascularized nerve graft has been tested experimentally and used clinically. Core necrosis can thus be prevented. But the clinical applications have so far been very limited. The paucity of nerves available for use as grafts, particularly when several are required, as in surgery of the brachial plexus, demands such a solution.

It is not inconceivable either that digits could be used as homografts, for a toe will always look like a toe and the disability that results from using the great toe as a transfer has been underestimated by the protagonists of this technique. Whether or not the aesthetic aspects of a digital homograft would be acceptable is open to question.

BONE GRAFTING

It is not often that large amounts of bone are needed in the hand, but there are circumstances in which the defects require consideration for methods more sophisticated than those in common use. The experience of Smith and Brushart (1985) in using the techniques developed by Henry Mankin in Boston, makes interesting reading and we can surely expect these methods to find a wider application. Just as with nerves so the problem in bones of slow and uncertain 'creeping substitution' can be prevented by using vascularized bones and even joints. To date the donor sites have been somewhat clumsy for use in the hand, but refinement and sophistication can again be expected here.

IMAGING

Conventional X-rays will be needed for the foreseeable future. Hand surgeons will benefit from further improvements in both computer tomography (CAT) scanning and nuclear magnetic resonance (NMR) methods. More particularly they will be helped by the miniaturization of image intensifiers, enabling them to be used as light hand-held tools, both in the consulting room and in the operating theatre. A few such devices already exist, but most need improvements in image quality and image storage facilities. Such improvements seem inevitable.

DISEASE CONTROL

Medical treatment of rheumatoid arthritis will improve and a 'cure' will probably be found. There will remain for many years, though, a 'bottomless pit' of patients suffering from the ravages of the disease upon the hand who will need our help.

The remarkable efficacy of immunization against poliomyelitis will hopefully be sustained and those pockets of resistance which still exist successfully dealt with. The treatment and eradication of leprosy poses a monumental challenge. Let us hope that it will soon be met. Better antenatal and perinatal care should continue to decrease the number of cases of cerebral palsy. The continued scope for intrauterine detection of musculoskeletal abnormalities may diminish the incidence of congenital abnormalities. Nor will we wish to see a repetition of the thalidomide disaster. At the other end of the age scale it is likely that treatment for skin cancer of the hand will be less surgically oriented in the future.

PAINFUL CONDITIONS OF THE HAND

The contribution by Wynn Parry and Robins (Chapter 11 of this volume) has highlighted the significant recent advances that have occurred in the management of these difficult and distressing conditions. One can envisage new methods evolving from an ever-increasing knowledge of neurophysiology allied to the inexorable advances in electronic engineering. Such perhaps that minute implantable electrodes will become used to modify the electrical environment and performance of groups of cells. Perhaps it may even become possible to produce locally those chemical substances that are involved in, or modify, the transmission of painful stimuli, rather than using systemic preparations. An understanding of the mechanisms by which the syndrome that we describe as 'the hysterical hand' occurs would be valuable. Its roots are probably deep within the brain.

CONTROL OF INFECTION

Happily the incidence of postoperative sepsis is low, following elective hand surgery. But it is not zero. We should not be complacent in this area and strive to use all methods by which the incidence may be further lowered. Nor should we forget those principles learnt, and painfully relearnt, in conditions of warfare. The removal of dead and devitalized tissues and the elimination of foreign material. These remain at the heart of practical management of contaminated wounds. Antibiotics are not a universal panacea for the eradication of infection in these circumstances.

DATABASES

It has been pointed out above that information will increasingly be stored electronically. Agreement is urgently needed in our specialty in terms of the hardware and software to be used. Standardization must soon be achieved so that the information may be made widely available and easily accessible to practitioners. A working party has already been set up under the auspices of the International Federation for Societies for Surgery of the Hand with this is mind. This will involve expertise and endeavour. It must be oriented towards both the collection of data relating to diagnosis and to that of treatment outcome, if it is to be generally accepted. There is an understandable fear of accountability amongst sections of the profession which may hamper progress here.

These databases will be linked to other practitioners as well as to the substantial mainframes on which are already stored much of the bibliography of our specialty.

PREVENTION

Last, but by no means least, of the topics discussed is that of prevention and yet this 'Cinderella' of roles has been woefully neglected. The virtual eradication of smallpox from the face of the earth must be one of the greatest medical triumphs of the century. Only recently have significant initiatives been taken to incorporate the formal advice of those whose practice involves the care of the injured hand into the design and operation of industrial machinery. Again, the role of the International Federation of Societies for Surgery of the Hand will be an important one here in terms both of communication and enforcement. As the industrial world veers inevitably towards more mechanization serious industrial hand injuries should become less frequent. Indeed there is already a wide discrepancy, even within the 'developed' world, in the incidence of such injuries. Where Health and Safety at Work Acts, or their equivalent, are on the statute books, and are properly enforced, the reduction has been dramatic. But machines with moving and heated parts remain a serious trap for the unwary. Notorious hazards will continue, for example the high pressure injection grease and solvent gun. But serious injuries do not always result from industrial accidents. Agricultural machinery is often dangerous. Illiteracy and inadequate instruction in the use of machines contribute to the hazards. Nor is the home free of danger. The bottles in which British people continue to demand that their milk is delivered are a constant source of serious lacerations, particularly amongst children. As leisure time increases so we can expect a different crop of problems to grow resulting from new pursuits and crazes.

CONCLUSION

Though we can anticipate the elimination of some of the conditions which now present to us, the need for expertise in the field of hand surgery will continue for the foreseeable future. Indeed, as the population becomes better educated in medical matters the expectations of our patients will increase. In this we can, and should, be pleased to be involved. The need for a large number of surgeons to deal skilfully with the various affections, injuries and infections of the hand that confront us is obvious. The practical and technical nature of this work cannot be overemphasized. For it will be in response to such demands, and in the light of improved results by such surgeons and their medical colleagues, that the specialty will continue to grow, and further substantiate the claims made for its proper recognition by our pioneering forebears, teachers, friends and colleagues.

References

HORNE, D. and HUESTON, J. T. (1985) The personality of hand surgeons. *Journal of Hand Surgery*, **1**, 5–7
SMITH, R. J. and BRUSHART, T. M. (1985) Allograft bone for metacarpal reconstruction. *Journal of Hand Surgery*, **10A**, 325–334

Index

DATE DUE

DEC 0 4 1999			